# Principles of Long-Term Health Care Administration

**Peter J. Buttaro, MSHA, JD, FACHE**
Director
HCF Educational Services
Aberdeen, South Dakota

**Emily L.H. Buttaro**
Editor

AN ASPEN PUBLICATION®
Aspen Publishers, Inc.
Gaithersburg, Maryland
1999

Library of Congress Cataloging-in-Publication Data

Buttaro, Peter J.
Principles of long-term health care administration / Peter J. Buttaro.
p.  cm.
"An Aspen publication."
Includes index.
ISBN 0-8342-1371-0
1. Long-term care facilities—Administration.   2. Nursing homes—Administration.   I. Title.
[DNLM: 1. Long-Term Care—organization & administration—United States.   2. Long-Term Care—legislation & jurisprudence—United States.
3. Nursing Homes—organization & administration—United States.   WX 162 8988p   1999]
RA999.A35B879   1999
362.1'6'068—dc21
DNLM/DLC
for Library of Congress
99-14786
CIP

Orders: (800) 638-8437
Customer Service: (800) 234-1660

**About Aspen Publishers** • For more than 35 years, Aspen has been a leading professional publisher in a variety of disciplines. Aspen's vast information resources are available in both print and electronic formats. We are committed to providing the highest quality information available in the most appropriate format for our customers. Visit Aspen's Internet site for more information resources, directories, articles, and a searchable version of Aspen's full catalog, including the most recent publications: **http://www.aspenpublishers.com**
**Aspen Publishers, Inc.** • The hallmark of quality in publishing
Member of the worldwide Wolters Kluwer group.

Editorial Services: Ruth Bloom
Library of Congress Catalog Card Number: 99-14786
ISBN: 0-8342-1371-0

*Printed in the United States of America*

1 2 3 4 5

# TABLE OF CONTENTS

# Acknowledgments

This publication is the result of input from and interaction with many individuals. Over the past 25 years, this text has been used extensively in the long-term care industry by individuals preparing for the NAB licensure exam. I am grateful to my wife, Emily, for the time and effort she has given me in editing and revising the book over the years. Without her help and assistance, this publication in its present form would not be available. I am grateful also to Aspen Publishers for their guidance in preparing this 1999 edition.

*Peter J. Buttaro*

# INTRODUCTION

Since early mankind, every society or country has had its own tradition of care for those who cannot care for themselves (such as the needy, chronically ill, aged, disabled or mentally ill), reflecting the demands of the particular culture. Churches and various levels of government have provided financial assistance to institutional (shelters, hospitals, workhouses) and non-institutional (home) settings according to which method was considered to produce the most care for the least cost at a particular time.

Around 300 AD, a Roman emperor directed the Christians to build facilities and care for the sick, helpless, poor and aged who congregated on the streets. These facilities were attached to bishopries, monasteries and cathedrals, and were financed by voluntary almsgiving by those who believed their donations assured them a place in heaven. Management was appointed by rulers and bishops; untrained clergy and religious orders provided food, shelter, comfort and care, especially dressing sores and wounds.

Until the late 19th and 20th centuries, little distinction existed between a long-term care facility and a hospital. Management of these facilities moved toward local citizens, sometimes with a board of directors. Physicians had little or no involvement in providing medical care; such care was given to those who could pay in their homes or private clinics. Communities were to provide cash and in-kind help to enable those who could not care for themselves to remain in their homes. Gradually, programs to assist those without means in their own homes, the elderly, the chronically ill, and the disabled followed suit. Almshouses and workhouses were established in an attempt to provide food, shelter and human comfort at less cost, with residents performing chores and assisting with their upkeep.

Public workhouses had infirmaries for medical functions; resident physicians were appointed to the staffs. In the early 20th century, physicians became more involved in providing medical care in institutions as significant scientific advancements in illness detection and treatment enabled long-term care facilities and hospitals to move toward cures and effective restorative care. Sanatoriums provided care for individuals, for instance, with tuberculosis or mental conditions, requiring long-term care. Death rates due to disease and infection started dropping dramatically. As the health care institutions assumed specialized roles and accepted only certain categories of patients, they began evolving into acute care and long-term care groupings. The roles of the hospital for short-term acute care and the long-term care facilities for long-term care gradually emerged. As this system of care evolved, the basic elements of nursing home administration emerged and were identified as compassion, sick or disabled persons, the need for long-term care, a caretaker, a facility, treatment and funding.

## GOVERNMENT INFLUENCE

During these years, our society had changed from an agrarian form where the home and workplace were closer and the workers more self-sufficient to an industrialized form where the home and workplace became more separate and economic conditions moved beyond the workers' influence. This industrialization has brought more urbanization and increased problems of survival for the aged and those unable to care for themselves. Until the Great Depression of the 1930s, care for the aged, chronically ill and disabled was largely in the public workhouses and infirmaries funded by states, cities and counties. As the Depression progressed, it left 50% of the aged indigent by 1935; this increased to 66% by 1940. Public pressure mounted for support for this population. States provide cash support to elderly persons in their homes who needed economic help; these payments usually were not enough to support full-time care in an institutional setting. As life expectancy increased, pressure increased to develop a care system for the growing older populations who no longer were able to pay cost of living out of savings. The states, cities and counties no longer were willing or able to assume this economic burden.

The federal government passed the Social Security Act in 1935 that created a cash assistance program intended to enable the aged to stay in their homes. Payments to the elderly receiving care in institutions were excluded; the states, counties and cities continued to fund this long-term care. However, the act did provide federal dollars under Old Age Assistance for up to half of the costs of noninstitutional care for those age 65 or older.

Toward the middle of the 20th century, as cures and treatment for various illnesses progressed, the aged—as they lived longer—wanted appropriate care and treatments, freedom from pain, and life quality in their declining years. The costs and levels of living rose; both husband and wife needed to be employed to survive. Some older people retired from work with incomes from business and other retirement programs, investments, Social Security, and other personal income. In addition, many chronically ill and disabled aged needed 24-hour care that could no longer be provided by young parents or older couples in their homes. In response to heavy pressure for a federal role in meeting the needs of the elderly, more of the traditional duties of family and church shifted to the government and private enterprise for the care and protection of both children and infirm elderly.

In response to requirements of noninstitutional care under the Social Security Act, many ill and blind aged began to leave state and county institutions and reside in boarding homes where their basic needs were met. The boarding homes became small nursing homes that evolved into today's variety of facilities providing varying levels of long-term care. Federal legislation, integrating systems of financial support by the individual and by society as a whole, expanded both federal and state financial support for care and institutions (under the Social Security Act of 1935) and care in the community (under the Older Americans Act of 1965). Social Security checks and reimbursement of Medicare and Medicaid bills for residents are an essential part of today's nursing facility industry. To ensure that adequate care is provided as intended, federal and state governments have developed guidelines, or regulations and enforcements that make this industry one of the most highly regulated in the United States. Since the 1970s, the trend has been to contain the related costs and services reimbursed: hospital stays have shortened, shifting post-acute care to nursing facilities.

The following chapters explain the basic concepts and provide the essential information at the foundation of long-term care administration.

# CHAPTER 1

# Governance and Management: Legislation and Regulation

## REGULATION AND LEGISLATION

Nursing facility care is regulated by both the federal and state governments. The federal government establishes standards that must be met by nursing facilities receiving Medicare and Medicaid payments. These standards are contained in the Code of Federal Regulations (42 CFR, Parts 430 to end). State governments supervise nursing facility care through each state licensing authority and work with the federal Medicaid program. Many states impose additional guidelines; when a conflict exists between the federal and state guidelines, the more stringent usually applies.

## FEDERAL GOVERNMENT REGULATORY AGENCIES

- **Department of Health and Human Services** (HHS) is one of the major departments of the federal government. Overall decisions regarding health and welfare are made by the Secretary of HHS.
- **Health Care Financing Administration** (HCFA) is part of HHS and is responsible for the administration of Medicare, Medicaid, and any related guidelines. The Medicare/Medicaid Final Requirements, published in the Federal Register on the September 21, 1991, specify the wide range of requirements (including the rights of the residents) that must be met by facilities receiving these funds.

- **Public Health Service** (PHS) is under HHS and gives financial aid and technical assistance to state and local public health agencies.
- **Administration on Aging** is within HHS and is responsible for the administration of activities and programs under the Older Americans Act.
- **Drug Enforcement Administration** is concerned with medications, drugs (particularly narcotics), their use and any breach of the law concerning that use.
- **Food and Drug Administration** is concerned with misrepresentation and other advertising assertions made relative to food and drugs used by the public. The agency has initiated many legal actions against companies accused of misrepresentation and fraud regarding products that have been put on the market.

## LEGISLATION RELATING TO NURSING FACILITIES

### Social Security Act—1935

The Social Security Act of 1935 was passed by Congress to assist those aged persons who could not pay the cost of living. It contained 11 titles which enacted the program, authorized supporting taxes and set up its administration. The Act intended to enable the aged, chronically ill, and disabled to remain in their homes or to enter the small nursing homes that were becoming available. It did not include payments to institutionalized persons or for home health care programs. Because the states had to fund institutional care, both state and local governments began to place those in need of long-term institutional care in private boarding homes that were eligible for federal reimbursement. As the federal government began to pay substantially for this long-term institutional care, the nursing home industry expanded and developed into an influential element of health care in the United States. By 1980, nearly 7 out of 10 older persons relied on Social Security for half of their incomes; a year later 1 out of 5 relied almost exclusively on Social Security for their entire incomes.

The Social Security Act of 1935 has been amended many times. In 1950, permanently and totally disabled persons were added as beneficiaries, and federal money was made available to states to help pay for the medical care of persons on public assistance. In 1960, the Kerr-Mills Act provided Medical Assistance to the Aged (MAA) by offering 50% to 83% in matching funds to states depending on each state's per capita income. The 1967 amendments mandated licensed nursing home administrators and recognized the intermediate care facility category. In 1974 in-home services to the elderly were supported, and in 1977 anti-fraud amendments were enacted to minimize abuse of the Social Security program.

## Civil Rights Act—1964

The Civil Rights Act is landmark legislation prohibiting discrimination on grounds of age, sex, race, religion or national origin in any program or activity receiving federal financial assistance.

Under Title VI of the Civil Rights Act, those nursing facilities participating in Medicare, Medicaid and other federally assisted programs must submit assurances to HHS that any program will be conducted in compliance with all requirements of this title. It is required that the public be notified of this compliance. A policy statement similar to the following example should be officially adopted and implemented. A copy should be given to each individual and organization referring residents to the facility and one should be prominently posted in the facility; such a statement also should be contained in written and media informational materials (referral agencies, marketing, admissions packets).

It is the policy of the _____(Name)_____ nursing facility to admit and treat all residents without regard to age, sex, race, religion or national origin. The same requirements for admission are applied to all, and residents are assigned within the facility without regard for age, race, religion or national origin. There is no distinction in eligibility for, or in the manner of, providing any resident service by this facility or by others in or outside the facility. All services and facilities are available without distinction to all residents and visitors regardless of age, sex, race, religion or national origin. All persons and organizations having occasion to refer individuals for admissions or to recommend the _(Name)_ nursing facility are advised to do so without regard to the individual's age, sex, race, religion or national origin.

Title VII of the Civil Rights Act created the Equal Employment Opportunities Commission (EEOC) to implement its provision prohibiting discrimination in employment. Personnel policies and procedures are shaped by the provisions, amendments, court decisions and subsequent federal legislation, and areas of employment: interviews and selection, written tests, training, promotion, pregnancy, firing and retirement. Affirmative action is a review of hiring practices to check adherence to these civil rights laws.

## Americans with Disabilities Act—1990

The Americans with Disabilities Act provides clear, consistent and enforceable standards to prohibit discrimination against qualified disabled individuals in employment, housing, education, transportation and public accommodations. This is a complex act which covers people with physical disabilities of any type and with psychological disabilities (such as depression or retardation). Alcoholics, drug abusers, bisexuals, homosexuals, AIDS patients and others are not protected.

Title I of the act covers employment and prohibits discrimination in the areas of application, firing, training, promotion, salary and wages, discharge and other employment privileges. Title III states that reasonable accommodations (not imposing undue hardship on the operation of the business) must be made for job applicants with disabilities. Such accommodations include modified work schedules, necessary equipment, alterations, and training materials.

The federal government is central to monitoring and enforcing this act. The EEOC monitors some of the related programs. Actions considered discriminatory in the area of employment include:

1. Using the term "handicapped"; "disabled" is appropriate.
2. Telling an applicant that disabled persons are not hired.
3. Inquiring as to the nature and severity of the disability.
4. Focusing the interview on the disability rather than on the ability to perform tasks.
5. Refusing to hire a disabled person because it would increase insurance costs.

## Medicare and Medicaid (Public Law 89-97)

In 1965 and 1966, two major amendments were added to the Social Security Act—Title XVIII (Medicare) and Title XIX (Medicaid).

**Medicare (Title XVIII)** is a social insurance program that pays providers of health care for some services to certain people. Covered services include: inpatient hospital, outpatient, physician and other health care services provided to the elderly (65 or older who are enrolled in the Social Security program and eligible for cash benefits) and some disabled (under 65 who have received Social Security disability benefits for 2 years). Any person may buy Medicare Part A and/or Medicare Part B whether or not he or she has paid into the program. The program is administered by the federal government through fiscal intermediaries. It is funded through Social Security payroll taxes and enrollee premiums. Nursing facilities must comply with the Code of Federal Regulations (42 CFR, Parts of 430 to end) to receive reimbursement for the services provided Medicare recipients.

**Medicaid (Title XIX)** is a complex public assistance program that pays various medical expenses for low-income medically indigent persons meeting the eligibility standards involving incomes and assets, age and disability. The program is jointly funded by general state and federal tax revenues and administered by the individual state departments of social services under federal guidelines. Generally low-income persons who are aged, blind, disabled, medically indigent and/or recipients of Aid to Families with Dependent Children are eligible for this program. The amount of payment and types of services covered vary from state to state and generally cover: inpatient and outpatient services, lab and X-ray services, skilled nursing services (for persons 21 and over), home health services (if eligible for skilled nursing services), physician services, family planning services, Medicare premiums, deductibles and co-insurance. States may require some copayments for prescriptions and some health care visits but cannot require deductible payments. No residency requirements may be imposed for eligibility to receive services. Facilities must meet the Code of Federal Regulations (42 CFR, Parts 403 to end) and state regulations to receive reimbursement for services to Medicaid residents.

Facilities receiving Medicare and Medicaid reimbursement must be certified. This is accomplished through surveys by state agencies and usually involves inspection of the physical aspects of the facility, conformance with the Code of Federal Regulations (42 CFR, Parts 403 to end), review of resident charts, drug regimens, care plans and activities, and resident interviews and observation. Sanctions (fines, revocation) may be imposed for facilities not meeting certification standards. The facility may be decertified or limited on the number of Medicare and Medicaid residents it may admit if it does not meet certification standards. Usually a grace period is granted for time to address deficiencies and come in line with standards.

## OBRA—1987 (Public Law 100-203)

The Omnibus Budget Reconciliation Act of 1987 (OBRA) is a national law relating to nursing facilities that seeks to establish consistent standards for facilities throughout the country by spelling out various conditions they must meet to receive Medicare and Medicaid funds. (The current Code of Federal Regulations [42 CFR, Parts 430 to end] are collated into the applicable chapters of this text.) Part of this act consists of comprehensive amendments to the Social Security Act and are termed Nursing Home Reform, Title C. This law emphasizes that nursing facility residents must receive services that help them attain or maintain their "highest practicable physical, mental and psychosocial well-being" in such a manner and environment as to "promote maintenance or enhancement of the quality of life of each resident." The skilled nursing facility and intermediate care facility classifications were combined into a single classification termed nursing facility, thus indicating that both would be held to the same standards under Medicaid.

## Older Americans Act—1965 (Public Law 89-333)

The Older Americans Act (OAA) came into existence in 1965 in response to long-time pressure for federal assistance in addressing the needs of older persons not requiring institutional care but experiencing the difficulty of performing daily activities that come with aging. Generally, the goals of this act are to provide equal opportunity to every older individual for:

1. Adequate incomes, employment and retirement with health and dignity.
2. Best possible physical and mental health without regard to economic status and restorative services.
3. Community services, such as low-cost transportation, living arrangements and social service assistance.
4. Independence and freedom to exercise individual initiative to plan and manage one's own life and to pursue civic, cultural, educational and recreational activities.

The funds for implementing the activities under this act come from federal government appropriations, community support, state funds and participant donation. It is administered by the Administration on Aging in the Department of Health and Human Services through local area agencies on aging. Some broad categories of activities that are legislatively approved include health services (such as education, screening, physical exercise, counseling or specialist referral), transportation to and from services, housing (obtain, maintain, adapt to disabilities), services to avoid institutionalization (home health, meals, homemaker, shopping, escort), legal services, job and career planning, and ombudsman service for long-term care complaints.

### *Ombudsman Program*

Favorable public response to previous ombudsman program demonstration projects lead to formal adoption under the 1978 amendment to the Older Americans

Act. This amendment required that every state plan and office on aging must include a long-term care ombudsman program to assure that nursing facilities and board and care homes observe the laws and provide good quality care. The broad purpose of the program is to provide advocacy for individual nursing facility residents. Ombudsmen have authority to bring the clout of public opinion into the facilities and to concerned citizens. They refer complaints to state licensing and certification agencies or provide residents with appropriate information if legal action against a facility may be warranted.

The ombudsman office is required to:

1. Investigate and resolve complaints by, or on behalf of, residents in nursing and board and care facilities. They represent residents and negotiate with the facility management and staff.
2. Prepare an annual report relative to problems and complaints found and recommend changes in laws, regulations and policies to remedy these.
3. Monitor, analyze and make recommendations concerning the development and implementation of local, state and federal laws.
4. Provide information to public agencies, legislators and others relating to the problems and concerns of nursing facility residents.
5. Train staff and volunteers and promote development of local citizens' organizations and a state-wide network to participate in the program.
6. Establish a state-wide reporting system and procedures to assure confidentiality of resident files (unless written permission is granted by the resident, his or her legal representative, or court order).

Many states have enacted ombudsman legislation that establishes the program's authority, responsibilities and funding. Each state must assure:

1. No liability for representatives of the ombudsman program for good faith performance of duties under the act.
2. Access to long-term care facilities and residents.
3. Access to review social and medical records with permission of the resident or his or her legal guardian, or by other appropriate access if the resident is unable to consent to review of the record and has no legal representative.

4. No retaliation for reprisals by the facility or other entity to any resident or employee for filing a complaint or giving information to the ombudsman office.

## FACILITY LICENSURE, CERTIFICATION AND ENFORCEMENT OF STANDARDS

All state governments require nursing facilities to be licensed as to the level(s) of care provided for a specific period of time in accordance with their particular state statutes. The state licensure programs try to protect consumers (especially those in private-pay-only facilities) by establishing acceptable business practices and by ensuring that adequate levels of desirable services exist. Certificates of need and construction approvals may be required before construction or modifications can begin. Determination of the category for nursing facility accreditation purposes is based on the primary function of the facility as determined at the time of survey. A facility must be licensed before it is eligible for federal certification.

### Facility Licensure

Basically these safeguards consist of enabling legislation and the rules and regulations adopted under the enabling legislation. Such legislation is developed on a broad basis, giving wide latitude to the regulatory agency to establish and revise the rules, regulations and specific standards. The basic purposes of enabling legislation are to provide a means of regulating the establishment, maintenance and operation of facilities, and offering education and consultative services to meet or exceed the minimum requirements is established. To carry out these purposes, the legislation usually provides a nursing facility advisory council and prescribes its powers; a requirement for periodic licensing inspection of the nursing facilities; the development, establishment and enforcement of any rules and regulations adopted by the licensing agency; and for injunctive and other necessary matters. The legislation also establishes an effective date, using approximately the following phraseology: "After (date and year) no person or persons shall establish, advertise, offer, operate or maintain a nursing facility in (state, county or city) without a license issued by (licensing authority) pursuant to this Act."

### Definitions and Terms

The exact meanings of legal and legislative terms are extremely important. Clear identification of essential terms in the enabling legislation and the pertinent rules and regulations will aid in compliance and enforcement. For instance, reference to *nonrelatives* is to permit individuals to care for relatives without being subject to licensure. *Nursing facility resident* means certain types of individuals usually are excluded from nursing facilities (unless there are special provisions for their care); these include individuals with active contagious diseases, under a certain age or requiring mental institution confinement, maternity care or treatment for alcoholism or narcotic addiction.

The arrangement of phrases in a definition is also important. The nursing facility is required to meet standards for providing a particular kind of care. The term *providing accommodations* implies room and board. Along with the term for *24 hours or more*, it exempts physicians' offices, day care centers and other similar facilities. The term *or unit thereof* is used because some nursing facilities may not be a complete facility but are clearly identifiable units of other facilities (such as hospitals).

Following are some terms that may be defined in the licensing rules and regulations. This list is not complete; it remains for each agency to select and define the terms most applicable to its particular situation. Qualifying adjectives (such as adequate, proper, safe, sufficient, satisfactory, suitable) mean the degree of completeness of performance determined by the Licensing Board to be maintained by the nursing facilities.

- **Administrator**—The person responsible for the management of a nursing facility.
- **Advisory Council**—A group of individuals officially appointed to advise the regulatory authority having jurisdiction.
- **Applicant**—The person who submits an application for a license or licensure renewal to operate a nursing facility.
- **Approved**—Refers to approval by the regulatory authority having jurisdiction.
- **Bed Capacity**—The maximum number of residents for which the nursing facility is licensed to care at one time.
- **Board of Directors**—A group of individuals officially appointed and legally responsible for the administration of the facility.

- **Combination Facility**—A facility that has identifiable sections in reasonable proximity and under the same overall management in two or more of the following categories: hospitals, nursing facilities, homes for the aged and/or residential facilities. Licensing of a *combination facility* poses certain difficulties because each of the units is designated, staffed and equipped to provide a particular level of care. No one set of standards is applied to such a facility as a whole; instead applicable standards are applied to each constituent unit. One inspector or one team of inspectors usually will inspect the entire facility and issue the necessary licenses.
- **Home for the Aged**—A facility designated, staffed and equipped for the care of individuals who do not need hospital or nursing care but do need assistance with everyday essential activities while living in a protected environment.
- **License**—The license for operation of a nursing facility issued by the regulatory agency having jurisdiction.
- **Licensed**—Duly licensed by the authority having jurisdiction.
- **Licensee**—The person to whom the license is issued and who is responsible for the maintenance and operation of the facility.
- **Nursing Facility**—An institution, building, residence, private home or other place, part or unit thereof, however named, for profit or not, including facilities operated by the state or a political subdivision thereof, that is advertised, offered, maintained or operated by the ownership or management for a period of more than 24 hours, whether for consideration or not, for the express or implied purpose of providing accommodations and care for 2 or more individuals not related to the owner or manager by blood or marriage within the third degree of consanguinity and who need nursing care and related medical services that are prescribed by or performed under the direction of persons licensed to provide such care or services in accordance with the laws of the state.
- **Person**—A natural person(s), firm, partnership, association, corporation, company or organization of any kind.
- **Resident**—Any individual residing in and receiving care in a nursing facility.

- **Resident-Facility**—This term includes hotels, motels, apartment houses, boarding homes or other types of accommodations for individuals who do not need the degree of care given in a hospital, nursing facility or home for the aged.

HHS uses the following definitions in surveys and inventories of nursing facilities and related facilities:

- **Skilled Nursing Facility**—A specially qualified facility providing 24 hours of skilled nursing care performed by or under the supervision of licensed nursing personnel only, rehabilitation services and related health services. The skilled nursing facility (SNF) accommodates individuals who no longer require hospital care but still need extensive nursing care. State standards are complied with. Compliance with the federal Code of Federal Regulations (42 CFR, Parts 430 to end) is required for participation in the Medicare and Medicaid programs.
- **Nursing Facility**—An institution that is maintained and equipped to accommodate individuals who are unable to properly care for themselves but are not acutely ill and do not require hospital or skilled nursing care. Supervised nursing care is provided with licensed personnel in accordance with state statutes. Rehabilitation and other related services are provided at a lesser degree than those provided by the SNF. State standards are complied with. Compliance with the federal Code of Federal Regulations (42 CFR, Parts 430 to end) is required for participation in the Medicare and Medicaid programs.
- **Supervised Living Facility**—A facility providing domiciliary care and simple nursing care for individuals who are not acutely ill or in need of skilled or moderate nursing care, but require supervision and/or medication.

### Application for License

Application for a license is made on the forms provided by the licensing agency and requires information necessary to identify the applicant and the type of license desired, and to affirm the applicant's ability to meet the relevant laws, rules and regulations. The licensing fee, method of calculation, handling of monies received and exceptions are usually clearly stated in the enabling legislation and rules and regulations.

### Issuance and Renewal of License

Annual (or more frequent) surveys are done by the state department of health relicensure. The enabling legislative act and implementing rules and regulations include:

1. A requirement for posting the license in a conspicuous place on the premises.
2. Prohibition of license transfer or assignment without the written approval of the licensing agency. The license is valid only for the licensee and premises for which it is issued.
3. A provision for the issuance of temporary/provisional licenses for a six-month period pending final action by the agency or board concerned.
4. Provisions concerning licensure renewal requirements.
5. Provisions for fees and other charges.

### Denial or Revocation of License

The legislation authorizes the licensing agency to deny, suspend or revoke a license in any case where it finds substantial failure to comply with the established requirements. A notice prior to any such action will be sent by registered mail or personal service to the applicant or licensee and specify the reasons for their proposed action and a date within 30 days for a hearing. Procedures in accordance with rules promulgated by the licensing agency govern the hearings, and a complete record is kept. Both parties may subpoena witnesses. The licensing agency will make a decision based on the hearing or if the licensee or applicant defaults. A copy of the decision specifying the findings of fact by the licensing agency and the conclusions of law is sent to the licensee or applicant by registered mail or personal service. The decision becomes final after 30 days unless the licensee or applicant appeals in accordance with the provision for judicial review.

### Rules, Regulations and Enforcement

A blanket requirement specifies that all nursing facilities comply with all applicable laws, ordinances and other requirements. The licensing agency may adopt, command, promulgate and enforce any additional rules, regulations and standards that accomplish the purposes of the enabling legislation. Nursing facilities operating on the effective date of new or amended regulations are not required to make unreasonable extensive building alterations and are given adequate time to comply with other regulations.

OBRA 1987 attempted to have nationally consistent standards. Although encouraged to establish higher standards than the minimum set at the federal level, state laws and regulations still vary. If a state requirement is stronger than a federal one, state regulation applies.

### Reports and Information

The licensure agency usually requires annual and other reports at specified intervals and on forms it may prescribe. Information received by the licensing agency through filed reports, inspection or other authorized means is confidential and is not disclosed publicly in such a manner as to identify individuals except in a legal proceeding involving the question of licensure.

### Inspections and Consultations

The licensing agency is empowered and provided with sufficient staff to:

1. Make yearly inspections and investigations as it deems necessary, with the nursing facility receiving appropriate written reports. They may coordinate inspections of other state and local agencies.
2. Provide consultation and aid in assisting nursing facilities to meet and exceed the requirements established by law.
3. Delegate to local agencies any duties and powers other than issuance of licenses.
4. Enforce regulations for and approve alterations in licensed facilities.
5. Use the injunctive process when advisable.

### Penalties

It is a misdemeanor to establish, maintain or operate a nursing facility without a license. Other penalties are established for violations of the laws, rules and regulations. Each day of a continued violation is considered a separate offense.

## Medicare and Medicaid Certification

The federal government purchases health care services from nursing facilities and pays for the cost of the services through the Medicare and Medicaid programs. After a **provider of care** applies, the federal government arranges to purchase services through a contract called a **provider agreement** whereby the nursing facility agrees to provide services at a minimal level set by federal standards termed **Long-Term Care Facility Requirements**. These requirements are established by HCFA and can be augmented or strengthened by the individual states.

## Nursing Facility Surveys

The federal government contracts with each state to conduct a survey/inspection program of nursing facilities to determine the extent of compliance with the federal regulations. Many states combine the annual state licensure survey with this survey. (By federal law, the government reimburses the state 75% of Medicare survey cost.) Inspections occur on a survey cycle of every 9 to 15 months.

Current survey or emphasis has shifted from inspection of written records to ascertainment of actual resident care outcomes. Surveyors interview a sample of residents and meet with the resident council. They also talk with the state ombudsman and family members, and watch and visit with residents who are eating, participating in activities, and receiving medication and other services. **Interpretive Guidelines** are issued for surveyors, requiring comprehensive training for implementing the standards and understanding the survey procedures.

If the state certifies that the facility is in substantial compliance with the federal standards, the provider contract is renewed. If the nursing facility has deficiencies in performance, the inspectors or surveyors complete a **Statement of Deficiencies** report. The facility must respond with a **plan of correction**, noting how the problem(s) will be corrected and by what date. The survey reports must be posted in the facility and are available from the state health department.

## Remedies for Noncompliance

OBRA 1987 established enforcement measures for when a provider is not in compliance with standards. State and federal governments must have levels of sanction severity to respond to degrees of noncompliance. The remedies for noncompliance are:

1. **Denial of Payment**—The government may stop Medicare and Medicaid payments for new admissions until the facility is in substantial compliance with the standards.
2. **Civil Monetary Penalty**—The government may collect fines for each day a facility is out of compliance. These are more severe for repeated or uncorrected deficiencies. There is no maximum amount for state fines; the maximum federal fine is $10,000 per day.
3. **Temporary Management**—When a facility is being closed or making improvements to bring it into compliance, a temporary manager may be appointed by the government. This temporary management stays until the state finds that the facility has complied with the standards.
4. **Termination of Provider Contract or Closing the Facility**—If it is determined that the health and safety of the residents is in immediate jeopardy, the government may terminate the provider agreement and close the facility.
5. **Other Solutions**—The states may use other remedies if these are "as effective in deterring noncompliance and correcting deficiencies" as the ones prescribed by OBRA 1987.

By law, the state and federal governments are to establish criteria for enforcement of the above remedies that will:

1. Indicate when and how the remedies are available.
2. Determine the amounts of fines and severity of remedies.
3. Expedite the time between the imposition of a remedy and the identification of the deficiency. Denial of payment, temporary management and facility closure may occur during a hearing; civil fines may not occur during a hearing.
4. Provide more severe fines for repeat and uncorrected deficiencies.

## LICENSURE OF NURSING HOME ADMINISTRATORS

Nursing home administrators are one of the few professional managers who are required to be licensed by both state and federal governments.

The Social Security Act was amended in 1965 (Section 1902) to require that nursing home administrators be licensed by the state provisionally by July 1, 1970, and by examination after July 1, 1972. A nursing facility could only provide Medicare or Medicaid services when under the supervision of a licensed nursing home administrator. By further amendment in 1967, the states were required to appoint and establish a licensing board of examiners who were to develop, impose and enforce standards; monitor the performance of nursing home administrators; issue, revoke or suspend licenses; and conduct studies to improve standards. All states make it a misdemeanor for an individual to practice without a license.

The educational requirements for licensure vary from state to state, ranging from a high school diploma to a bachelor's degree in health care administration. Many states require that the candidate for licensure also complete a 2-month to 3-year administrator-in-training (AIT) program under the supervision of a qualified preceptor. Finally, each state requires that the candidate pass an oral or written state exam relative to its laws and rules. After meeting a specific state educational requirement, each candidate also must pass a national examination.

OBRA 1987 felt that the educational background of nursing home administrators should be more uniform and required that the HHS secretary establish minimum federal standards for nursing facility administrators. In October 1990, Congress passed an amendment providing that the federal mandate for the licensure of administrators be repealed when the secretary's standard becomes effective.

In February 1992, HCFA published a proposed rule in the *Federal Register* recommending that candidates for licensure, such as nursing home administrators, must:

1. Have a baccalaureate degree.
2. Complete an internship.
3. Pass an examination.
4. Have 10 hours of continuing education per year.

Once these standards are published in the final form and become effective, the states are expected to incorporate them into their licensing requirements.

Other organizations that enhance the professional educations of nursing home administrators are the American College of Health Care Administrators, the American Health Care Association and the American Association of Homes for the Aging.

## LIFE SAFETY CODE

The nursing facility must meet the requirements of the Life Safety Code promulgated by the National Fire Protection Association (NFPA). This code, as it relates to health care occupancies, includes hospitals, nursing facilities, limited-care facilities and ambulatory health care facilities. In some states, standards set for fire and safety exceed those standards set by the Life Safety Code; parts of the Life Safety Code may be waived as long as the state codes are met in these cases.

Following is a summary of the requirements of the Life Safety Code (1988) as it relates to new health care occupancies.

### Fire Resistancy Construction

One-story buildings must adhere to the following types of construction: protective, noncombustible, fire resistant, protected ordinary construction, protective woodframe, heavy timber or unprotected noncombustible.

Buildings of two or more stories are required to be constructed of noncombustible materials with a minimum of a two-hour fire resistance rating. It is recognized that movement of residents may not be possible, and occupants of a health care facility may be required to remain in the structure for the duration of the fire. If an approved automatic extinguishing system is available, construction may be of a protected combustible type and rating of enclosure walls may be reduced to one hour. All interior walls and partitions must be of noncombustible fire resistant materials. Every exterior and interior wall and partition must be able to stop fire at each floor level, at the top story and at the roof supports. Unoccupied attics must have larger than 300 square feet. Concealed spaces must have fire-stop areas of not less than 1,000 square feet between ceiling and floor, or 3,000 square feet between ceiling and roof.

An outside door or outside window that can be opened easily from the inside without keys or tools must be provided in every sleeping room or room occupied more than 24 hours. Sill height must not be more than 36 inches above the floor, or more than 60 inches above the floor in special nursing care areas. Interior finishes must be approved for intended use for such factors as flame spread, type and amount of smoke generated, and fire retardant properties. No furnishings or decorations of an explosive or highly flammable character are permitted. The use of flame retardants is encouraged and the retardants should be renewed at intervals required to keep the necessary properties.

## Exits

At least two exits remotely located from each other must be provided for each floor or fire section of the building. At least one exit from each floor or fire section shall be: a door leading directly to outside the building, a stair, a smokeproof enclosure, a ramp or an exit passageway. Every habitable room shall have an exit access door leading directly to an exit access corridor.

Any resident sleeping room or suite that includes resident sleeping rooms of more than 1,000 square feet shall have at least two exit access doors remote from each other.

Exits should be placed so that the entrance door of every resident's room is not more than 100 feet from the nearest exit. No point in the resident's room and an access door of that room shall exceed 50 feet from the door. This travel distance may be increased by 50 feet in a building protected throughout by an approved supervised automatic sprinkler system.

Exits used by residents shall be marked by an approved sign readily visible from any direction of exit access. Signed placements shall be such that access from an exit is no more than 100 feet from the nearest visible sign.

Horizontal exits are considered a way of passage to a place of safety from the smoke and fire area until evacuation can be completed. The requirement for horizontal exits is that at least 30 net square feet per resident in a nursing facility shall be provided within the aggregate area of corridors, resident rooms, treatment rooms, or lounge or dining areas. A single door may be used in a horizontal exit if the exit serves one direction only; this door may be a swinging door or horizontal sliding door with a minimum width of 44 inches.

## Exit Signs

Every exit sign shall have the word "exit" in letters not less than 6 inches high with the principal strokes not less than ¾ inches wide.

Every sign shall be suitably illuminated by a reliable light source. Externally and internally illuminated signs shall be visible in both normal and emergency lighting mode.

## Stairs

Stairs must be a permanent construction as follows:

|  | New | Existing |
|---|---|---|
| Minimum width clear of all obstructions | 44" | 44" |
| Maximum height of risers | 7" | 7-1/2" |
| Minimum height of risers | 4" | |
| Minimum tread depth | 11" | 10" |
| Minimum head room | 6'8" | 6'8" |
| Maximum height between landings | 12' | 12' |

Stairways should have evenly spaced risers and treads. Treads should be solid and nonslip. Each stair landing must be constructed to carry a load of 100 pounds per square foot and be at least equal to the width of the stairway.

Each new stair with a slope exceeding 1 foot rise every 15 feet shall have handrails on both sides. Required handrails shall continue for the full length of each flight of stairs. The design of handrails and hardware for attaching handrails to guards shall be such that there are no projecting lugs on attachment devices or nonprojecting corners or members of grilles or panels that may engage loose clothing.

Handrails on new stairs shall not be less than 34 inches or more than 38 inches above the surface of the tread. Existing handrails shall not be less than 30 inches or more than 38 inches above the surface of the tread.

Stairways must be enclosed with noncombustible material having fire resistance of at least two hours.

Each stairway should be clearly marked "fire exit." Where the stair continues beyond the exit, it should have an effective means of interruption of travel.

When used as an exit, outside stairs must be permanently installed on the exterior of the building, meet the same requirements for the inside stairs, and be provided with guardrails and other devices to enable those who fear heights to use them. Exterior stairs on buildings of more than three stories must have screening arrangements at least four feet high. Such stairs may lead to roofs or approved fire resistance construction where a safe and continuous means of exit is located.

## Ramps

Because of the possibility of accidents, ramps of an extremely gradual slope are practical only for moving resident beds from one area to another where elevators may be unavailable and for permitting safe travel by wheelchair residents.

An interior or outside ramp may be used as a means of exit. Ramps are classified as A or B; ramps in nursing facilities shall be Class A with the following dimensions:

> Minimum width—44"
> Maximum slope —1' rise in 10'
> Maximum height between landings—12'

All existing Class A ramps and new ramps not exceeding a slope of 1 foot rise every 15 feet do not need to be provided with landings.

Outside ramps shall be separated from the interior and other parts of the building by walls with a fire resistance rating (1 hour in three-story or less buildings, and 2 hours in four-story or more buildings) with fixed or self-closing opening protectives. This protection shall extend at least 10 feet upward or to the roofline, whichever is lower, and at least 10 feet horizontally and downward to the ground level.

Outside ramps shall be so arranged as to avoid any handicap to their use by persons having a fear of high places. For ramps with more than 3 stories in height, any arrangement intended to meet this requirement shall be at least 4 feet in height.

These ramps shall be constructed of noncombustible or limited combustible material. Floors and landings shall be solid with a slip-resistant surface and without perforations. Ramps and intermediate landings shall continue with no decrease in width along the direction of exit travel.

## Corridors

Nursing facility corridors should have exits or open into corridors that have exits. All resident rooms should open directly into a corridor or the exterior. Dead end corridors are undesirable and preferably should not be permitted. In no event should an exit access corridor have a dead end exceeding 30 feet.

Handrails are required on both sides of the corridors used by the residents. They should be of an approved type and securely mounted to the wall at an approved height. Signs of an illuminated type must be mounted in all corridors showing the way to the nearest exit.

All interior walls and partitions must be of a noncombustible material with one-hour fire-resistance rating, and be of continuous construction from the floor slab (through any concealed space) to the underside of the floor above or roof. Corridors used for exit access must have an unobstructed width of at least 8 feet (nursing facilities), or at least six feet (residential-custodial homes). Openings to the corridor must have 1¾ inch solid bonded core wood doors of 20-minute fire-resistance rating (except when an exit or to a hazardous area) and may have approved fixed wire glass windows. Vision panels of wired glass no larger than 1,296 square inches in approved steel frames are also allowed in corridor walls.

Partitions with approved doors may be used to separate corridors from use areas where an approved automatic extinguishing system is available throughout the building.

## Waiting Areas

Waiting areas (maximum 250 square feet) on sleeping floors may open directly to the corridor, providing there is an approved automatic smoke detector and direct supervision by the staff. Large waiting areas (maximum 600 square feet) on other than sleeping floors also may open directly to the corridor under the same conditions, providing no obstruction blocks the exits. Other spaces that may open to the corridor include charting, communications and clerical areas.

## Fire-Resistant Elevators

A facility with residents housed on floors other than those at street level shall have at least one elevator equipped with automatic floor devices and be large enough to accommodate the wheeled stretcher and an attendant. Shafts for elevators must be of noncombustible construction of two-hour fire resistance. All openings must be equipped with doors having a self-closing device and a positive latch. The installation and maintenance of all elevators shall comply with all applicable state and local regulations. Regular compliance inspections shall be posted.

## Doors

Doors (including doorway, frame and door hardware) are to be constructed so that the direction of exit travel is easily understood. Doors must swing easily in the direction of exit travel to provide full use of the doorway and should at no time interfere with the full use of stairs or landings. Floors of both sides of the door must be level for at least the width of the door, although there may be a step of up to eight inches lower than the floor level when the door exits to the outside. As to width, no single door should be less than 28 inches or more than 48 inches wide. (Forty-four inches are required in new construction.) Thresholds of doorways should be flush with the floor.

The door latches should have single releasing devices (knob, handle or panic bar) that are easily understood and used. If there are locks, simple operation by means other than key must allow exit from the building or resident's room into a corridor. Approved panic hardware must be able to be released by a force of less than 15 pounds in the direction of exit travel, placed at suitable heights (30 inches to 44 inches above the floor), and incapable of being locked when pressure is applied to the bar.

Doors that normally are kept closed should have a self-closing mechanism and be marked as such: "Fire door—Please keep closed." For practical purposes of resident observation and efficiency, doors and fire separations, horizontal exits and smoke partitions may be held open with electrical hold-open devices arranged to activate self-closing by the approved fire and smoke detection systems. Interior doors, except for closets on corridors, should not swing into corridors. No doors to rooms used by residents shall be equipped with locks or other devices designed to bolt or bar them, except doors leading directly to the outside of the building which are not a means of egress. Doors, which are a means of egress, may be equipped with a latch or lock which does not require a key or other tool to unlock the door from the egress side.

## Smoke Partitions

The NFPA recognizes that smoke may be produced before a fire is extinguished with automatic sprinklers and may create a panic hazard. Every floor used by residents (sleeping or treatment) or occupied by 50 or more persons must be divided into at least two compartments no larger than 150 feet in length or width. The smoke partition must be constructed of noncombustible materials, be continuous from outside wall to outside wall and from floor slab to floor slab, and have a fire resistance rating of one-hour minimum. Doors must be able to swing in opposite directions, be self-closing, have wired glass windows and a fire protection rating of at least 20 minutes.

## Hazardous Areas

Hazardous areas must be enclosed with construction having a minimum rating of one hour fire resistance or have approved automatic fire protection with not more than six sprinklers served by one piping. These areas include boiler and heater rooms, laundries, kitchens, handicraft shops and gift shops.

Both fire-rated construction and automatic fire protection must be used in severe hazard areas, including soiled linen rooms, paint shops, trash collection rooms, repair shops and the rooms or spaces used for storing combustible supplies and equipment in quantities considered hazardous by the authorities having jurisdiction.

Self-closing or automatic fire doors are required for openings to hazard areas of both types. Thin glass windows or other approved vents must be provided to the outside of the building in an explosion hazard area. A separate building may house hazardous operations or materials far enough away to not cause danger to occupants in the main building, with only such protection as required for those working there.

## Fire Protection Systems

According to the Life Safety Code, there are three major parts of a protective signaling system:

- **Initiating devices** used manually or automatically to initiate an alarm signal.
- **Control panels** receive the alarm signal and send it to the indicating device.
- **Indicating devices** audibly and visually warn occupants and personnel of an alarm situation.

Signaling systems and component devices (pull stations, smoke detectors, alarm and sprinkler systems) must be:

- Approved for their specific purpose.
- Operated, maintained and tested regularly by qualified personnel.
- Tested periodically as specified by the authority having jurisdiction.
- Installed to not interfere with the operating of manual fire alarm boxes.
- Returned to normal as soon as possible after fire alarm or drill.

The signaling system also may automatically initiate release of self-closing or self-opening doors, shutting off gas, fuel oil and electricity supplies, and switching on emergency lights, so long as these functions do not interfere with the power for lighting and operating elevators.

### Manual Electrically Supervised Fire Alarm System

A manual electronically supervised system is required in all nursing facilities and residential-custodial care facilities. The fire alarm boxes are located within convenient reach of all areas of the facility, so that the alarm may be sent without leaving the area of activity, fire or those in the immediate vicinity. The alarm should connect with the fire station and be uniquely, distinctly and effectively audible and visual in any interior part of the facility. This permits assistance to be requested for immediate removal of the physically helpless and otherwise handicapped occupants. Each section where a division is made by a firewall or other adequate safeguard against the spread of smoke and fire is considered a separate building.

Manual fire alarm boxes of the same general type should be located in paths of escape from fire or near exits and where they can be easily seen and reached. Additional boxes must be used so that a box is available in a maximum of 200 feet in all directions on the same floor. These boxes may only be used for fire, with no difference in signals used for drills or actual alarms.

Approved automatic smoke detection and alarm initiating systems—properly installed and electronically interconnected with the manually operated fire alarm system—must be placed in all corridors no further apart than 30 feet on centers or 15 feet from any wall. Corridor systems are not required where each sleeping room is protected by a smoke detection system with a local detector at the smoke partition.

Approved fire detector and alarm initiating systems may be located in required areas on the ceilings or on the side walls near the ceilings as determined by an engineering survey.

Supervisory signal initiation devices—which monitor water pressure, valves, water level, water flow, temperature pumps and other functions necessary for the fire extinguishing system—must be provided on all extinguishing systems with an audible signal different from the fire alarm. These must be installed so that the device can be operated both automatically and manually.

All audible alarms must have unique and distinct sounds, be used only for fire alarm purposes and be located so as to be clearly heard above the usual maximum noise levels in the facility. Visual alarms should activate simultaneously with the audible alarms.

### Sprinkler Systems

The NFPA recommends complete standard automatic sprinkler systems (such as carbon dioxide, dry chemical phone or water spray) as the most effective means of safeguarding against loss of life and property by fire physically and by minimizing possible panic. Properly designed automatic sprinkler systems provide both automatic alarm and automatic extinguishment. A standard extinguishing system of another type may be installed with the approval of the authority having jurisdiction in those areas where another type would be more effective.

Approved standard automatic sprinkler systems must be installed and maintained throughout all nursing facilities and custodial care facilities, except in buildings of fire-resistance construction or one-story protected noncombustible construction, and must have a water flow alarm device. The system must be ready to operate at all times, tested and inspected periodically, and electrically interconnected with the fire alarm system. The main sprinkler control valve must be electronically supervised so a local alarm (at least) will sound when the valve is closed. Sprinkler piping may be directly connected with domestic water supply having pressure of 9.15 gallons per minute per square foot of floor area of the building.

## *Portable Fire Extinguishers*

Portable fire extinguishers (PFEs) of a type approved by the NFPA are required in all nursing facilities. Extinguishers of a type, capacity and number adequate to meet the needs of the facility and to comply with state and local codes must be located on each floor and adjacent to special hazard areas (such as kitchens and shops). No extinguishers using toxic vaporizing liquids, such as carbon tetrachloride, are permitted. They must be located so that a person will have to travel no more than 75 feet (Class A) or 50 feet (Classes B and C) from any point to reach the nearest extinguisher and should be located low enough for persons of short stature to reach comfortably. Portable fire extinguishers are used for the following types of fires:

- **Class A**—This extinguisher is symbolized by $\triangle$ and is used on ordinary combustibles such as wood, cloth, paper, rubber and some plastics. The background symbol is metallic or green. It always will be found on water and multipurpose dry chemical extinguishers.
- **Class B**—This extinguisher is symbolized by $\boxed{B}$ and is used on flammable or combustible liquids, flammable gases, greases, or similar materials. The background symbol is metallic or red. It always will be found on dry chemical, carbon dioxide and foaming extinguishers.
- **Class C**—This extinguisher is symbolized by $\copyright$ and is used on fires involving energized electrical equipment. The background of this symbol is metallic or blue. It always will be found on multipurpose dry chemical and carbon dioxide extinguishers.
- **Class** $\triangle$ , $\boxed{B}$ , $\copyright$ —This extinguisher is a multipurpose dry chemical type that can be used on Class A, B or C type fires. (These extinguishers are very practical for home use; they are flame interrupting and, in some cases, cooling agents.)
- **Class D**—This extinguisher is symbolized by $\textcircled{D}$ and is used on certain combustible metals such as sodium, magnesium and potassium. The background of the symbol is metallic or yellow. It is always found on special dry powder extinguishers. (These fires are rare in a home or office.)

Fire extinguishers must be kept in perfect working condition at all times and should be checked quarterly by the fire department and recharged or serviced annually by a qualified agency. A tag should be attached to each extinguisher after inspection or servicing to indicate the date that it was done.

## Emergency Power

Emergency power of at least 1 hour duration must be automatically and continuously provided with no noticeable interruption (a maximum delay of 10 seconds) of lighting.

Maintenance on the emergency power system includes: (1) a weekly check, (2) monthly tests under a full load for 30 minutes and (3) proper documentation.

## AMERICAN NATIONAL STANDARDS INSTITUTE BUILDING SPECIFICATIONS FOR THE PHYSICALLY HANDICAPPED

This standard applies to all buildings and facilities used by the public and to temporary, emergency and permanent conditions. The federal government requires that the following standards promulgated by the American National Standards Institute (ANSI) be adhered to by nursing facilities.

### Purpose

The specifications in this standard are intended to make buildings and facilities accessible to and usable by people with such disabilities as: inability to walk, difficulty in walking, reliance on walking aids, blindness and visual impairment, deafness and hearing impairments, incoordination, reaching and manipulation disabilities, lack of stamina, difficulty in interpreting and reacting to sensory information, and extremes of physical size. Accessibility and usability allow a physically handicapped person to approach, enter and use a building or facility.

This standard can be applied to the following: (1) the design and construction of new buildings and facilities, including both spaces and elements, site improvements and public walks; (2) remodeling, alteration and rehabilitation of existing construction; and (3) permanent, temporary and emergency conditions.

## Definitions

These terms have the following meanings for the purpose of this standard.

- **Access Aisle**—An accessible pedestrian space between elements (such as parking spaces, seating and desks) to provide clearances appropriate for the use of the elements.
- **Accessible**—Describes a site, building, facility or portion thereof that complies with this standard and that can be approached, entered in used by physically handicapped people.
- **Accessible Route**—A continuous unobstructed path connecting all accessible elements and spaces in a building or facility that can be negotiated by a person with a severe disability using a wheelchair and that also is safe for and usable by people with other disabilities. Interior accessible routes may include corridors, floors, ramps, elevators, lifts and clear floor space at fixtures. Exterior accessible routes may include parking access aisles, curb ramps, walks, ramps and lifts.
- **Adaptability**—The capacity of certain building spaces and elements (such as kitchen counters, sinks and grab bars) to be altered or added so as to accommodate the needs of persons with different types and degrees of disability.
- **Administrative Authority**—A jurisdictional body that adopts or enforces regulations and standards for the design, construction or operation of buildings and facilities.
- **Assembly Area**—A room or space accommodating a number of individuals as specified by the authority having jurisdiction and used for religious, recreational, educational, political, social, amusement, or consumption of food and drink purposes. It includes all connected rooms or spaces with a common means of egress or ingress. Such areas as conference rooms would have to be accessible in accordance with other parts of this standard, but would not have to meet all of the criteria associated with assembly areas.
- **Automatic Door**—A door equipped with a power-operated mechanism and controls that open and close the door automatically upon receipt of a momentary actuating signal. The switch that begins the automatic cycle may be a photoelectric device, floor mat, sensing device or manual switch mounted on or near the door itself.
- **Clear**—Unobstructed.
- **Common Use**—Refers to those interior and exterior rooms, spaces or elements that are made available for the use of a restricted group of people. For example: residents of an apartment building, occupants of an office building or the guests of such residents/occupants.
- **Curb Ramp**—A short ramp cutting through a curb or built up to it.
- **Detectable**—Perceptible by one or more of the senses.
- **Detectable Warning**—A standardized surface texture applied to or built into walking surface or other elements to warn visually impaired people of hazards in the path of travel.
- **Disability**—A limitation or loss of use of a physical, mental or sensory body part or function.
- **Dwelling Unit**—A single unit of residence that provides a kitchen or food preparation area in addition to rooms and spaces for living, bathing, sleeping and the like. A single-family home is a drawing unit; dwelling units are to be found in such housing types as townhouses and apartment buildings.
- **Egress, Means of**—A path of exit that meets all applicable code specifications of the regulatory building agency having jurisdiction over the building or facility.
- **Element**— An architectural or mechanical component of a building, facility, space or site that can be used in making functional spaces accessible. For example: telephone, curb ramp, door, drinking fountain, seating or water closet.
- **Facility**—All or any portion of a building, structure or area, including the site on which such building, structure or area is located, wherein specific services are provided or activities are performed.
- **Housing**—A building, facility or portion thereof (excluding inpatient health care facilities) that contains one or more dwelling units or sleeping accommodations. Housing may include, but is not limited to: one-family and two-family dwellings, multifamily dwellings, group homes, hotels, motels, dormitories and mobile homes.
- **Physically Handicapped Person**—An individual who has a physical impairment, including im-

paired sensory, manual or speaking abilities, that results in a functional limitation in gaining access to and using a building or facility.

- **Power-Assisted Door**—A door used for human passage with a mechanism that helps to open the door, or to relieve the opening resistance of the door, upon the activation of a switch or the use of a continued force applied to the door itself. If the switch or door is released, such doors immediately begin to close or close completely within 3 to 30 seconds.
- **Principal Entrance**—An entrance intended to be used by the residents or users to enter or leave a building or facility. This may include, but is not limited to, the main entrance.
- **Public Use**—Describes the interior and exterior rooms or spaces that are made available to the general public. Public used may be provided at a building or facility that is privately or publicly owned.
- **Ramp**—A walking surface in an accessible space that has a running slope less than 1 foot for every 20 feet.
- **Running Slope**—The slope of a pedestrian way that is parallel to the direction of travel.
- **Service Entrance**—An entrance intended primarily for delivery or service.
- **Signage**—Verbal, symbolic or pictorial information.
- **Site**—A parcel of land bounded by a property line or a designated portion of a public right-of-way.
- **Site Improvements**—Landscaping, pedestrian and vehicular pathways, outdoor lighting, recreational facilities and the like added to the site.
- **Sleeping Accommodations**—Rooms in which people sleep. For example: dormitory and hotel or motel guest rooms.
- **Space**—A definable area. For example: toilet room, hall, assembly area, entrance, storage room alcove, courtyard or lobby.
- **Tactile**—Describes an object that can be perceived using the sense of touch.
- **Temporary**—Applies to facilities that are not of permanent construction but are extensively used or essential for public use for a given (short) period of time. For example: temporary classrooms or classroom buildings at schools and colleges or facilities

around a major construction site to make passage accessible, usable and safe for everybody. Major construction, such as portable toilets, scaffolding, bridging, trailers and the like are not included.

- **Vehicular Way**—A route intended for vehicular traffic, such as a street, driveway or parking lot.
- **Walk**—An exterior pathway with a prepared surface for pedestrian use, including general pedestrian areas such as plazas and courts.
- **Walking Aid**—A device used by a person who has difficulty walking. For example: a cane, crutch, walker or brace.

## Accessible Elements and Spaces

### Accessible Route

- Accessible routes within the boundaries of the site shall be provided from public transportation stops, accessible parking and accessible passenger loading zones, and public streets or sidewalks to the accessible building entrance they serve.
- The minimum clear width of an accessible route shall be 36 inches except at doors. If a person in a wheelchair must make a turn around an obstruction, the minimum clear width must be areas of 36 × 36 × 36 inches or 42 × 48 × 42 inches.
- If an accessible route has less than 60 inches clear width, then passing spaces at least 60 × 60 inches shall be located at reasonable intervals not to exceed 200 feet. An intersection of two corridors or walks also shall be considered a passing space.

### Alarms

- Audible emergency alarms shall produce a sound that exceeds the prevailing equivalent sound level in the room or space by at least 15 decibels or exceeds any maximum sound level with a duration of 30 seconds by 5 decibels, whichever is louder. Sound levels for alarm signals shall not exceed 120 decibels.
- Visual alarms shall be flashing lights arranged to flash in conjunction with the audible emergency alarms. The flashing frequency of visual alarms shall be approximately 1 Hz. Specialized systems using advanced technology may be substituted if

equivalent protection is provided for handicapped users of the building or facility.

- Auxiliary or sensory alarms provided for persons with hearing impairments shall be connected to the building emergency system or there shall be a standard 110 volt electrical receptacle into which any alarm unit can be connected to be activated by the building alarm system. Instructions for use of the auxiliary alarm or connections shall be provided.

- Detectable warning textures on walking surfaces shall consist of exposed aggregate concrete, cushioned surfaces made of rubber or plastic, raised strips or grooves. Textures sharp contrast with that of the surrounding surface. Raised strips or grooves shall be ¾ inch to 2 inches wide, ¼ inch to ¾ inch apart and ⅛ inch high, slant away from the hazardous area and be used indoors only.

- Doors that lead to areas that might prove dangerous to a blind person (doors to loading platforms, boiler rooms, stages and the like) shall be made identifiable to the touch by a textured surface on the door handle, knob, pull or other operating hardware. This textured surface may be made by knurling, roughening or applying materials to the contact surface. Such textured services shall not be provided for emergency exit doors or any doors other than those to hazardous areas.

- All stairs (except those in dwelling units, enclosed stair towers or set to the side of the path of travel) shall have a detectable warning at the top of the stair runs.

- If a walk crosses or adjoins a frequently used vehicular way and no curbs, railings or other elements are detectable by a person who has a severe visual impairment separating the pedestrian and vehicular areas, the boundary between the areas shall be defined by a continuous detectable warning texture that is 36 inches wide.

- The edges of reflecting pools shall be protected by railings, walls, curbs or detectable warnings.

### Controls and Operating Mechanisms

Controls and operating mechanisms in accessible spaces, along accessible routes or as part of accessible elements (light switches, dispenser controls) shall comply with the following.

- Clear floor space allowing a forward or parallel approach by a person using a wheelchair shall be provided at controls, dispensers, receptacles and other operable equipment.

- The highest operable part of all controls, dispensers, receptacles and other operable equipment shall be placed within at least one of the forward or side-reach ranges, except where the use of special equipment dictates otherwise. Electrical and communications-system receptacles on walls shall be mounted no less than 15 inches above the wall.

- Controls and operating mechanisms shall be operable with one hand and shall not require tight grasping, pitching or twisting of the wrist. The force required to activate controls shall be no greater than 5 pounds-force (lbf).

### Crutches

- Individuals 5 feet 6 inches tall require an average of 31 inches between crutch tips in the normally accepted gaits.

- Individuals 5 feet 9 inches tall require an average of 32.5 inches between crutch tips in the normally accepted gaits.

### Curb Ramps

- The minimum width of a curb ramp shall be 36 inches, exclusive of flared sides.

- Curb ramps shall be located or protected to prevent their obstruction by parked vehicles.

### Doors

- Doorways intended for user passage shall have a minimum clear opening of 32 inches with the door open 90 degrees as measured between the face of the door and the stop.

- Thresholds at doorways shall not exceed ¾ inch in height for exterior residential sliding doors or ½ inch for other types of doors. Raised thresholds and floor level changes at accessible doorways shall not be beveled with a slope of greater than 1 foot for every 2 feet.

- Hardware such as handles, pulls, latches, locks and other operating devices on accessible doors shall have a shape that is easy to grasp with one hand and does not require tight grasping, tight pinching or twisting of the wrist to operate. They shall be mounted within reach ranges as specified for wheelchairs. Lever-operated mechanisms, push-type mechanisms and U-shaped handles are acceptable designs.

- If a door has a closer, the sweep period of the closer shall be adjusted so that from an open position of 90 degrees, the door will take at least 3 seconds to move to an open position of approximately 12 degrees.
- The maximum opening force, expressed in lbf, for pushing or pulling open a door shall be as follows:

| Fire Doors | Minimum force allowable by the appropriate administrative authority |
|---|---|
| Exterior Hinged Doors | 8.5 lbf |
| Interior Hinged Doors | 5 lbf |
| Sliding/Folding Doors | 5 lbf |

These forces do not apply to the force required to retract latch bolts or disengage other devices that may hold the door in a closed position.

### Drinking Fountains and Water Coolers

- Spouts shall be no higher than 36 inches as measured from the floor or ground surface to the spout outlet.
- Wall-mounted and post-mounted cantilevered units shall have a clear knee space between the bottom of the apron and the floor or ground at least 27 inches high, 30 inches wide and 17 inches to 19 inches deep. Such units shall also have a minimum clear floor space 30 inches to 48 inches to allow a person in wheelchair to approach the unit facing forward.

### Elevators

- Elevator operations shall be automatic. Each car shall be equipped with a self-leveling feature that will automatically bring the car to floor landings within a tolerance of ½ inch under rated-loading to zero-loading conditions. This self-leveling feature shall be automatic and independent of the operat-

ing device and shall correct for overtravel or undertravel.
- Call buttons in elevator lobbies and halls shall be centered at 42 inches above the floor. Such call buttons shall have visual signals to indicate when each call is registered and when each call is answered. Call buttons shall be a minimum of ¾ inch in dimension. The button designating the up direction shall be on top.
- Elevator car control panels shall have the following features: raised, flush or recessed control buttons at least ¾ inch in dimension and arranged with numbers in ascending order reading from left to right and tactile and visual indicators by raised standard alphabet characters for letters and arabic characters for numerals or standard symbols.

### Entrances

- Entrances to a building or facility that are part of an accessible route shall comply with the specifications for accessible routes. Such entrances shall be connected by an accessible route to public transportation stops, to accessible parking and passenger loading zones, and to public streets or sidewalks if available. They also shall be connected by an accessible route to all accessible spaces or elements within the building or facility.

### Grab Bars

These specifications apply to all grab bars and tub and shower seats in accessible toilet or bathing facilities.

- The diameter or width of the gripping services of a grab bar shall be 1¼ inches to 1½ inches or equivalent. If the grab bars are mounted adjacent to a wall, the space between the wall and the grab bar shall be 1½ inches.
- The bending stress in a grab bar or seat induced by the maximum bending moment from the application of 250 lbf shall be less than the allowable stress of the material of the grab bar or seat.

### Ground and Floor Surfaces

- Ground and floor surfaces along accessible routes and in accessible rooms and spaces (including floors, walks, ramps, stairs and curb ramps) shall be stable, firm and slip resistant.

- If carpet or carpet tile is used on a ground or floor surface, it shall be securely attached, have a firm cushion, pad or backing or no cushion or pad, and have a level loop, textured loop, level cut pile or cut/uncut pile texture. The maximum pile height shall be ½ inch. Exposed edges of carpet shall be fastened to floor surfaces and have beveled (maximum 1 foot rise for every 2 feet slope) trim along the entire length of the exposed edge if the carpet pile height is between ¼ and ½ inch.
- If gratings are located in walking surfaces, they shall have spaces no greater than ½ inch wide in one direction. If gratings have elongated openings, they shall be placed so that the long dimension is perpendicular to the dominant direction of travel.

### Lavatories, Sinks and Mirrors

- Lavatories shall be mounted with a clearance of at least 29 inches from the floor to the bottom of the apron.
- Sinks shall be mounted with the counter or rim no higher than 34 inches from the floor. Each sink shall be a maximum of 6½ inches deep.
- A clear floor space 30 × 48 inches allowing accessibility by wheelchairs shall be provided in front of a lavatory or sink to allow a forward approach.
- Hot water and drain pipes under lavatories or sinks shall be insulated or otherwise protected if they abut the clearance areas indicated.
- Mirrors shall be mounted with the bottom edge of the reflecting surface no higher than 40 inches from the floor.

### Parking Spaces and Passenger Loading Zones

- Parking spaces for physically handicapped people shall be at least 96 inches wide and shall have an adjacent access aisle at least 60 inches wide. Accessible parking spaces shall be designated as reserved for physically handicapped people by a sign showing the symbol of accessibility. Such signs shall not be obscured by a vehicle parked in the space.
- Passenger loading zones shall provide an access aisle at least 48 inches wide and 20 feet long

adjacent and parallel to the vehicle pull-up space. A minimum vertical clearance of 108 inches shall be provided at accessible passenger loading zones and along vehicle access routes to such areas from site entrances.

### Protruding Objects

- Objects protruding from walls (such as telephones) with their leading edges between 27 inches and 80 inches above the finished floor shall protrude no more than 4 inches into walks, halls, corridors, passageways or aisles. Objects mounted with their leading edge at or below 27 inches above the finished floor may protrude any amount. Freestanding objects mounted on posts or pylons may overhang 12 inches maximum from 27 inches to 80 inches above the ground or finished floor. Protruding objects shall not reduce the clear width required for an accessible route or maneuvering space.
- Walks, halls, corridors, passageways, aisles or other circulation spaces shall have 80-inch minimum-clear headroom. If vertical clearance of an area adjoining an accessible route is reduced to less than 80 inches nominal dimension, a guardrail or other barrier having its leading edge at or below 27 inches above the finished floor shall be provided.

### Ramps

- The least possible slope shall be used for any ramp. The maximum slope of a ramp in new construction shall be 1 foot rise for every 12 feet. The maximum rise for any ramp run shall be 30 inches.
- Ramps shall have landings at the bottom and top of each run. The landings shall have the following features: the landings shall be at least as wide as the widest ramp run leading to it, the landing length shall be a minimum of 60 inches clear, and if ramps change direction at landings, the minimum landings size shall be 60 × 60 inches.
- If a ramp run has a rise of greater than 6 inches or a horizontal projection greater than 72 inches, handrails will be available on both sides. Handrails are not required on curb ramps. Handrails shall have the following features:
  1. Be provided along both sides of ramp segments. The inside handrail on switchback or dogleg ramps shall always be continuous.

2. If handrails are not continuous, they shall extend at least 12 inches beyond the top and bottom of the ramp segment and shall be parallel with the floor or ground surface.

3. The clear space between the handrails and wall shall be 1½ inches. Handrails may be located in a recess if the recess is a maximum of 3 inches deep and extends at least 18 inches above the top of the rail.

4. Gripping surfaces shall be continuous and the diameter or width of the gripping surfaces of a handrail shall be 1¼ to 1½ inches. The top of the handrail gripping surfaces shall be mounted between 30 and 34 inches above ramp surfaces.

Outdoor ramps and their approaches shall be designed so that water will not accumulate on walking surfaces.

### Seating, Tables and Work Surfaces

- Accessible seating for people in wheelchairs at tables, counters and work surfaces shall have knee spaces at least 27 inches high, 30 inches wide and 19 inches deep.
- The tops of tables and work surfaces shall be from 28 to 34 inches from the floor or ground.

### Shower Stalls

- Shower stall size and clear floor space shall be accessible to wheelchairs. The shower stall may be 36 × 36 inches or fit into the space required for a bathtub.
- All shower stalls must have grab bars.
- A shower spray unit shall be provided with a hose at least 60 inches long that can be used as a fixed shower head or as a hand-held shower. If an adjustable-height shower head mounted on a vertical bar is used, the bar shall be installed so as not to obstruct the use of grab bars.

### Signage

The following specifications apply to all signage that provides emergency information, general circulation directions or identifies rooms and spaces.
- Letters and numbers on signs shall have a width-to-height ratio between 3:5 and 1:1 and a stroke-to-height ratio between 1:5 and 1:10; the uppercase "X" is used for measurement.
- Raised letters and numbers for identification shall be on the wall between a height of 4½ feet and 5½ feet.
- Characters and symbols shall contrast with their background—either light characters on a dark background or dark characters on a light background.
- Characters, symbols or pictographs on tactile signs shall be raised at least 1/32 inch. Raised characters or symbols shall be sans serif uppercase characters. Raised characters or symbols shall be at least 5/8 inch high and no higher than a nominal 2 inches.

### Stairs

- On any given flight of stairs, all steps shall have uniform riser heights and uniform tread depth. Risers shall be a maximum of 7 inches in height and stair treads shall be no less than 11 inches in depth as measured from riser to riser. Open risers are not permitted on accessible routes.
- Stairways intended for public use or as specified by the authority having jurisdiction shall have handrails at both sides of all stairs meeting the same general specifications as those for ramps.

### Storage

- A clear floor space at least 30 × 48 inches, to allow either a forward or parallel approach by a person using a wheelchair for accessibility to the storage facilities, must be provided.

### Telephones

The specifications apply to accessible public telephones and related equipment.
- Clear floor or ground spaces at each accessible public telephone shall be at least 30 × 48 inches and shall allow either a forward or parallel approach by a person using a wheelchair.
- For hearing-impaired people, telephones shall be equipped with a receiver that generates a magnetic field in the area of the receiver cap. Volume control should be available in any building or facility containing a bank of telephones with an accessible telephone.

- Accessible telephones shall be equipped with a minimum handset cord length of 29 inches.

### Toilet Stalls

- The size and arrangement of toilet stalls shall be accessible and usable by persons in wheelchairs. Toilet stalls with a minimum depth of 56 inches or 66 inches shall have wall-mounted water closets. If the depth of the toilet stalls is increased at least 3 inches, a floor-mounted water mounted water closet may be used. The approach may be left-hand or right-hand.

### Urinals

- Urinals shall be stall type or wall hung with an elongated rim at a maximum of 17 inches above the floor.
- A clear floor space 30 × 48 inches shall be provided in front of urinals to allow forward approach. This clear space shall adjoin or overlap an accessible route and be of the size to accommodate wheelchairs. Privacy shields allowing less than 30 inches clear width shall not extend beyond the front edge of the urinal rim.

### Water Closets

- Clear floor space for water closets not in stalls shall allow for operation of a wheelchair and be arranged to allow for either a left-hand or right-hand approach.
- The height of water closets shall be 17 inches to 19 inches as measured to the top of the toilet seat. Seats shall not be sprung to return to a lifted position.
- Flush controls shall be hand-operated or automatic and shall be operable with one hand and not require tight grasping, tight pinching or twisting of the wrist. The force required to operate the controls shall be no greater than 5 lbf. Controls for flush valves shall be mounted for use from the wide side of the toilet stall and shall be no more than 44 inches above the floor.

### Wheelchairs

- The minimum clear width for a single wheelchair passage shall be 32 inches at a point and 36 inches continuously.

- The minimum width for two wheelchairs to pass is 60 inches.
- The space required for a wheelchair to make a 180 degree turn is a clear space of 60 inches diameter or a T-shaped space.
- The minimum clear floor or ground space required to accommodate a single, stationary wheelchair and occupant is 30 inches by 48 inches. The minimum clear floor or ground space for wheelchairs may be positioned for forward or parallel approach to an object. Clear floor or ground space for wheelchairs may be part of the knee space required under some objects.
- If the clear floor space allows only forward approach to an object, the maximum high forward reach allowed shall be 48 inches and the minimum low forward reach shall be unobstructed and no less than 15 inches above the floor.
- If the clear floor space allows parallel approach by a person in a wheelchair, a maximum high side reach shall be 54 inches and the low side reach shall be no less than 9 inches above the floor.

## OCCUPATIONAL SAFETY AND HEALTH ACT AND ITS APPLICATION TO HEALTH CARE FACILITIES

The Occupational Safety and Health Act (1970) applies to all types of facilities and became effective April 28, 1971. Its administration is within the Department of Labor. The general purpose is to ensure safe and healthful work conditions for working men and women by:

1. Developing mandatory job health and safety standards.
2. Authorizing the enforcement of the standards developed under the Act.
3. Assisting and encouraging the states in their efforts to ensure safe and healthful working conditions.
4. Providing for research, information, education and training in the field of occupational safety and health.
5. Establishing "separate but dependent rights and responsibilities" for both employers and employees.

6. Maintaining a recordkeeping and reports system to monitor job-related illness and injury.

The act aims to provide a working environment where no employee will suffer material impairment to his or her health or functional capacity no matter how long he or she remains on the job and to reduce loss of production and wages, medical expenses and disability compensation carried by commerce. It is based on the federal power granted in the Constitution to regulate interstate commerce and thus work-related injuries and deaths that would affect it.

The act applies to all employers except the federal government, state government or state political subdivisions, self-employed persons, most religious groups, farms employing immediate family members only and workplaces protected by other federal agencies. Coverage is provided directly by the Occupational Safety and Health Administration (OSHA) or by approved state programs.

## Administrative Functions

### Area Directors

The Act is administered through 10 regional offices that may be subdivided into several area and district offices and field stations. The professional judgment, discretion and knowledge of the OSHA standards are extremely important in the intermediary role the regional and area directors play in evaluating adjustment and gravity factors of accidents, violations and penalty recommendations. What citations are to be issued or penalties recommended are determined by the area director after the findings of an inspection. The area director may enter into settlement agreements revising citations and penalties to avoid prolonged disputes. A regional solicitor provides consultation on more serious violations, enforcement and legal problems.

### State

No states can enforce laws concerning occupational safety and health that are inconsistent with OSHA provisions, but may enforce those laws where no federal standard is in effect. Congress anticipated that all the states eventually would administer OSHA to workers within their own boundaries. Therefore, once a state

has developed similar or better standards, rules and regulations than those promulgated by OSHA and an effective enforcement plan, its legislation will apply. OSHA retains the power to step and if the state's administration of its plan becomes ineffectively enforced. In any case, employers remain answerable to OSHA for general duty provisions and in areas where no standards are set up by the state.

### National Institute for Occupational Safety and Health

The National Institute for Occupational Safety and Health (NIOSH) was established by the act as an HHS agency. It is authorized to conduct research and provide technical assistance to OSHA. It also recommends standards for adoption. While conducting its research, NIOSH may make inspections, issue citations, obtain testimony, grant variances and require medical examinations, especially in the investigation of toxicity.

### Secretary of HHS

The secretary of HHS is responsible for the research programs under NIOSH, appoints the director and makes the regulations concerning implementation of the functions of NIOSH.

### Secretary of Labor

Under OSHA, the labor secretary is responsible for and has the sole power to promulgate, modify or revoke standards, rules and regulations for occupational health and safety and for enforcing their terms by inspections and investigations of working conditions, the issuance of citations and penalties for violations and the authority to bring legal action if necessary. It is the secretary's duty to be vigilant and issue safety and health standards in keeping with modern industrial and chemical developments. The secretary presents reports and recommendations to the President and must submit progress reports to regular sessions of Congress.

The labor secretary's duty is largely limited to seeing that OSHA rules and regulations are followed; the secretary has no discretion over the issuance of citations that are mandatory for all violations (except *de minimis* offenses) of the act. The secretary has sole discretion to decide when and under what circumstances a violation exists and, if so, the exact nature of the charge. In Occupational Safety and Health Review Commission proceedings, the truth of the violations must be proved by the secretary under the standard concerned or the general duty clause.

### Occupational Safety and Health Review Commission

The Occupational Safety and Health Review Commission (OSHRC) was created under the act and empowered to review acts of the labor secretary concerning the enforcement of OSHA. This Review Commission has three members who are charged with ensuring objective administration and judging substantial compliance with standards. It is an administrative agency with quasi-judicial powers to arbitrate contests between the labor secretary and the employer. Administrative judges are assigned by the chairman with duties to conduct a fair and impartial hearing, assure relevant facts are fully brought out, and adjudicate issues and generally avoid delays. A judge can dismiss contests where there is refusal to testify, follow his or her directives or file pleadings when due. The Review Commission does not have the power to enforce its orders or punish for contempt; these actions must be taken to court.

The Review Commission generally judges the employer's substantial compliance by the facts in each individual case and by what a reasonable person of ordinary prudence would do under the same circumstances—that the employer was reasonably diligent under the circumstances in protecting employees. Another important factor taken into consideration for penalty assessments—and at hearings for contests, abatements or variances—is the good faith of the employer regarding implementation of OSHA rules and standards.

### Compliance Officer

The compliance officer is the representative of the Labor Department with whom most employees come in contact; he or she and any accompanying staffers carry credentials bearing a photograph and serial number. The compliance officer must have a well-grounded understanding of industrial processes, of standards and regulations to be interpreted, applied and enforced; and of the sophisticated equipment used. The primary concern of the compliance officer is whether or not the employer is meeting applicable OSHA standards and the general duty clause. He or she does not have the authority to waive or release employers from the OSHA violations found upon inspection or from any penalties that have resulted from previous inspections. If the compliance officer fails to act in imminent danger situations and injuries result, the injured employee may bring an action forcing the officer as a public official to perform his or her duty.

### Employer

Employers have certain rights and responsibilities under the act; following is a summary of these.

Under the **general duty clause** of OSHA, the employer must provide a place of employment that is "free from recognized hazards that are causing or are likely to cause death or serious physical harm to his [or her] employees." Employers must be well-informed as to the hazards of their particular industry. It is their responsibility to be aware of applicable standards, to judge if the standards apply to operations and, if so, how to apply them. This is difficult because no definite outlines or criteria are available to follow, particularly when dealing with horizontal standards. Consulting services are available at OSHA's regional or area offices, and the use of this service will not lead to an inspection.

Not only does the employer examine workplace conditions, investigate immediate hazardous situations and lay down rules and regulations under OSHA, but the employer must follow up, supervise and enforce them. It is the employer's duty to see that employees comply with safety and health rules and regulations and to consistently discipline those who do not. Adequate follow-up measures include instruction and training in the proper use of equipment and machinery and seeing that protective equipment is worn. So that employees will follow safety and health requirements, the employer must keep them informed of mandatory OSHA standards and related operational procedures; rights and responsibilities; access to records of work-related injuries and illnesses; warnings of potential hazards, citations and any actions or proceedings; and OSHA-required medical examinations by training, posters in conspicuous proper places and supervision.

The employer also must meet the requirements of the **Chemical Hazards Communication Standard** and the guidelines regarding **Bloodborne Pathogens Standards**. The standards are covered in detail at the end of this section.

Though employers are strictly accountable for the safety and healthful conditions of their workplace, they are not liable if the employees disregard simple routine safety rules. Employers can be held liable and citations issued if lack of due care on their part contributes to the injury of employee. Employers are not responsible for ensuring the conduct of employees and all their acts.

The employer has a right to participate in the industry association and in OSHA standard advisory committee involvements in job health and safety. Regarding inspections, employers can receive identification of the compliance officer immediately prior to inspection, be advised of the reason for the inspection, participate in an opening and closing conference, and be assured of the confidentiality of trade secrets. The employer can apply to OSHA for permanent or temporary variances from standards and file a notice of contest concerning citations and proposed penalties.

### Employees

Because the effectiveness of the act depends upon positive employee participation, OSHA advises that employees must comply with the standards and rules applicable to them. Employee responsibilities include: reviewing applicable OSHA regulations, reporting hazardous workplace conditions and/or job-related injuries or illnesses to the supervisor, and cooperating with compliance officers during inspections. Although no provisions exist for citations or penalties to be issued for noncompliance, an employee must obey such health and safety requirements of the employer as are necessary and reasonable to meet OSHA requirements or risk discipline and/or discharge. Negligence on the part of the employee can be considered a defense to an employer charged with violation of his or her general duty.

Employees have the right to representation by an authorized collective bargaining representative, a fellow employee with written authority to represent them under the act, or an employee where a maximum of three employees work in the same place for the same employer. Substantive and procedural rights provide that the employee:

- Or the employee representative may accompany the compliance officer on inspections of the workplace.

- May request toxicity rulings.
- Is protected against reprisals and discrimination by the employer, employment agencies, trade associations, etc., if engaged in employee activities such as complaining to the employer, OSHA or union about job safety and health hazards; filing grievances; participating in workplace or union health and safety committees; or participating in inspections.
- May review OSHA standards and be informed on hazards, safety precautions and procedures in the workplace, OSHA actions regarding complaints, variance applications, and job-related injuries and illnesses records.
- Is protected from being fired for refusal to work if danger is imminent, the employer has been asked to eliminate it, a reasonable person in the same circumstance would agree that real danger or death or serious physical harm exists, and no other reasonable alternative is available.

The employee representative or lawyer also may lodge a complaint with OSHA (in writing and signed) and request an inspection when imminent danger or violations threatening physical harm exists. The employer must be charged with a violation of the act substantiated with a description of the hazardous condition. The complaint is submitted to the regional director with a copy to the employer. (This does not have to be signed by the employee.) Upon substantiation, an inspection of the entire workplace will be scheduled.

### Standards

OSHA is responsible for promulgating legally enforceable standards under the act; therefore, the labor secretary has issued rules, regulations and standards requiring conditions, practices, methods and processes to provide safe and healthy employment and worksites. Before 1970, many safety standards and regulations had been worked out by federal agencies, private organizations having highly qualified personnel and technicians, and other interested institutions connected with specific industries or areas of operation. So long as these met the criteria, the act took them and gave them the force of the law.

The labor secretary must follow specific procedures when promulgating or modifying standards. This starts with the publishing of the intent to modify, revoke or promulgate a new standard in the *Federal Register* and provides specific time for interested persons to file objections or call for a hearing. Other standard-setting and revision procedures are started on OSHA's initiative or in response to petitions from the HHS secretary, states and their agencies, standards-producing organizations, employers and employees, and by standing and ad hoc advisory committees. The final text of the standard and the date it becomes effective is published in the *Federal Register*.

All standards are presumed valid and remain in force so long as the labor secretary has followed the correct procedure in their adoption. When conflicting standards emerge, those giving the most protection to the employee take precedence. If the standard is vague, an employer's application will be judged on whether its interpretation was reasonable and in accordance with keeping the workplace as safe and healthful as possible.

If any employer finds it impossible to comply with a standard, he or she must work out other acceptable safety measures and have them approved through a variance petition to OSHA. A summary of each variance petition must be posted with a notice of employee rights to express their views or arguments. Interim orders may be issued to allow the employer to operate under existing conditions until a variance decision is made. Variances are usually granted where the purposes of the act are not frustrated. Temporary variances apply for up to one year where the employer shows he or she is complying safely and as soon as possible after the effective date of the standard. A permanent variance is granted when the employer shows that an alternative—while not following the letter of the standard—has the same effect.

## Recordkeeping

To provide information necessary for gauging and solving work-related problems where there have been previously few and inadequate records on causes, results and prevention, OSHA requires employers, including nursing facilities (with 11 or more employees), to maintain records of industrial casualties, injuries and illnesses, and to respond to OSHA random surveys. All occupational illnesses must be recorded regardless of severity. They must be recorded if they result in death (regardless of time elapsing between injury and death),

one or more lost workdays, restriction of work or motion, loss of consciousness, transfer to another job or medical treatment other than first aid. On-the-job fatal or serious multiple accidents (five or more hospitalized) must be reported by the employer within 48 hours to the nearest OSHA office in person, or by telephone, telegraph, facsimile or e-mail. An explanation of the circumstances, the number of fatalities and/or the extent of injuries are minimum required information. An inspection of the occurrence may follow at the regional director's discretion. Small employers (no more than 10 employees during the calendar year) need not follow the recordkeeping requirements but must report fatalities and accidents resulting in fatalities or hospitalization and must respond to any statistical surveys requested by the Bureau of Labor Statistics (BLS).

The following records are maintained on a calendar year basis and must be kept current. These are not filed with OSHA but remain on the premises and stored for five years at each establishment. These are to be available for inspection and copying by OSHA, HHS, BLS or designated state agency. The employer may apply to the regional BLS for a variance to keep his or her records in a manner other than required by OSHA:

- **OSHA #200** (Log and Summary of Occupational Injuries and Illnesses)—Each recordable occupational injury or illness must be recorded within six working days from when the employer learns of it. If the log is prepared at a central location (automatic data processing), a copy current to within 45 calendar days must be in the establishment at all times. Substitutes for this form are permitted if they are equally detailed and understandable.

  A copy of the totals and information (even if there are none during the year) following the fold line on the last page of this form must be posted at each establishment along with customary employee notices not later than February 1 and remain posted until March 1 of the following year.

- **OSHA #101** (Supplementary Record of Occupational Injuries and Illnesses)—This form goes into detail regarding each injury or illness and must be completed within the same time period as OSHA #200. Worker's compensation or insurance forms may be used—providing all the required information is available.

- **OSHA #2203** (Workplace Poster)—This informs employees of their rights and responsibilities and must be permanently posted within the workplace.

## Inspections

To enforce and carry out its standards, OSHA is authorized to carry out inspections of workplaces. In recent years, OSHA has been increasing its survey of nursing facilities. This is a broad power enabling the compliance or health officer, who usually makes the inspection, to enter the premises without delay during regular working hours or at other reasonable times in a reasonable manner that does not unduly interrupt normal business procedures. The officer must present his or her credentials to the owner or owner's agent in charge at the time. No advance notice of the inspection is made unless authorized by OSHA. Advance notice of not less than 24 hours may be given in imminent danger situations, for after-hours or special preparations, to ensure presence of certain personnel or to produce a more effective inspection. The compliance officer will check to ascertain that OSHA standards, rules and regulations are being followed; the employer is complying with the general duty clause; notices informing employees of their rights and obligations are posted; recordkeeping requirements are met; and notice of the inspection was given to employees where the employer had been notified in advance.

Inspections are made from the following sources in order of priority: imminent danger situations, catastrophe or fatalities, employee complaints, target high-hazard industries, follow-up and general inspections on a random basis. Not all major accidents are necessarily investigated. Generally, accidents will be investigated when they involve previous complaints of imminent danger, fatalities where there have been willful or repeated violations, hospitalizations of numerous employees, and extensive property damage where the possibility of death or injury existed if employees had been present.

The following are points to be considered when an OSHA inspection of the facility occurs:

1. The compliance officer must be allowed to enter upon presentation of his or her credentials. This right to enter is limited only by conditions that may be injurious to his or her health and safety.

2. The employer is obligated to inform the employees or their representative promptly of the inspection and of the steps taken thereafter in the enforcement process.

3. The compliance officer must discuss the scope of the inspection at an opening conference. The officer will provide the employer with a copy of the complaint (if applicable), request records be made available and determine the employees' representative.

4. During the walk-around inspections, the employer and employee representative have a right to accompany the compliance officer. The compliance officer may question and confer with employees to obtain information material to pending action, the employer's compliance attitudes, and the health and safety of their workplace. If the employer interferes or tries to limit any important aspect of the inspection, the inspection will be terminated and warrant obtained.

5. At the conclusion of the inspection, the compliance officer is required to have a closing conference with the employer and the employee representative where all the conditions and practices that may violate OSHA are discussed. The officer will give the employer copies of the laws, standards and rules applicable to the operation; point out those violated; and provide provisionary protective measures until conditions can be corrected. The time and the cost necessary to abate any violations and to obtain loans if needed also will be considered at this time. Pending citations and penalties will not be considered here.

6. In imminent danger situations, the compliance officer will inform the employees involved and immediately contact the employer to initiate the corrective measure and follow up by inspection within 24 hours. The danger can be abated immediately by eliminating the procedure or removing employees from the area. Should the employer refuse to voluntarily abate the imminent danger, temporary restraining orders will be obtained from the nearest U.S. District Court upon verification, petition and testimony from the compliance officer. A court order is necessary to shut down a facility in whole or in part.

At the request of the employer and/or employee representative, informal conferences may be held with the area director to discuss issues raised by the inspection. Issues can be settled as long as the settlement is consistent with provisions and objectives of OSHA. The area director may issue a *de minimis* notice describing violations that are not directly related to OSHA standards or the general duty clause. This is sent to the employer with a copy to the complaining employee (if applicable). No posting requirements or penalties are made, and it is up to the employer to determine whether or not he or she wishes to take corrective action.

## Citations

Citations are issued by the OSHA area director for violations of OSHA standards or the general duty clause found at the time of inspection. They are mandatory for both serious (including willful and repeated violations) and nonserious violations. The employer is not under any legal obligation to correct unsafe conditions until he or she is formally informed of their existence by a citation.

The citation contains a detailed description of the violation, the standard or general duty involved and how it was violated, measures to abate the hazardous situation, and the date by which the violation must be abated. The citation is issued, generally within 72 hours of the completion of the inspection, and usually is served upon the employer by certified mail. It includes a transmittal letter informing the employer that violations exist as described in the citation, the citation must be posted where involved employees will see it until the violation is abated (three days maximum), violations must be abated within the specified time, the labor secretary will inform the employer of any penalties within a reasonable time, and the employees have a right to bring the citation before the Review Committee. No citation may be issued after six months from the occurrence of a violation which has been corrected.

If less than 30 days is given for abatement, the employer must let the area director know when the corrective action was taken and completed; OSHA then will reinspect the premises. If the employer has not complied within the allotted time, penalties will be imposed. The employer will be informed of any failure to abate by certified mail. This becomes a new claim against the employer—apart from the citation it rests on—and becomes final if no contest is made within 15 days.

## Penalties

On or about the time a citation is issued, the labor secretary must follow up with a notice of proposed penalty if there is to be any within a reasonable time. The act provides both civil and criminal sanctions with wide latitudes in the penalty amounts.

Civil penalties in the form of monetary assessment are imposed upon the employer with notification by certified mail. They fall into the two classes of serious and nonserious including violations of the employer's general duty and any applicable OSHA standards, rules and regulations. These penalties are either mandatory or discretionary. Their intention is to ensure a safe workplace by inducing the employer to comply with OSHA—not to harass or punish financially. To assure some uniformity regarding penalties and the nature of violations, OSHA has proposed guidelines, definitions, classifications and a system of adjustments for nonserious violations.

The penalties usually are proposed at the local level by the area director before going to OSHA. These are judged on a case-by-case basis considering the following criteria:

1. The gravity of the situation considering such factors as the likelihood of an injury or disease that could result, the severity of the injury or illness that did result, and the extent to which the standard is violated (such as percentage of work area involved or frequency of violation).
2. The size of the employer's establishment and the effect the penalty would have on his or her business.
3. The employer's attitude as determined during the inspection and his or her good faith in keeping a safe and healthful workplace. This could be evidenced by such factors as: adequate and effective safety and training programs, the degree to which supervisory personnel are safety conscious, current maintenance of OSHA records, voluntary installation and use of safety devices, and prompt correction of hazardous conditions as they arise.

4. The history of previous violations under OSHA and their abatement.

The following is a brief listing of both fixed and discretionary penalty amounts:

1. The penalty for willful ($5,000 minimum) or repeated violations is up to the Review Commission's discretion and may be up to $70,000 for each violation.
2. For other serious violations, the penalty is up to $7,000 each at the Review Commission's discretion. A serious violation may be reduced to a nonserious violation if the labor secretary fails to prove the evidence of a serious violation. An additional penalty will be assessed up to $1,000 per day for each day a serious violation continues after the abatement period has ended.
3. For nonserious violations, all matters relating to the penalty of up to $7,000 per violation are discretionary. This includes the Review Commission setting the amount of or waiving the penalty. Such fines can apply to violations such as posting requirements, recordkeeping, accident reports or employee notification of inspections. For failure to abate these violations within the time limit, an additional penalty of up to $7,000 per day will be imposed.

The act defines four acts as criminal, and imposes sanctions for violations. The Review Commission does not have jurisdiction to conduct proceedings under these sections. Cases concerning these are taken directly to court.

1. If the employer willfully violates an OSHA regulation and that violation results in the death of an employee, the first conviction carries a fine of up to $250,000 ($500,000 for a corporation) and/or imprisonment of up to 6 months.
2. To the employer and informant, if advance notice of an inspection is made without the authority of the labor secretary or agent, the penalty imposed can be up to $1,000 and/or 6 months in prison if convicted.
3. The employer or employee who knowingly prepares, certifies and files false OSHA documents may be fined up to $10,000 and/or imprisoned for 6 months if convicted.

4. Assaulting, intimidating or interfering with a compliance officer in the performance of duty is subject to a maximum fine of $5,000 and maximum imprisonment of 3 years. A single penalty of imprisonment for any term of years or for life is imposed upon one found guilty of murder or manslaughter of an officer or employee of the Department of Labor or the Department of HHS in the performance of investigative, inspection and enforcement functions.

## Appeals and Contest

If a citation seems uncertain and inadequate to an employer, he or she may confer with the area or regional director for clarification. The employer may request an informal meeting to reach settlements revising citations and penalties to avoid prolonged legal disputes. If the employer is making an effort in good faith but cannot correct violations within the abatement time due to factors beyond his or her control, a petition may be filed with OSHA to modify the date.

The employer has the right to contest the citation to the Review Commission and the right to require that the labor secretary prove the truth of the charges in connection with the citation, the penalty notice and/or the abatement period. The employer must file the notice of contest in writing to the OSHA area director within 15 days after receiving the notice. Although the notice can be a letter, regulations address form and content. However, the issue (such as citation or proposed penalty) that the employer intends to contest should be clearly stated. The employer must inform employees of the contest to the citation by posting a copy of the notice or giving it to the employee representative. A contest stays the running of the abatement period in the citation, which then starts when the order of the Review Commission becomes final, unless again stayed by a court order. Penalties are imposed in cases in which employers contest for delay or avoidance of penalties and in bad faith.

The OSHA area director forwards the case to the Review Commission for assignment to an administrative judge on the Review Commission. The hearings are held in accordance with federal statutes outlining procedures to ensure due process—usually in the district where the employer's facility is located. Although representation by an attorney is not required by the act, it is probably best to hire a lawyer to assure the hearing is based upon the issues and not upon the knowledge of complex rules and technicalities. At the hearing, each party has a right to present his or her case, produce witnesses and cross-examine. Rules of evidence are generally followed; a summation of facts and statement of supporting law are presented by each side at the conclusion. The judge will make the conclusion of fact and issue his or her decision, whereupon his or her power in the contest ceases. The judge's decision affirming, modifying or nullifying the citation or proposed penalty becomes a final order of the Review Commission 30 days after it is issued. Further motions may be presented during the 30 days to the Review Commission, which retains jurisdiction and can direct that the decision be reviewed. If review is not forthcoming, the Review Commission's jurisdiction ends with the final order.

Any party has the right to have the final decision of the Review Commission reviewed by a U.S. Court of Appeals after using all available administrative remedies. The labor secretary may go to the U.S. Court of Appeals for a decree ordering the employer's compliance with the final orders of the Review Commission or be cited for contempt of court and imprisonment until compliance is achieved.

## OSHA-ENFORCED STANDARDS

Among the standards enforced by OSHA are the Chemical Hazard Communication Standard and the Bloodborne Pathogens Standard with which nursing facilities must comply. Following are summaries of the purpose and requirements of these standards.

### Chemical Hazard Communication Standard

The basic goal of this standard is to make sure that both employers and employees are informed about chemical work hazards and how to protect themselves. Employees have the need and right to know the identities, hazards and protective measures prior to exposure concerning physical and health chemicals to which they are exposed at work.

The rules in this area are performance-oriented, allowing judgment in implementing programs to address what is done in each particular facility. Generally, the employer must:

1. Develop a written plan, covering chemicals present at the site, the person(s) responsible for the various aspects of the program, how relative informational materials are available to employees.
2. Identify and list hazardous chemicals in the facility.
3. Obtain material safety data sheet (MSDS) and labels for each hazardous chemical.
4. Communicate the information concerning the recognition and avoidance of exposure to chemical hazards to employees (mostly in housekeeping and maintenance).

OSHA compliance inspectors will look at the facility's written program for sufficiency and implementation of labeling, the current MSDS for each chemical in the plant as required, access of employees to MSDS sheets and employee training.

Lists of the hazardous chemicals used or stored at the facility are maintained, updated and available to employees at each jobsite. A MSDS for each chemical used and stored must be retained at the facility (i.e., notebooks at each work area or computer terminal access). The hazards of each chemical are determined, and the MSDS is developed or obtained by manufacturers and importers who are responsible for the accuracy (including updates) of the information on these sheets. Procedures should be in place to ensure that distributors supply the properly prepared MSDS. A labeling system also is established (i.e., using those provided by supplier, labels stenciled and fixed to the container, or placards where labels are not feasible) with written alternatives for labeling any in-plant containers and procedures for review and update of information as necessary. Every container of hazardous material must be labeled, tagged or otherwise marked with the identities of the material and appropriate warnings. All labels must be legible and prominently displayed.

Each employee who may be exposed to hazardous materials in the workplace must be provided with information and training prior to any such actual or potential exposure. Labeling and the MSDS for each chemical are available at all times and give substance-specific information. Employees are to: be aware of exposures to hazardous materials for routine and nonroutine work;

know how to read and use labels and material safety data sheets; recognize there are appropriate protective measures; and keep up to date on any new hazard information. The training program must be written and include the format of the program (i.e., classroom, audiovisuals), locations and explanations of the written program lists, lists of hazardous materials, MSDS, labeling, appearance and odor of chemicals, emergency procedures, and cleanup of leaks and spills. Employer records must show tasks analysis (what actual and potential hazards pertain to each particular job) and how employees are trained to minimize injury to themselves and others. Records of such training should be kept in employee files.

The Chemical Hazards Communications Standard is a continuing program. It is, therefore, necessary to assign responsibility for the ongoing related activities necessary for compliance with the rule. Personnel are designated to obtain and maintain the necessary MSDS; carry out labeling procedures for in-plant, newly purchased and shipping containers; conduct the training programs; and ensure compliance and other areas (such as spills or nonroutine work).

## Bloodborne Pathogens Standard

The Bloodborne Pathogens Standard covers the protection of health care workers against infection from the human immunodeficiency virus (HIV) and hepatitis B virus (HBV) that may result from contact with blood and other potentially infectious materials. OSHA requires that nursing facilities establish a written bloodborne pathogens exposure control plan. The plan must be available to workers and OSHA representatives, reviewed and updated as necessary (at least annually) and must:

1. Identify job classifications where there is exposure to blood and other potentially infectious materials.
2. Explain protective measures in effect and methods of compliance and implementation, such as hepatitis B vaccination and post-exposure follow-up, prevention of hazard communication, personal protective equipment, housekeeping and recordkeeping.
3. Establish procedures to evaluate circumstances of an exposure incident.

Exposure determination is based on occupational exposure without regard to personal protective clothing and equipment. Job classifications where all employees have such exposure include: physicians, nurses, nurse aides, lab technicians and emergency personnel. Job classifications where some employees' specific tasks and procedures put them at risk of occupational exposure are: people handling blood or infectious specimens and housekeeping staff.

Training programs must be provided to all employees with occupational exposure at no cost and during working hours at the time of initial assignment to tasks where such exposure may take place. These programs must be conducted annually thereafter. The programs must include:

1. An explanation of symptoms of bloodborne disease, transmission of bloodborne pathogens, preventive measures and control of transmission of HBV and HIV, recognition of occupational exposure and emergency procedures for exposure incidents.
2. Information on availability and benefits of free hepatitis B vaccinations, post-exposure evaluations and follow-up.
3. Description of the selection, use, decontamination and disposal of personal protective equipment; use and limitations of safe work practices (engineering control); and use of labels, signs and color-coding.
4. Provision of copies of the written exposure control plan and regulations.

The employer or designated health care professional must see that the necessary materials and equipment are available and maintained and that relative policies and procedures are in place to prevent and control exposure to bloodborne pathogens and other infectious materials. The single most important measure to control transmission of HBV and HIV is to observe the universal precautions to prevent contact with infectious materials by treating all body fluid types as potentially infectious, especially those that are difficult to identify.

Engineering controls isolate the hazard from employees and include color-coded leak-proof containers to discard, store and reprocess sharps or transport specimens. Work practice controls reduce exposure by the manner in which a task is performed and include handwashing when gloves are removed, immediate eye irrigation, and proper use and disposal of needles. Personal protective equipment is selected as to quantity and type of exposure expected and is used to prevent blood or potentially infectious materials from passing through to the workers' clothing, skin or mucous membranes. Proper housekeeping, laundry and waste control methods must be used to prevent exposure to bloodborne pathogens and infectious materials.

The bloodborne pathogens standard requires two types of records in addition to the OSHA Recordkeeping Form Numbers 200, 101 and 2203:

- A medical record, which is confidential and separate from other personnel records, must be established for each employee with occupational exposure. This record includes hepatitis B vaccinations status, occupational exposure documentation, results and post-evaluation. These records must be maintained 30 years past the last date of the worker's employment.
- A training record must document the date, content, outline, trainer's name and credentials, and names and job titles of persons who attend each training session. These are to be kept three years.

These records are passed on to any new owners of the facility or to OSHA if the business ceases operations.

These records are available to the employee on written request.

## BIBLIOGRAPHY

Allen, J.E. 1992. *Nursing home administration*, 2nd ed. New York, NY: Springer Publishing.

American National Standards Institute. 1986. American national standard—physically handicapped, A117.1. New York, NY.

Code of Federal Regulations, *Hazard communication standard*, Title 29, Part 1910.1200.

Code of Federal Regulations, *Bloodborne pathogens*, Title 29, Part 1910.1031.

Davis, W. 1994. *Introduction to health care administration*, 4th ed. Bossier City, LA: Publicare Press.

Department of Labor, Occupational Safety and Health Administration. 1992. *All about OSHA* (publication 2056). Washington, DC.

Department of Labor, Occupational Safety and Health Administration. 1992. *Bloodborne pathogens and acute care facilities* (publication 3128). Washington, DC.

Department of Labor, Occupational and Safety Health Administration. 1992. *Chemical hazard communication guidelines for compliance* (publication 3084). Washington, DC.

National Board of Examiners for Nursing Home Administrators. 1997. *NAB study guide*, 3rd ed. Washington, DC.

National Fire Protection Association. 1984. *NFPA: Health care facilities*. Quincy, MA.

National Fire Protection Association. 1988. *NFPA: Life safety code*. Quincy, MA.

# Appendix 1–A

## Glossary of OSHA Terms

*De minimis* **violation**—Violation of a standard that is not directly or immediately related to occupational safety and health, for which there is no penalty.

**Employee**—A person or organization of persons employed in a business affecting commerce.

**Employer**—A person or entity (not including the federal government, state governments, or political subdivisions) engaged in a business affecting commerce who has employees.

**Established federal standards**—An operative occupational safety and health standards established by any agency of the United States, currently in effect or contained in any federal statute in force when OSHA was enacted.

**Establishment**—A workplace, a physical location where business is conducted or a place where services or industrial operations are performed; each distinctive separate activity at a single location being considered an establishment or where employees report to work or are paid from.

**General duty clause**—Impels the employer through sanctions to furnish each of his or her employees employment and a safe workplace free from recognized hazards that could cause or are likely to cause death or serious physical harm.

**Hazard communication standard**—Requires that the employer establish a written comprehensive hazard communication program.

**Health hazard**—Any condition likely to cause death or injury to employees in their employment or workplace.

**Horizontal standard**—Standard of broad application applying to widely diversified employments.

**Imminent danger**—Any condition or practice in a workplace causing danger that could reasonably be expected to cause death or serious physical harm immediately or before correction through regular OSHA enforcement procedures.

**Initial standards package**—Original standards issued by the labor secretary in 1971, including national consensus standards and established federal standards.

**National consensus standards**—Any occupational health and safety standard or modification thereof that has been promulgated by nationally recognized standards-producing organizations and substantially adopted by affected persons, formulated with consideration of diverse views and designated as a standard by the labor secretary.

**Nonserious violation**—A violation where a direct and immediate relationship occurs between the condition and occupational health and safety—but not such as to cause death or serious physical harm.

**Occupational illness**—Abnormal condition or disorder that is not an injury caused by exposure to environmental factors of employment, involving, for instance, inhalation, absorption or direct contact with toxic substances or harmful agent.

**Occupational injury**—Cut, fracture, sprain or amputation resulting from work-related accidents or exposure involving an incident in the work environment.

**Permanent variance**—Allowed by OSHA where the employer proves that the facility or method of operation provides protection at least as effective as the OSHA standard.

**Proprietary standards**—Safety regulations, practices, equipment and materials produced by professional organizations connected with specific industries or spheres of operation—some of which have become OSHA standards.

**Reasonable diligence**—That degree of care a reasonable person would exercise in the same position and circumstances as the employer.

**Reasonable time**—The time taken to correct a hazardous condition after it is brought to the employer's attention, involving judgments such as to the extent of injuries employees could sustain, the number of employees exposed, or the time needed to correct the condition.

**Reasonably prudent employer**—An employer who is safety conscious and possesses the technical expertise normally expected of an employer similarly engaged.

**Recognized hazard**—One of common knowledge or wide general recognition in the particular industry where it occurs, and detectable by the senses or by generally known and accepted tests.

**Repeated violation**—Where the employer violates the same standard previously violated.

**Serious physical harm**—Harm to the degree where the employee cannot function normally, permanently or for extended and substantial periods of time; also causes temporary disability requiring in-patient hospital treatment.

**Small business concerns**—Those businesses that are independently owned and not dominant in their field of operation.

**Substantial probability**—Proof that the consequence of an accident resulting from a violation of a particular standard will be death or serious physical harm.

**Time to abate**—A specific date fixed in a citation by which a violation must be corrected.

**Vertical standard**—A standard applicable only to practices, methods or operations found in a specific employment.

**Willful violation**—Exists where the employer committed an intentional, voluntary and knowing violation of the act or of a standard commonly recognized in his or her industry as hazardous or violative; when the employer fails to act when a peril has been brought to his or her attention.

# Appendix 1-B
## Glossary of Chemical Hazard Terms

**Hazard Warning**—Words, pictures, symbols or combination thereof appearing on a label or other form of warning on a container, conveying any chemical hazards.

**Hazardous Chemical**—A chemical that is a physical or health hazard.

**Health Hazard**—Chemical that may cause acute or chronic health effects to exposed employees, as determined by at least one study conducted in accordance with established scientific principles (such as rashes or lung damage).

**Label**—Written, printed or graphic material affixed or displayed on containers.

**Material Safety Data Sheet (MSDS)**—Contains written or printed materials concerning a hazardous chemical in accordance with the standard.

**Physical Hazard**—Combustible liquid, compressed gas, explosive flammable chemical, organic peroxide, oxidizer, unstable (reactive) or water reactive chemical.

# Appendix 1-C
## Glossary of Bloodborne Pathogens

**Bacteria**—Generally, free-living single-celled organism capable of surviving independently.

**Bloodborne**—Pathogen is found in the blood and can be transmitted to other persons by contact with the contaminated blood.

**Contaminated**—The presence (or reasonable anticipated presence) of blood or other potentially infectious materials on an item or surface.

**HBV**—Virus that causes hepatitis B.

**HIV**—Human immunodeficiency virus. A virus that causes acquired immunodeficiency syndrome (AIDS).

**Occupational Exposure**—Reasonably anticipated skin, eye, mucous membrane or parenteral contact with blood or other potentially infectious materials that may result from performance of work duties.

**Pathogen**—Any micro-organism (bacteria, virus, fungus) that is able to cause disease.

**Parenteral**—Piercing mucous membrane or skin by human bites, needlesticks, cuts or abrasions.

**Personal Protective Equipment**—Specialized clothing or equipment worn for protection against a hazard.

**Regulated Waste**—Liquid or semiliquid blood or other potentially infectious materials; contaminated items that can release blood or other infectious materials if compressed or handled; and pathological and microbiological wastes containing blood or other potentially infectious materials.

**Virus**—Biological agent consisting of DNA and protein, which must reside in a cell to survive. Virus can be transmitted by contact with human cells in the blood containing the virus within them.

# CHAPTER 2

# Governance and Management: Community Interrelationships

## COMMUNITY SUPPORT ORGANIZATIONS AND PROGRAMS FOR LONG-TERM CARE

Long-term care is provided in communities by coordinated providers to the home, in the community and in institutions. This system is sporadically interconnected by individual case management efforts of caseworkers employed by state departments and area agencies on aging. Following are brief descriptions of some of the agencies, programs and services involved.

### Hospitals

The standards of the Joint Commission on Accreditation of Healthcare Organizations (Joint Commission) define a hospital as an institution that:

1. Is engaged primarily in providing inpatient diagnostic, therapeutic and rehabilitation services for medical diagnoses, treatment and care of the injured, disabled or sick.
2. Maintains health or clinical records on all patients.
3. Has an organized medical staff with appropriate constitution and bylaws (ratified and approved by the governing body) to be followed by all staff physicians.
4. Requires that every patient must be under the care and supervision of a physician.

5. Provides continuous (24 hour) nursing service, rendered or supervised by a registered professional on duty at all times. Some exceptions are made for rural hospitals.
6. Has a hospital utilization review plan in operation.
7. Is duly licensed by applicable law or approved by the agency licensing hospitals in its state.

With hospital stays becoming shorter due to the diagnosis-related groups (DRGs) reimbursement, persons needing subacute care (such as restorative care after strokes or care after surgery) are discharged to nursing facilities under home-based, community-based and institutional care.

### Physicians

Physicians practicing in a community are in the following categories relative to their mode of practice:

1. **Sole Practitioner**—Practices as an individual.
2. **Group Practice**—A number of physicians consolidate and have common billing and administrative procedures. The group practice organizational structure may or may not include a partnership practice.
3. **Partnership Practice**—A number of physicians who have a formal or informal partnership agreement. These physicians usually share common

facilities for administrative purposes and distribute their profits in accordance with the partnership agreement.

4. **Professional Medical Corporation**—Corporate structures licensed according to the laws of their respective states. Usually one or more physicians are licensed to practice. It is a requirement that all corporate members of the professional medical corporation be licensed.

## Outpatient and Diagnostic Clinic Facilities

These are service organizations primarily engaged in establishing the diagnosis of patients. Some well-known facilities in the United States are The Mayo Clinic in Rochester, Minn., and The Leahy Clinic in Mass. These diagnostic and outpatient facilities are usually associated with one or more hospitals in the area. In the event the patient needs to be hospitalized, there is usually a formal working agreement with the hospital.

## Health Maintenance Organizations

A health maintenance organization (HMO) is a health managed care delivery system organized and sponsored by medical foundations, community groups, labor unions, governmental units, or by profit and non-profit community groups associated with an insurance company or other financial institution. An HMO may be part of a hospital, medical school or a free-standing facility.

Preventive medicine and discovery of early complaints are its primary goals. Checkups, surgery, doctors' visits and lab tests are provided for a fixed charge. Usually one primary care physician is chosen by the enrollee to provide care and make treatment recommendations and referrals to specialists. Although several types of HMOs exist, the enrollee is limited to using the plan's doctors and hospitals and must get approval for treatment and referrals outside the particular HMO network.

Four basic elements are included in an HMO:

1. An organized system of health care bringing together or arranging for the provision of inpatient and outpatient facilities for preventive, diagnostic and acute care.

2. Comprehensive health maintenance and treatment services of physicians and other health care professionals to provide emergency, acute inpatient and rehabilitative care for chronic and disabling conditions.

3. A voluntarily enrolled group of persons in a specific geographic area who contract with the HMO to receive needed services and agree that the HMO will be the primary source of any health care required.

4. Payment by the enrollee according to a prearranged schedule for various services received.

## Committees on Aging

These are community-sponsored committees whose purpose is to study the needs of older persons, stimulate planning and development of programs for the aging, seek better coordination of all services on behalf of the aging, and provide information for legislation beneficial to the aging. The committees on aging are catalyst groups designed to obtain action within the community for the benefit of the aging.

## Adult Services and Aging

Adult Services and Aging (ASA) programs are a component of long-term care, enabling the elderly to remain in their own homes for as long as possible. This service is available in larger metropolitan areas; its greatest value is assistance to families to secure services for the elderly. Priority is given to those with the greatest economic or social needs. Social workers conduct a needs assessment and evaluation with individuals requesting services. The services offered are considered supplemental to those already provided by family, friends and other community resources. Services available include: case management, counseling, community placement, protective services, ombudsman, health screening, respite care, adult foster care, legal services, personal care, homemaker/home health aide services, nutrition and community resource development. The programs are funded by Older Americans Act funds and individual cost sharing.

## Central Information and Referral Service

This service is designed to assist individuals needing help in various problem areas to access private and public services. The agency is staffed by a professional social worker who understands the purposes and functions of the participating agencies. Types of participating agencies are health agencies (hospitals, nursing facilities and clinics), churches, clubs, fraternal organizations, educational institutions, welfare and social agencies, and law enforcement and fire protection agencies.

Files are kept with information on the purposes of each participating agency, services rendered, fees (if any) and conditions for eligibility. The social worker screens incoming calls, provides interviews or refers the individual requiring service to the appropriate agency.

## Home Health Agency

Home health is a major alternative care service to entering a nursing facility. It provides nursing, personal and rehabilitative services to the homebound. There has been a great increase in a wide variety of certified providers of the necessary services and equipment in the last 20 years.

A professional nurse may provide nursing care after hospitalization or help with and teach self-care to the disabled shut-in. Physical, occupational and speech therapies as ordered by the attending physician are furnished. Home health care is funded through Medicare Parts A and B, Medicaid under the Social Security Act, or from the area agencies on aging under the Older Americans Act.

The organizational structure for home health services are affiliated with a voluntary, nonprofit organization (hospital or community organization), the city or county health department, or with a combination of voluntary and/or governmental supported agencies.

## Home Health Aide

If an older person is receiving Medicare services at home for a specific illness or injury, home health aides are provided to perform health-related tasks (such as administering medicines or changing dressings). Funding is received from Medicare and Medicaid.

## Medical Transportation Services

This community service provides rides to and from hospitals, clinics, day care centers, doctors' offices and nursing facilities within the city or area limits. Provision is made to accommodate wheelchair participants accompanied by an escort. This service is mostly utilized by the needy living at home; nursing and other long-term care facility residents also may use it. The service can be funded by medical centers, the United Way, contributions from the riders, Medicare or Medicaid.

## Meals-on-Wheels Program

This program for the elderly shut-in or disabled person who cannot prepare his or her own meals or go to a restaurant provides a well-balanced hot meal for a nominal fee based on cost and income. The program is provided by a local council on aging and is usually connected with a voluntary, nonprofit corporate structure, such as a senior citizens center, nonprofit hospital or nonprofit nursing facility.

## Congregate Meals

Senior nutrition programs provide a single well-balanced and nourishing meal, nutrition education and socialization for people age 60 or older on a donation basis. Area agencies on aging give subcontracts to groups (schools, hospitals, nursing facilities) who serve such meals five or more days a week.

## Homemaker Service

This program, sometimes referred to as home maintenance service, provides assistance to the elderly disabled or shut-in to keep his or her residence or domicile clean. Included are such services as laundry, cleaning floors, washing windows, dusting, vacuuming, dish washing and other essential household tasks. This program is supported by the area agencies on aging under the Older Americans Act.

## Foster Care Program

A foster care program is usually connected with a senior citizens center and involves the elderly person who is capable of taking care of daily living activities, but needs support with homemaking and socialization. Similar to a foster care program for children, an elderly or aged person is adopted by a private family and lives with them.

## Hospice

This is a public agency or private organization that offers supportive care, symptom management and pain relief to terminally ill people and their families. There are hospice centers for inpatients, but such care is usually provided in the home. Medicare Part A pays a large proportion of such costs when the conditions are met.

## Senior Citizens Center

This organization is designed to provide recreational, social and educational programs for the elderly person. It may be financed through the Older Americans Act through state, county or municipal organizations or as a private voluntary corporation. The senior citizens center provides a variety of programming; typical services are meals-on-wheels, homemaking, friendly visiting and the foster parent program.

## Activity Centers

Activity centers are more formal than social clubs and are unique because they are open daily, allowing a person to visit them at various times. These centers offer cafeteria-style programs that enable the individual to choose the activities that appeal to him or her such as games, arts and crafts, physical exercise, lectures on problems of the aging, reading and dramatic groups. Some provide low-cost noon meals and personal counseling services. Older persons also may become involved with community activities such as visiting shut-ins, preparing toys for institutionalized children and making bandages for hospitals.

## Social Clubs

These organizations sponsor activities strictly of a social nature and are connected with churches, public agencies or other service clubs. They meet weekly or monthly and provide the opportunity for social get-togethers, singing, games, travel, talks, and so on.

## Adult Day Care Centers

Day care centers provide the elderly person with special help and recreational and social activities during the day or after working hours. This type of service helps fill the gap for companionship and care for the impaired or disabled person in a protective supervised environment while the caregiver is at work or away from home. Such services often are provided by hospitals or nursing facilities. Health or support services may be offered or obtained for individuals in need of them.

## Service to the Blind or Visually Handicapped

Assistance for the blind or visually handicapped is provided by state schools for the visually handicapped or by the state welfare department under the program of categorically needy of aid to the blind. Services include brailling, cane and guide dog training, mobility training and talking books.

## Lions Club

The purpose of this community-oriented social and service club for men is to aid the blind and visually handicapped through fund-raising programs. The Lions Club pays for eye examinations, glasses or possible eye operations. They maintain cornea banks and financially assist those individuals requiring such transplants.

## Masonic Temple

This is a service, social and fraternal organization. Known as the Shriners, this club maintains children's hospitals and burn treatment centers around the country.

## Moose Lodge

This charitable fraternal organization maintains a community for the care and education of orphaned and/

or disadvantaged children near Chicago, Illinois, and a retirement community near Jacksonville, Florida, for aged members of the Moose Lodge.

## HOUSING AND LIVING ARRANGEMENTS FOR THE ELDERLY

It has been estimated that 7 out of 10 elderly (aged 65 and older) persons (couples, widows, widowers, divorcees) maintain their own households in private homes, apartments or rooming houses scattered throughout the community. The concept of continued independence for the able aging person is an emerging pattern in our society.

As persons age, one of the greatest needs is to have special housing adapted to the associated psychological and physiological changes. Reduced vision and hearing, unstable movement and forgetfulness accentuate the need for better safety features in the construction and design of housing for the elderly. Housing should be easily maintained and located close to shopping centers and community social, service and health facilities. Some accommodations and housing for the elderly are:

- **Residential Apartments**—These complexes usually are built by private community groups with the assistance of the Federal Housing Administration (FHA) and are geared to the lower income levels.
- **Retirement Villages**—These are geared to higher income, older, retired or semi-retired persons who are able to purchase the single or attached homes that are built in an entire area or subdivision. The villages are located outside of the larger cities in warmer climates and contain stores, recreational and health care facilities. Such villages may be privately owned or incorporated into a city. Sun City, Arizona, and Sun City, Florida, are examples of these retirement communities.
- **Mobile Trailer Park Retirement Villages**—These are privately owned trailer complexes where the land, some services and social and recreational activities are included in the rental fee for the trailer or trailer space.
- **Low Rent Retirement Hotels**—Older hotels are converted to meet the needs of the elderly and usually have private or semi-private accommoda-

tions and community dining rooms. Guests take care of their own rooms.

- **Continuing Care Retirement Communities (CCRCs)**—This is a retirement (life care) community that guarantees the resident by contract: housing, health care and meals for the remainder of his or her life. Additional services and activities (transportation, recreational facilities) may be available. One usually enters the community in an independent living situation and progresses to various units as the need arises for more protective care, assisted living, or full-time nursing care. Usually this arrangement entails meeting certain age, health and financial requirements, an entrance fee, and monthly charges for various service packages (such as two meals a day, cleaning, linens, utilities, recreation).
- **Board and Care Homes**—These are sometimes termed adult homes, personal care homes or rest homes. The homes may or may not be licensed. They provide rooms, meals, some protective supervision and assistance below the level of nursing care, although many states do allow assistance with medications.
- **Assisted Living Centers**—These centers are somewhere between home care and nursing facility care. Tenants are categorized as the frail elderly, averaging 83 years of age, needing assistance with activities of daily living (ADLs) and medication monitoring. The emphasis is on individual autonomy and independence in a safe, nonregimented, homelike setting. Centers generally supply 24-hour care and services by center employees to meet each tenant's functional and cognitive incapacities; three meals a day including special dietary needs; procedures for doctors and/or nurses to meet medical emergencies; and procedures to handle and administer medications. Tenants leave these centers as needs increase for higher levels of ADL assistance, protective oversight, behavior management, and/or nursing care of illness, hospitalization or death.
- **Nursing Facilities**—Prior to nursing home reform regulations included in the Omnibus Budget Reconciliation Act (OBRA) of 1997, residents were placed in a federally defined intermediate or skilled nursing facility. OBRA eliminated the federal differences in levels of care, but retained a separate

payment program for Medicare skilled nursing facilities (SNFs). The primary difference between a SNF and other nursing facilities is that SNFs have more restrictions on the waivers for professional nursing care.

A nursing facility (NF) is an extended care facility for persons needing extensive medical attention (but no hospitalization) as prescribed by a physician. Although other persons (mentally retarded, stroke victims, accident/brain damaged victims, those with congenital deformities) requiring long-term care reside in nursing facilities, over 50% of this population is elderly. Both NFs and SNFs are designed and staffed to provide 24-hour nursing and related care by a licensed and other qualified personnel according to each resident comprehensive care plan in areas including ADLs, vision and hearing, pressure sores, urinary incontinence, range of motion and rehabilitation, mental and psychosocial functioning, nutrition and hydration, drug therapy, and special needs. Care is geared toward obtaining or maintaining best practical physical, mental and psychosocial well-being of each resident.

Sub-acute care is another level of care often provided by SNFs; this involves medical and rehabilitative care in a variety of areas including ventilator care, intravenous therapy, wound care, head trauma and rehabilitation therapy. This level of care, which is outcome-focused and utilizes a professional team to deliver a determined course of complex medical care, has developed in response to a reimbursement system that focuses on diagnosis-related groups (DRGs), causing shorter stays in hospitals, growth of the geriatric population, and growth of managed care systems.

Some of the factors that cause people to enter nursing facilities include:

1. A greater level of chronic disability as they age.
2. Lack of family members to provide help when needed.
3. Deterioration in mental and cognitive functioning.
4. Advancing age.
5. Increased time spent in a hospital.

### Continuum of Post-Acute Care Services

These services range from very little assistance to those who reside in apartments, to helping with ADLs in the assisted living facility, to rendering nursing care to those in a nursing facility. The concept of rendering all of these services on a single campus helps the resident to transfer to each facility without the trauma involved in moving to a new location in town or to a new area completely. Because of the availability of managed care and the lesser costs involved in alternative living to nursing facilities, managed care programs are looking at this concept favorably.

## PROFESSIONAL ORGANIZATIONS

### Joint Commission on Accreditation of Healthcare Organizations

This is a voluntary nonprofit corporation located in Oakbrook, Illinois. Its bylaws indicate the following purposes:

1. Conduct an accreditation program that will encourage physicians, hospitals and long-term care facilities to take care of patients efficiently.
2. Establish standards for hospitals and long-term care facilities.
3. Recognize compliance with the standards by issuance of certificates to accreditation.
4. Assume other responsibilities and conduct activities that are compatible with the accreditation program.

The membership includes: the American College of Surgeons, the American College of Physicians, American Society of Internal Medicine, American Hospital Association, American Medical Association, American Health Care Association, and the American Association of Homes for the Aging.

The Joint Commission offers a voluntary accreditation program for both hospitals and long-term care facilities and generally has outlined the following policies and procedures regarding accreditation for the long-term care facilities. They must meet the definition of either:

- **Long-Term Care Facility**—A facility providing medical, preventive, rehabilitative, social, spiritual and emotional care to both long-term and convalescent inpatients. There is an organized medical staff, medical director or equivalent, and continuous medical service with a director of nurses.

- **Resident Care Facility**—A facility providing safe, hygienic living arrangements and supportive services, including preventive, rehabilitative, social and emotional care, on a regular basis. Regular and emergency health services are available.

In addition, the facilities must have been in operation under the same ownership for at least six months prior to survey; have a current license to operate as required by the state; and complete an application, pay a fee, and pass an accreditation inspection survey.

Inspection surveys for accreditation are conducted by surveyors of the staff of the Joint Commission. If an institution complies substantially with the standards, it will be given a certificate of accreditation for two years. If it is in substantial compliance (weak in some areas), a one-year accreditation will be granted. If the institution does not comply, it will either be denied a certificate or, in the case of a previously certified institution, it will be given provisional accreditation of one year until it complies with the standards set forth.

These administrative regulations apply to long-term care facilities with SNFs, NFs and SNF and NF (swing) beds as licensed by the state.

## American Health Care Association

This association located in Washington, D.C., is an advocate serving a membership that includes both proprietary, corporate and not-for-profit institutions. The focus is on issues affecting quality, consistency, affordability and availability of long-term health care. It publishes the *Provider* magazine. Some goals are:

1. Gain public understanding by communicating the dedication and contributions of nursing facility owners, administrators, nurses and other personnel to the nation's media, all levels of government and the American public.
2. Demand enforcement of adequate standards by the government and elimination of unlicensed facilities.
3. Oppose oppressive and unrealistic regulations that are adverse to the interests of the resident and detrimental to good resident care.
4. Support health care programs that intend to solve the problems of American senior citizens and other individuals requiring long-term care.

5. Improve the educational level of all nursing facility personnel by:
   a. Developing and recommending new educational techniques.
   b. Surveying and recommending educational systems and training aids.
   c. Providing educational workshops to the affiliated state associations.

## American College of Health Care Administrators

This is a national professional society for long-term health care administrators and is located in Alexandria, Virginia. Its primary purpose is to enhance the knowledge and skills of professional administrators through voluntary credentialling, accreditation and self-regulating programs, and thus promote high quality of life and care for nursing facility residents. The college does not provide lobbying services, but offers such quality assurance activities as:

1. Fostering, developing, conducting and sponsoring programs and related opportunities to promote professional education in nursing facility administration.
2. Publishing appropriate educational materials and *The Journal of Long-Term Care Administration*.
3. Certifying as fellows those members who adhere to its code of ethics and standards of performance.
4. Convening an annual convention presenting matters of interest, opportunities for interaction and furtherance of education related to nursing facility administration.

Membership is nonrestrictive and open to persons who are actively engaged in the practice of nursing facility administration or directly related areas. Categories of membership are:

1. **Active** (voting member)—Individual with qualified experience and training to practice long-term health or residential care administration.
2. **Associate**—Individual interested (not actively engaged) in long-term care administration.
3. **Faculty**—Individual teaching full-time in long-term health care or related educational programs.
4. **Student**—Individual enrolled full-time in a long-term health care related degree program.

## American Association of Homes for the Aging

The American Association of Homes for the Aging (AAHA) is an industry trade association located in Washington, D.C., and is open to all nonprofit facilities and corporations representing concerns in long-term care and aging (independent housing, continuing care retirement communities, community service programs for the aging). It publishes a newsletter and other educational materials and is an advocate for the membership. Some areas of concern are:

1. **Tax Exemption**—Seeks to maintain tax-exempt status for nonprofit "charitable" institutions. AAHA's legal section provides an information exchange and consultation service for legal counsel representing nonprofit facilities.
2. **Medicare**—Protects the rights of residents entitled to Medicare and the special interest of those facilities participating in the Medicare program (i.e., "spell of illness," levels of care, reimbursement, audit and certification procedures).
3. **Medicaid**—Represents the nursing facility's concern for high standards of care regardless of reimbursement source (i.e., skilled nursing care regulations, intermediate care policies, reimbursement and inspecting policies).
4. **Licensing**—Recommends giving nonprofit facilities a voice on state governing boards and maintaining high standards and qualifications of administrators.
5. **Housing**—Supports legislation and appropriation bills for programs of the Department of Housing and Urban Development (the prime source of federal funds for housing for the elderly) specifically designed to meet the special needs of the aging.
6. **Representation on the Joint Commission on Accreditation of Healthcare Organizations**— Gives the nonprofit facility a voice in accreditation and certification procedures.

## National Fire Protection Agency

The National Fire Protection Agency (NFPA) is a nonprofit voluntary membership organization whose sole objective is the reduction of fire waste of lives and property. Located in Quincy, Massachusetts, and organized in 1896, its stated functions are to: promote the science and improve the methods of fire protection and prevention, obtain and circulate information on these subjects, and secure the cooperation of its members and the public in establishing proper safeguards against loss of life and property by fire.

The association has two classes of members: organizational (trade, professional, and public service associations) and associate (organizations or individuals from industry, commerce, government agencies at all levels, the military forces, insurance companies, architects, engineers, the professions, hospital, nursing home and school administrators, and others who have vocational or avocational interest in fire control). The bulk of the members come from the United States, with sizable representation from Canada, and a scattering of members in other countries.

The basic function of NFPA is the preparation of standards and codes. These are developed by technical committees that are made up of widely representative parties who may be affected. Case histories of fires are gathered from many sources; NFPA staff people investigate significant fires, especially those involving substantial loss of life. This data is carefully analyzed to show factors that contributed to the fire spread and fire deaths, which in turn may point up the need for additional protective measures. For nursing facilities, the single most important NFPA standard is the Life Safety Code (NFPA No. 101).

The standards and codes are developed in a quasilegislative process; official adoption is by vote of members assembled at the association's annual meeting. NFPA has no power to legislate or enforce its standards and codes, but they are widely adopted as the bases of laws and regulations, and are extensively used as the basis of good practice.

The education informational functions of the association are carried out by publication of a wide range of technical, information and educational literature.

## National Association of Boards of Examiners for Long-Term Care Administrators

Established in 1971, this is a membership organization for state boards which is located in Washington, D.C. Objectives are to enhance the effectiveness of the state boards of long-term care administrators in meeting their statutory and regulatory duties and responsibilities to protect the health and welfare of the public. It oversees nursing home administrator licensure and relicensure programs, and writes the federal licensure examination and an examination for residential and assisted living administrators. The primary purpose is to ensure that candidates for licensure demonstrate competence at entry-level administration.

### National Citizens' Coalition for Nursing Home Reform

This organization, located in Washington, D.C., supports positive models of quality nursing facility care. It offers a monthly technical assistance series for both consumers and providers to present current information on regulatory concerns. *Quality Care Advocate* is the organization's bimonthly newsletter.

### National Senior Citizens Law Center

The center is located in Washington, D.C., and provides technical assistance regarding the prevention of discrimination against Medicaid recipients.

### National Institute on Aging

Established in 1974, this organization conducts and supports biomedical, social and behavioral research and training on the aging process and common problems of older persons. It is one of the National Institutes of Health (NIH) in Bethesda, Maryland.

### National Eldercare Institute on Long-Term Care

This institute provides general information on long-term, community-based, institutional services. Located in Washington, D.C., and funded by the Administration on Aging, it is operated in collaboration with Brandeis University.

### National Eldercare Institute on Elder Abuse and Ombudsman Services

This institute is operated by the National Association of State Agencies on Aging in cooperation with the National Citizens' Coalition for Nursing Home Reform and the American Public Welfare Association. It is located in Washington, D.C., and funded by the Administration on Aging.

### Alzheimer's Association

This membership organization, located in Chicago, Illinois, provides family members, professional caregivers and researchers with educational materials and technical assistance regarding the care of persons with Alzheimer's disease and related disorders.

## GENERAL TRENDS IN CURRENT LONG-TERM CARE

Increased emphasis on alternatives to institutionalization, coupled with government encouragement, supports the trend toward allowing needy persons to function in their own homes with health care and other assistance. Public expenditures are reduced as the individual and/or family share the financial burden. Currently, there is a deceleration of expenditures for hospital stays and long-term care by Medicare and Medicaid. Recent increases of 25% to 35% in Medicare spending, indicate a shift toward funding for nursing facilities and home health and hospice services. Figures for 1996 providers and suppliers of long-term care seem to support this trend as both inpatient and short-stay hospital beds have decreased and the number of SNFs and home health agencies have increased.

Average life expectancy has increased to 75 years; greater numbers of people are reaching 65. In turn, this population is growing older. Most of the elderly (65 years or older) live outside of institutions. However, over 50% of nursing facility populations are elderly; the greater percentage of this group is 85 years old or more. The U.S. Census Bureau projects an increase in the over-85 population to more than 10.7 million between 2000 and 2050, with accelerated growth in the last 25 years. This indicates a need for more than double the current nursing facility beds, according to the long-term care industry. Alternatives to institutionalization only will accommodate a small portion of this demand to meet the needs for institutional-type care.

January 1996 figures show 5,252 short-stay hospitals, 13,444 skilled nursing facilities and 8,437 home health agencies providing long-term health care. With the more restrictive reimbursement for hospital stays, hospitals are treating more persons on an outpatient basis. As occupancy rates drop, hospitals also are seeking needed revenue from long-term units, hospice, home care services and other health related out-reach programs.

Increasing costs and needs for long-term care are presenting challenges for future funding. Medicare and Medicaid enrollees are increasing along with Medicaid recipients (35% over a six-year period ending in 1996). However, the out-of-pocket payment portion of funding has been increasing during the late 1980s and early 1990s. In 1997, the growth of spending per Medicare enrollee was decreasing and the growth of spending per private insurance enrollee was increasing, indicating the narrowing of the gap between Medicare and private health insurance (personal) expenditures for health care for persons over age 65. These expenditures for the elderly are projected to triple by 2020.

In 1992, the costs of nursing facility care were paid as follows: 42.9% directly by individuals and their families, 47.6% by Medicaid, 4.6% by Medicare, 1% by private insurance, and 3.9% by other sources, with a total expenditure of $65 billion. Although the cost of nursing facility care differs widely, the average comes to $31,000 per year ($84 a day). Home care with one visit per day by a skilled professional costs about the same as a day of nursing facility care. Home aides and other paraprofessionals needed three to five times a week would cost approximately $20,000 per year.

As Medicare and Medicaid spending is shifting toward managed care, the future of long-term health care seems to be in providing a continuum of care in an affordable manner. Health care providers (hospitals, nursing facilities, assisted living, home health care) may link into this continuum.

**BIBLIOGRAPHY**

Allen, J.E. 1992. *Nursing home administration*, 2nd ed. New York, NY: Springer Publishing.

American Association of Retired Persons Gerontology Research Center. 1988. *Acronyms in aging*. Washington, DC.

American College of Health Care Administrators. 1991. *The long-term care administrator*. Bethesda, MD.

Davis, W. 1994. *Introduction to health care administration*, 4th ed. Bossier City, LA: Publicare Press.

Department of Health and Human Services, Mental Health Administration. *Health maintenance organizations: the concept and structure* (publication HIM 11). Washington, DC.

Department of Health and Human Services, Health Care Financing Administration. 1996. *1996 HCFA statistics*. Baltimore, MD.

National Board of Examiners for Nursing Home Administrators. 1997. *NAB study guide*, 3rd ed. Washington, DC.

Quality care for life. 1992. *Provider Magazine*.

South Dakota Department of Social Services, Adult Services and Aging. 1991. *Adult services and aging*. Pierre, SD.

# Appendix 2–A

## Acronyms

| | | | |
|---|---|---|---|
| AAA | Area Agencies on Aging | MDS | Minimum Data Sheet |
| AAHA | American Association of Homes for the Aging | MSDS | Material Safety Data Sheet |
| | | N4A | National Association of Area Agencies on Aging |
| ADA | Americans with Disabilities Act | | |
| ADL | Activities of Daily Living | NAB | National Association of Boards of Examiners—LTCA |
| AHCA | American Health Care Association | | |
| ANSI | American National Standards Institute | NAHC | National Association for Home Care |
| AOA | Administration on Aging | NCOA | National Coalition on the Aging |
| AGS | American Geriatrics Society | NF | Nursing Facility |
| ASA | Adult Services and Aging; American Society on Aging | NFPA | National Fire Protection Association |
| | | NIA | National Institute on Aging |
| CASPA | Complaint about State Program Administrator under OSHA | NIH | National Institutes of Health |
| | | NIMH | National Institute of Mental Health |
| CCRC | Continuing Care Retirement Community | NHA | Nursing Home Administrator |
| CMHC | Community Mental Health Center | OAA | Older Americans Act; Old Age Assistance |
| CON | Certificate of Need | | |
| CRCF | Certified Residential Care Facility | OBRA | Omnibus Budget Reconciliation Act |
| DNR | Department of Natural Resources | OHDS | Office of Health Development Services |
| DRG | Diagnosis-Related Group | OSHA | Occupational Safety and Health Administration; Occupational Safety and Health Act |
| EEOC | Equal Employment Opportunity Commission | | |
| EPA | Environmental Protection Agency | OSHRA | Occupational Safety and Health Review Commission |
| FCA | Federal Council on Aging | | |
| FHA | Federal Housing Administration | PASSAR | Preadmission Screening and Annual Resident Review of Mentally Ill and Mentally Retarded Individuals |
| HBV | Hepatitis B Virus | | |
| HCFA | Health Care Financing Administration | | |
| HCS | Hazard Communication Standard | PMA | Petition for Modification of Abatement under OSHA |
| HHA | Home Health Agency | | |
| HHS | Department of Health and Human Services | PPE | Personal Protective Equipment |
| | | PPS | Prospective Payment System |
| HIV | Human Immunodeficiency Virus | PRO | Peer Review Organization |
| HMO | Health Maintenance Organization | RAI | Resident Assessment Instrument |
| HUD | Department of Housing and Urban Development | SNF | Skilled Nursing Facility |
| | | SSA | Social Security Administration; Social Security Act |
| LTC | Long-Term Care | | |
| MAA | Medical Assistance to the Aged | SSI | Supplemental Security Income |
| MCO | Managed Care Organization | VA | Veteran's Administration |

# CHAPTER 3

# Governance and Management: Business and Management

## INTRODUCTION TO BUSINESS

The creation and distribution of goods and services plays an important role in our society. The consumer, for the most part, influences the type of goods to be produced and the distribution of those goods. Because consumers operate in a somewhat free society, they may buy what they please and from whom they please. The producer must know what goods consumers want and they produced them at a price consumers can afford. Out of the interplay of consumer and producer evolves a complex group of organizations and functions. This is a business system. This study of business will be concerned from a general viewpoint with how this system operates. In order to understand the system adequately, there should be an understanding of the people who operate in the system: the producer who produces goods and services for others, the consumer who buys the goods, and the workers who are employed by the business to do the work.

### Business Systems

A business is defined as a person or group of people who produce or distribute goods or services. These people or groups of people may take the forms of proprietorships (a single person operating a business), partnerships (two or more people who enter into a verbal or written agreement to produce goods or render services such as law, medicine or engineering) or cor-

porations (at least one person who organizes a corporation under the statutes of a state that usually has a board of directors and stockholders). In order to classify as a business technically, the organization must experience as its objective a profit and take the risk of a loss. Some examples of business under this category are grocery stores, manufacturing plants and banks.

On the other hand, the operation of a hospital or university is not technically a business enterprise because the primary motive is not for profit. Normally, the primary goal of such institutions is to provide services—whether it be taking care of sick patients or attempting to educate students. So-called nonprofit organizations very often make a surplus (i.e., they have more income than expenses at the end of the year). Many businesses are nonprofit not because they intended it that way, but because that is the way it happened. Generally, an essential difference between a nonprofit and a profit organization is that the true business distributes its profits to its partners or shareholders. A nonprofit organization, if it has a surplus, uses the money to improve the quality of the service it provides. If a nonprofit health care facility makes a profit, the money is not paid to the governing body but is used for buying better equipment and hiring better help to provide a better quality of service to the resident.

### The Consumer

In a basic or primitive society, the consumer wants the necessities of life: food, tools to get food, clothing and shelter. Because of our standard of living in the United States, we want the best food, the nicest clothing and the most elaborate shelter. We continually attempt to upgrade our needs. This is essential to our ever expanding economy because unless people demand bigger and better gadgets, new corporations would not come into existence and our older corporations would not expand. An element of risk is involved in producing these items, for example, suppose the consumer is not ready to accept them. In that case, the business will suffer a loss rather than a profit. Without the changing attitudes of consumers, a group of unemployed people would exist: the market researchers. These people study the market and help business make future plans by predicting changes in demand for goods and services.

### The Worker

A very important person to business is the worker—the one who gives skills and labor for a stipulated wage or salary. Very often management is placed in a conflicting pattern because of the desires of the consumer and those of the worker. The consumer is interested in buying the product at the lowest possible price; however, management has to demand a sufficient price in order to pay the workers an adequate salary and still earn a profit.

### The Producer

In order to meet the needs of both the consumer and the worker, a person with keen skills and judgment is required. In our complex society, this person is the manager. Basically two types of managers exist: the owner-manager, who also may be called the proprietor or a partner in a small group, and the professional manager, who has undertaken special studies and is usually employed by a corporation.

For example, in the health care field not many years ago, the manager or administrator of a hospital was a clergyman, doctor, nurse or social worker without any specialized skills in management techniques. As the facility became more complex, trained administrators were required to operate and direct its activities. Many have a masters degree in science, public health or business administration. By the same token, in order to operate any business successfully, the specialized skills of a trained manager are necessary.

### Owner-Manager vs. Professional Manager

Some basic differences are found between an owner-manager and a professional manager as to motives and objectives in operating a business. The goals the typical proprietor hopes to obtain are independence in operating a business and maximum earnings. Independence is never completely acquired by anyone; we are all somewhat dependent on each other—the doctor upon the whims of his or her patient, the lawyer upon the attitudes of his or her client, or the business upon the practices of its customers. To this extent, even the owner of a business is dependent.

Relatively speaking, the owner does have more freedom in establishing policy and operating business than the professional manager. If profits are made in a sole proprietorship, they usually go to the owner. This may not be entirely the case in a corporate structure. The owner also receives greater monetary benefits from his or her ideas; the professional manager must share ideas with the corporation employing him or her and will receive only a part of the monetary return on an invention or idea. Of course, the owner-manager usually puts in long hours of work during the first 10 years of the business; the professional manager has somewhat stabilized hours.

## Business and the Social System

American business is based on the concept of capitalism. In a capitalistic society, the production and distribution of goods is planned by private individuals so that they can make a profit. Exceptions occur even in our society. Certain businesses are operated by state and municipal government authorities (i.e., a cement plant operated by a state, or the water and electrical services operated by a municipality). The three basic traits underlying our American business system are:

- **Private Property**—The property rights of an individual in our American society are guaranteed to us in the U.S. Constitution by the Fifth and Fourteenth amendments. The Fifth Amendment relates to the rights of individuals that are safeguarded from interference by the federal government. The Fourteenth Amendment safeguards the property rights of the individual from interference by the state. The due process clause of the Fifth and

Fourteenth amendments has become increasingly important in our modern society.

- **Freedom of Contract**—A contract is a very basic method of making agreements among suppliers, distributors, employers, and so on. Technically, it is a promise or set of promises between two or more people. When there is a violation of this promise by a person, the law gives the other contracting party a remedy (i.e., he or she may sue the breaching party in an action at law). Without the protection in law of contracts, our entire business system would disintegrate.

- **Free Enterprise**—This is the right of a person to enter into any business one chooses. Of course, these rights are subject to rules and regulations that are needed to safeguard the welfare of all citizens. Just as automobiles cannot be operated illegally, contracts that are illegal (gambling) or contracts that are against public policy may not be entered into.

### Competition in Business

It may be stated somewhat accurately that the most basic aspect of our American economic system is competition. Competition can be the rivalry between two organizations or individuals who produce the same goods or provide the same services, or it can be competition for a greater share of consumer spending. An example of the first type of competition is when two firms manufacture steel within the same price range. An example of the second type of competition is when all business organizations, regardless of type, compete for the consumers' dollars. Competition induces new methods and systems to be developed in business and encourages the production of new materials or products. The benefits of competition are reaped by the consumer. It tends to cause production of better merchandise; if two companies manufacture the same product, usually the company with the best quality goods will prevail for the consumer dollar. Competition also produces lower prices by increasing efficiency and keeping the cost down.

### BUSINESS ENVIRONMENT

A number of interrelationships exist between business and the community. The sum of these interrela-tionships is called the business environment. The business environment varies with the society in which the business is transacted. Two aspects of our society that influence business are the legal framework in which the business operates and the form of business ownership found in the society.

### Legal Framework

A law is a rule of conduct that society will enforce for the common good of a group of people in the society. The law determines the rights we have as members of the society and the obligations we owe to the society. There are two basic types of law:

- **Common Law**—In the Middle Ages, the laws were primarily customs of the society handed down from generation to generation. Much of our so-called case law in the United States today is this type of law. The courts in interpreting a set of facts may come to a conclusion based on *stare decisis* or customary law handed down from similar cases that have taken place before the particular case in question. This is known as common law. Much of our common law has been taken from the law of England.

- **Statutory Law**—Statutory laws are laws that are made or enacted by our legislators and are termed statutes. The statutes are compiled into volumes called general laws. All the laws in our country fall into two large categories—public law and civil law—depending upon the type of activity they regulate. Law that regulates conduct between the government, state or municipality and the individual is public law. The plaintiff who prosecutes the action in public law is the government, and the defendant is usually the individual.

When we have the consent of the government, there are cases in which an individual may sue the sovereign, and the government becomes the defendant. Such a case would be a taxpayer suing the government for illegally assessed federal taxes. Generally, the most common types of public law are constitutional law dealing with the relationship of the Constitution and the individual; administrative law dealing with regulatory bodies such as the worker's compensation board, labor board or other commissions created by the government; and criminal law dealing with individual conduct that offends the welfare of the state.

Civil law, on the other hand, is concerned with the relationship between individuals. The individual bringing the action is called the plaintiff, and the person against whom the action is brought is called the defendant. Some general areas of civil law are: torts or laws relating to civil wrongs such as negligence, defamation and civil assault and battery; sales and negotiable instruments law; corporation and agency law; and real property law. Perhaps the most important law to the business system is contract law.

Generally speaking, in order for a court to try a case, it must have legal jurisdiction over the subject matter of the case being tried. If a court has no jurisdiction, this can be grounds for a mistrial or for dismissal of the case. The federal government has jurisdiction over such matters as interstate commerce, espionage and treason. The state courts usually have jurisdiction over all activities that take place intrastate. Where both federal and state governments have jurisdiction, the federal law is supreme. The federal government is particularly interested in such areas as trade practices, labor laws and regulations, wages and hours of work.

## Forms of Business Ownership

Ownership is a legal relationship between a person and some object. The meaning of ownership (the rights which an individual may exercise over his or her possessions) is determined by law. Ordinarily the term ownership implies the exclusive right to possess and use property within the limits of the law. Ownership implies also the responsibility on the part of the owner for the activities of his or her property. The law may allow ownership of a pistol, but that does not carry with it the right to shoot another person. The owner of a business is responsible for its conduct—a responsibility the courts will enforce if necessary. In any business, establishing clearly who is the legal owner or owners is important. Ownership usually decides, for instance, who shares the profits or has the responsibility for illegal activities.

There are three basic forms of ownership in our country: proprietorship involving an individual owner, partnership involving legal relations between two or more owners, and corporation involving a special type of ownership characterized by the granting of a charter by the state. To be legal, business organizations must be sanctioned by laws that provide for them or do not prohibit them. Common or statutory laws sanction our forms of business ownership. Proprietorship and partnership are unique forms of ownership because documented sanction by a government is not necessary for their creation. They are common law forms of ownership. The most significant feature of these ownership forms is the fact that the business and the owner(s) are one and the same. Business assets and liabilities are personal assets and liabilities.

## Proprietorship

The word proprietorship describes business that is owned by individuals. The sole proprietorship is the oldest form of business ownership. It is also the simplest and can be established quite informally. There are more proprietorships in the United States than any other form of the business organization.

How does one start a proprietorship? Suppose a man named Thomas Simple is employed as an accountant in a large firm, but he wishes to go out on his own. He finds a number of people willing to employ him to handle their accounts, and he begins working on these accounts. Simple is now a sole proprietor; no legal action is necessary. There are no organizational expenses and no formal requirements for publicity. The business may be full time or part time.

However, if Simple wished to enter business under a different name, such as Dakota Accounting Service, he must record, usually at the town hall, the fact that this is his business. A small registration fee is charged for recording the name and then the business becomes a matter of public record. Some proprietorships cannot be established without a license or permit. Permits usually are required to sell tobacco products and alcohol. Professions like medicine, architecture and dentistry require a license as a matter of course. But these restrictions are placed on all forms of business ownership; they are not limited to proprietorships.

### Advantages of Sole Proprietorship

- **Simplicity of Formation**—All states have enacted laws affecting the various forms of business ownership, but the number applicable to sole proprietorship are at a minimum.

- **Freedom to Exercise Personal Judgment**—A sole proprietor makes the decisions in a business. If one wishes to add new products to the business, it may be done without the consent of associates. If one wants to raise a sizable amount of money in order to expand a business, the consent of stockholders is not necessary. Consequently, the proprietor can make decisions promptly, assuring maximum flexibility.

- **Ownership of All Profits**—No other form of organization permits one person to own 100% of the profits. In a partnership or corporation, the amount shared with others may be limited but some portion of the profits will be distributed to them.

- **Personal Satisfaction**—The successful businessman who owns and operates an established and profitable business is one of the most satisfied people in the community. One may achieve success through a combination of special skills, willingness to take risks, hard work and personal sacrifice. Knowledge that one alone is responsible gives the individual incentive for further accomplishment. The proprietor usually has all his or her personal capital invested and as a result works harder than a person on a salary.

- **Savings in Taxes**—As contrasted with corporations, special taxes are not levied against an individual as a sole proprietor. He or she must pay regular individual and business taxes such as those on income, property and payroll, but these are not considered special taxes against the form of business ownership. Furthermore, if profits are so high that they would be subject to federal income taxes higher than those that would be levied against a corporation, the Revenue Act of 1954 permits an election to be taxed as a corporation.

- **Prime Credit Rating**—Because the sole proprietor's liability for debts extends beyond business assets to personal assets, one usually enjoys an excellent credit rating. If there are unencumbered personal assets, he or she will enjoy better credit standing than a corporation with equal business assets as a rule. Interestingly enough, if a proprietorship becomes incorporated, its credit may drop because the possibility exists that unscrupulous stockholders might convert the business assets into personal

assets by voting themselves excessive salaries. Because the claims of creditors extend only to the corporation assets, they could not recover their loans from the stockholder's personal assets.

- **Secrecy**—Because the proprietor is simply an individual who has gone into business for himself or herself, there is no need to share confidential information with anyone else. If the success of the business depends upon a secret formula or a special technique known only to the owner, the sole proprietorship is the best form of organization to ensure that this information remains secret.

- **Ease of Dissolution**—No legal procedure is involved in dissolving a sole proprietorship. Should the owner of a clothing store decide to enter another business or retire, he or she need only sell the inventory and close the shop.

### Disadvantages of a Sole Proprietorship

- **Unlimited Liability**—This refers to the availability of a person's wealth beyond the amount invested in a business to satisfy the claims of the business creditors. In a sole proprietorship, this means that practically everything an individual owns is subject to liquidation for the purpose of paying business debts. Every year thousands of sole proprietorships discontinue operations either voluntarily or because of failure. In each case creditors expect to collect the amounts owed them either from the business itself or from the individual owner.

- **Limitation on Size**—The investment in a sole proprietorship is limited to the amount one person can raise by investing his or her own capital by borrowing or a combination of the two. If the business to be organized requires a substantial amount of capital, it may well be that the individual will find it necessary to choose another form of organization.

- **Difficulty of Management**—The typical proprietor may have to prepare a sales campaign, pack a rush order, assist the bookkeeper with the annual audit or negotiate with a union. The large amount of work in which one may become personally involved leaves little time for general management problems. Unlike executives in a big business, the sole proprietor can seldom call on experts to solve an immediate problem. Many proprietors are prone to spend more time than they should on the special business functions that interest them. The management problems of a sole proprietor may be solved in part if the proprietor elects to accept a franchise. Both the firm granting the franchise and the one accepting it agree to perform certain functions for each other under a franchise agreement. One of the important services the grantor often renders is management aid.

- **Lack of Permanence**—Death of the owner usually means the end of the proprietorship. If the business is sizeable, it may have to be liquidated in order to pay the inheritance tax. Some owners provide for this through an insurance program that will enable their heirs to pay the tax and carry on the business. There is also a similar problem of permanence if the proprietor becomes sick or emotionally unbalanced.
- **Lack of Opportunity for Employees**—If an employee of a sole proprietorship proves to be unusually able, he or she will not be satisfied to work indefinitely for the owner. The employee may be paid a bonus but generally has little opportunity to share in management or profits.

## Partnerships

A partnership is an association of two or more persons to carry on as co-owners of a business for profit. The partnership is based upon a legal agreement, written or oral, of a voluntary nature. Most partnerships are relatively small businesses. Of the three common forms of ownership, partnerships are the least popular. The vast majority of partnerships in this country consist of two persons. Most of the larger partnership firms in terms of members are in the professions of law, accounting and engineering.

No requirement exists that a partnership contract be written; it may be oral. However, the better procedure is to have a written contract to prevent ill will or misunderstanding in the future. Many problems may arise with an oral contract especially if profits and losses are to be divided on any basis other than equal shares because affirmative proof is required to overcome the presumption of equality among partners. Usually, articles of partnership are drawn up and signed by both

parties to a partnership. The fact that two people own property as joint tenants—tenancy in common or tenancy by the entirety—does not establish a partnership by itself even when such co-owners do or do not share in any profits made by use of the property. The sharing of gross returns by itself also is not sufficient to establish a partnership.

### *Advantages of a Partnership*

- **Larger Amount of Capital**—In a sole proprietorship, the amount of capital is limited to the personal fortune and credit of one individual. The capital can be doubled or trebled by bringing in additional partners to a partnership.
- **Credit Standing**—The partnership usually enjoys the highest credit standing of the three types of business ownership. The personal wealth of the owners is available to satisfy the business debts.
- **Combined Judgment and Managerial Skills**—Partners can consult each other about proposed actions. Of the partners in a partnership, one may be good at organization and one at sales; when they combine their skills, a more efficient operation will usually occur.
- **Retention of Valuable Employees**—If a person is a very important asset to a firm, he or she can be advanced to a partner in the organization.
- **Personal Interest in the Business**—Because each general partner is liable for the actions of the other partners as well as for his or her own in relation to the partnership, there is vital concern in every move made by the business.

### *Disadvantages of the Partnership*

- **Unlimited Liability of the Partners**—The law states that "Every partner is an agent of the partnership for the purpose of its business, and the act of every partner binds the partnership unless the partner so acting has in fact no authority to act for the partnership in the particular matter, and the person with whom he [or she] is dealing has knowledge of the fact that he [or she] has no authority."
- **All Partners are Liable**—If any one of the partners participates in a wrongful act in the course of business which results in a monetary loss to the

partnership, all of the partners are held liable for the loss incurred.

- **Lack of Continuity**—If a partner dies or withdraws from the business, the partnership dissolves. Also, if a partner becomes insane or takes out bankruptcy papers, the partnership dissolves. The more persons in a partnership, the greater are the chances that this will occur.

- **Frozen Investment**—For an individual who wishes to invest some money in a business, the partnership may be a poor choice from the standpoint of liquidation and transferability of ownership. For example, if a partner withdraws or dies, the firm is dissolved. A fair price is difficult to arrive at if the remaining partners or an outsider are unwilling to purchase the vacated interest.

## *Special Types of Partnerships*

- **Limited Partnership**—According to law, a limited partnership is a partnership formed by two or more persons under statute, having as members of one or more general partners and one or more limited partners. A general partner has unlimited liability for the debts of the firm. A limited partner does not assume responsibility for the debts of the partnership beyond the amount of his or her investment that may be cash or other property but not services. There are certain problems involved in a general or limited partnership limiting the use of this type of ownership. The major problems are unlimited liability for the owners, difficulty in transferring ownership, management problems, mandatory dissolution upon death of an owner and restriction of total capital available. To overcome one or more of these problems, other variations of partnership forms have become prevalent.

- **Limited Partnership Associations**—In a limited partnership association, all members have limited liability. It is necessary to adhere strictly to the law in forming such associations. They are permitted in only five states: Michigan, Virginia, Ohio, New Jersey and Pennsylvania. The laws in the various jurisdictions differ regarding these associations. One common requirement is that a copy of the articles of association must be filed in a public office. In Ohio, the life of the association cannot exceed 20 years, the number of partners cannot be less than three nor more than 25 and the management must be delegated to a small group of three to five individuals. In all states the name of the association must contain the word "limited" or "Ltd."; this is no relation to English and Canadian corporations.

- **Joint Ventures**—A venture is a special type of partnership formed for a single undertaking of a short duration. Members have unlimited liability. For example, a joint venture may be formed to share the cost of purchasing, outfitting and operating a vessel for a round-trip voyage. All profits are then distributed upon arrival of the vessel, and the venture is terminated. A joint venture is created by a contract signed by the partners, and the management is delegated to one partner. Partners cannot bind the partnership; only the designated manager may do so. Property owned is usually held in the name of one of the partners in trust for the benefit of the others. The death of a member does not terminate the business, and the ownership interest of the deceased passes to his or her estate.

- **Syndicates**—Syndicates are formed when a group of people or companies join together to accomplish a single purpose with limited liability. The most common use is an underwriting syndicate. For example, if a corporation desires to sell a large issue of stocks or bonds, it will do so through an investment bank. This bank will form an underwriting syndicate composed of a number of investment banks to help in disposing of the stocks or bonds. Each bank assumes a quota of the entire issue, and the liability of each is limited to the amount of its participation in the total amount. Management is vested in the investment bank that formed the syndicate.

- **Joint Stock Company**—A joint stock company is sometimes called a quasicorporation as it combines characteristics of partnership and corporation. There is limited liability; the ownership of the shares is transferable, and management is by a board of directors.

- **Mining Partnerships**—In a mining partnership, liability is unlimited. However, a partner may sell his or her interest to any willing buyer without the consent of other partners and without dissolving the partnership. The shares can be issued to facilitate a transfer of ownership. Profits are distributed in proportion to the shares held. Some of the western states allow this type of partnership for the express purpose of mining operations and oil drilling. Mining requires continuous operation; if a firm had to be dissolved upon the death or withdrawal of an owner, big problems could ensue.

### Types of Partners

- **Secret Partner**—A secret partner is active in the affairs of the partnership but is not known as a partner to the public.
- **Silent Partner**—A silent partner does not take an active part in management and is known as a partner to the public.
- **Dormant Partner**—A dormant partner does not take an active part in the management and is not known as a partner to the public.
- **Nominal or Ostensible Partner**—A nominal or ostensible partner is not actually a partner, but probably announces himself or herself as a partner or allows others to hold him or her out as a partner even though he or she does not actually share in the profits of the business or invest money in it. Some courts, however, have held that a nominal partner may obligate firm members by his or her acts or become liable for the debts of the partnership.

### Corporations

In the early days of the United States, it was necessary to establish banks and to form canal and road building companies. These enterprises were established as special private corporations. Each of these corporations was set up by a special act of the state legislature or by Congress at first. As business grew, the incorporation of new businesses became so frequent that state legislators found it expedient to set up general laws to handle incorporation (i.e., Uniform Corporations Act).

Today a group of people may set up a corporation to undertake any form of legitimate business enterprise provided they follow state statutes. The corporation is an artificial or fictitious organization created by law to function as an individual in the eyes of the law. It is a legal entity that is separate and apart from its owners. The corporation is without question the most important form of business ownership in the United States. Only 20% of businesses are incorporated; however, these incorporated firms account for 75% of the total receipts and 60% of all net profits in the business world.

There are two types of corporations. **Closed (or family type) corporations** have few owners and the stock is not normally open for general sales to the public. Its stockholders are relatives, friends or business associates. This type of corporation is conducted like a partnership. **Open corporations** sell stock to the public on a large scale. It has many owners or stockholders of whom nearly all take no active part in the operations and have very little to say in the management.

The **stockholders** are the owners of a corporation. The total ownership or capital of the corporation being represented by a designated number of shares of stock. Based on the number of shares owned, the stockholders vote for the board of directors, which is responsible for the operation and general conduct of the corporation. Shares of stock can be sold, bequeathed to heirs or given away. The new owner has all the rights in the corporation that his or her predecessor had. After the stockholder has paid for his or her shares, he or she has no further liability for the debts or actions of the corporation. Creditors only can look to the property of the corporation for payment of their claims. When the corporation makes a profit, the board of directors may distribute as much of this profit that it feels the corporation can spare among the stockholders in proportion to their holdings. The distribution of corporate earnings to the stockholders is known as declaring a dividend.

There are two types of stock in corporations. **Common stock** represents the basic ownership of the company. Stockholders of common stock have the right to vote at a stockholders meeting, to elect directors and vote on important changes. They receive in dividends as much of the corporation's earnings as the directors declare as dividends. **Preferred stock** is a special type of stock where the rate of dividends is fixed. Owners of preferred stock receive dividends before anything is given to the common stockholders. Preferred stockholders normally do not have the right to vote at stockholders meetings.

**Stock certificates** usually have printed on them a figure in dollars. This figure is called the **par value** and indicates the amount at which the firm was nominally financed. For example, if the corporation is capitalized at $10,000 and each share has a par value of $10, there will be 1,000 shares. The incorporators may have put that amount of cash or valuables such as real estate and merchandise into the corporation. Therefore, the par value is no indication of the actual cash value of the stock; some stocks are even termed "no par value." The significant value of a stock is its **market value**. The market value is the selling price for the stock on which buyers and sellers agree. This value may fluctuate from day to day depending upon supply and demand of the stock. The market value, therefore, cannot be printed on the certificate. The **book value** indicates the value of the corporation according to the books of the corporation and may be different from the actual value of the corporation. This happens when the actual appreciation or depreciation of fixed assets differs from the appreciation or depreciation of unfixed assets as determined by accounting procedures.

### Advantages of a Corporation

- **Limited Liability**—Each stockholder is liable only to the extent of his or her original purchase of stock.
- **Contracts**—Only designated officers can bind the corporation and contracts. No one owner can make a contract that will bind the company as a partner can do.
- **Continued Existence**—The corporation life is not affected by death, disability or disagreement of a stockholder.
- **Tremendous Growth Possibilities**—The public corporation can grow larger by selling securities to the general public.
- **Opportunity for Expert Management and Large Scale Economies**—The large public corporation can afford to hire skilled personnel and save money by large scale purchases.

### Disadvantages of a Corporation

- **High Taxes**—The corporation pays many special kinds of taxes, and its income is subject to double taxation.
- **Government Regulation**—The state and federal governments surround the corporation with many regulatory laws.

- **Credit Depends on Its Assets Alone**—A small corporation may find it difficult to borrow money because no owner is liable for its debts.

## GOVERNMENT AND BUSINESS

The proper role of government in business will depend largely upon your feelings, your political leanings, your philosophy and many other factors. There are those who feel that government is far too strong in our society; others believe that there should be a more active role in business affairs. It must be admitted, however, that in recent years the federal and state governments have had more regulation of business affairs. The basic reasons why governments (federal, state and local) feel that their activities are important is that they see themselves in the following roles: maintaining free competition, protecting public health and safety, protecting the public against fraud, producing revenue and ensuring adequate service at reasonable rates from those businesses deemed to be important to public welfare. To achieve these aims, governments collect taxes from businesses, forbid certain types of business activity, and set standards of quality and performance that businesses must meet when they sell their products or render services. The principal methods of government control are:

- **Statutes**—Government enacts laws which either prohibit or demand certain kinds of activities. Equal opportunity, minimum wage and overtime compensation are statutes affecting labor.
- **Charters and Franchises**—Government controls economic activities by requiring the owner to get a charter or franchise before going into business. Bus lines are usually operated under a franchise by the municipality. To get the franchise, the owner must meet certain standards of operation and may have to agree to provide a certain amount of service to an area at approved rates.
- **Administrative Agencies**—Specialized agencies control certain types of business activity. Some agencies have investigative powers only, and others have law enforcement powers. The following federal administrative agencies may oversee, control or regulate some aspects of business:

1. **Securities and Exchange Commission**—This agency regulates the sale of securities (stocks, bonds, etc.). The Securities Act protects the investor by requiring accurate, published information about traded securities. Securities traded in national security exchanges must be registered with the Security and Exchange Commission (SEC) together with information to evaluate these companies. The Securities Exchange Act regulates the operation of the stock market. The Federal Reserve Board has the power to fix the margin of credit (the down payment) in stock purchases.

2. **Federal Trade Commission**—The Federal Trade Commission (FTC) regulates and controls monopolistic practices forbidden by the antitrust laws. It regulates unfair methods of competition and deceptive trade practices. It investigates business activity and promotes self-regulation of business by holding practice conferences. The FTC can investigate business practices on its own initiative or at the request of the attorney general. When a corporation is ordered to cease particular operations by a court, the FTC may investigate to make sure that order is carried out. The FTC has power to prevent certain unfair competition methods, such as misleading advertising, mislabeling of fabrics, selling used goods as new and bribing buyers.

3. **Federal Communications Commission**—This agency is established to regulate all common carriers of messages sent by wire or wireless. Where wires are used, the Federal Communications Commission (FCC) establishes the locality that will be serviced and reviews that rates for the service. They require any individual or group wishing to engage in wireless broadcasting to have a license. It also allocates television channels and radio frequencies.

4. **Interstate Commerce Commission**—This commission originally had control over the railroads only. Today it controls all railway travel, coastal water transportation, trucking and shipping.

5. **National Labor Relations Board**—Labor practices are regulated by the National Labor Relations Board to protect workers against unfair practices by employers. The Taft-Hartley Act attempts to balance the relation between employer and employee by limiting the unfair practices of labor unions.

- **Federal Government Ownership**—The U.S. government owns the Tennessee Valley Authority, the Federal Crop Insurance Corporation and the Federal Deposit Insurance Corporation.

- **Municipalities**—Facilities such as transportation, water supply systems and state liquor stores may be owned and operated by municipalities.

- **State Government Ownership**—Corporate charters are governed by law with each state having its own laws. Most states define and limit the purpose for which corporations may be formed, the amount of capital required for incorporation and the representatives to state agencies. A corporation chartered in one state but wishing to do business in another state is called a foreign corporation.

## MANAGEMENT AND ADMINISTRATION

Management generally is the utilization of means to accomplish a specific goal. A manager supplies the environment and the means for the employees to work together to achieve a business goal. Customarily there are three levels (or echelons) of management:

1. **Top**—Comprised of the executive staff or administrator and assistant administrator(s).
2. **Middle**—Consisting of supervisors answering to managers over them while directing subordinate managers under them; usually department heads or floor supervisory managers.
3. **Line Comprising**—Consisting of those supervisors over employees or line workers and who are at the bottom of the management hierarchy (i.e., staff nurses).

The terminology used in the field of management is sometimes ambiguous. Very often, the word **management** is used to refer to a group of managerial personnel, including those who have supervisory responsibility (the right to direct and control) over others. The term management is also used to refer to the processes of management: planning, organizing, directing and controlling.

There is a difference between administration and management. *Administration* means the overall determination of policies, the setting of major objectives and the laying out of broad programs. **Management** essentially means the executive function of the direction of human efforts toward achieving the business goal and the "getting things done" concept with and through other people. Generally administration is responsible for the determination of the aims of the organization, and management directs and guides the operations of the organization in realizing its established aims.

Generally management and administration are not performed by two separate people. Each manager may perform both activities. All managers, regardless of their level, perform the same functions. The higher up in the hierarchy, the more time will be spent in the administrative activity and less in the management activity. Top management of an enterprise will devote most of its time to broad policy formulations and a lesser amount of time to directing and supervising those immediately under its command. In a nursing facility, most managers have a dual role—supervising others and performing the technical task themselves.

## Management: Science or Art?

Management is both an art and a science. Science is a body of systemized knowledge which is accumulated and accepted with reference to the understanding of general truths concerning a particular phenomona or object of study. This body of knowledge is objective; it is free of prejudice. Commonly it is classified to better understand it. Knowledge of management exists; it is used by all managers. This leads to the belief that there is a science of management. However, the science of management is neither as comprehensive nor as accurate as the physical sciences (i.e., chemistry or physics). Any process such as management that is so weighted down with variables and which can never be duplicated in exactly the same way in an experimental environment probably will not qualify as a physical science.

Art is the bringing about of a desired result through the application of skill. Arts is the application of knowledge or science in performance. Science teaches one to know (astronomy); art teaches one to do (navigation). Science and art are complementary fields of endeavor; they do not exclude each other. A physician acquires the knowledge of the sciences such as chemistry or biology, but excellence in applying this knowledge makes him or her an outstanding physician.

A manager needs a systematized body of knowledge that provides fundamental truths. At the same time, a manager inspires, cajoles, flatters, teaches and induces others to work together toward a given goal. Managers use skills. There are technical and managerial skills. Most managers use more technical skills at lower levels of the management scale; higher levels in the organizational structure use managerial skills to a greater degree. A good chief executive officer will draw upon the technical skills of the supervisor to help solve problems. Generally speaking, a manager at the lower levels who becomes a chief executive officer because of a specialty in a particular area will have to look beyond the specialty area to generalities.

## Universality of Management Concept

The management process has universal application. The manager uses the same basic managerial skills of planning, organizing, directing and controlling in each managerial position. Thus, management skills are applicable to any kind of enterprise where there is coordinated effort of human beings. The type of enterprise is not significant. Universality of management principles also means that the skills of management are transferable from one department to another regardless of their function in the other department. These skills also may be transferred from one level of management to another.

## MANAGEMENT AUTHORITY

The term authority is used with different meanings. This textual material will be concerned primarily with managerial authority.

Authority is the power or the right to act, to command or to exact action from others. Regardless of how a manager uses authority, it must be present; without it, the manager is helpless. Authority is the key to the managerial job. Implied in authority is the power to make decisions and to see to it that they are carried out. Compliance with the directives of the administrator or executive is included in authority. This compliance may be sought through persuasion, sanctions, requests, constraint or force. Although most administrators or managers would rather talk about the responsibility, tasks and duties the subordinate has than impose their authority, his or her authority does include the power and the right to take disciplinary action and, if necessary, to dismiss a subordinate.

## Source and Nature of Authority

Various schools of thought exist regarding the source of authority.

### Institutional or Formal Authority

Ownership of a business includes the right and power to put the property to use and to direct how it is to be used. The ultimate source of authority is, therefore, principally founded in the ownership of private property. In a corporate structure, the owners through the board of directors delegate their right and direction of how to use their property to the president of the company, who in turn delegates portions to major department heads.

In a modern corporate nursing facility, the administrator receives authority from the board of directors, and in turn delegates to department heads and supervisors. The same reasoning applies in the ownership of public property. The property is owned by the government that delegates its right to direct and manage the property to elected or appointed officials. The followers of the institutional or formal source of authority believe that authority is conferred on an individual by the position in the organization.

The effectiveness of a manager's formal authority may frequently fall short of what is desired by the manager or his or her subordinates. These failures can be attributed to inadequate delegation of authority or to lack of managerial competence.

### Subordinate Acceptance

The behavioral school of management theory essentially does not agree with the formal authority theory point of view, stating that the true source of authority comes to its holder through acceptance by the subordinates of the manager's decision making and decision enforcement. Under this theory, a manager has no authority until it is conferred upon him or her by subordinates.

This theory emphasizes leadership, the importance of a manager winning, not ordering, support and the recognition by the subordinate that someone in the group must make decisions. The subordinate acceptance theory is considered "bottom-up management." The manager encourages his or her employees to contribute ideas and suggestions for improving procedures, save time and effect positive working conditions. The success of bottom-up management depends in a large measure upon the kind and amount of authority that each employee accepts and uses. The subordinate acceptance approach is premised on subordinate approval without any sanctions.

From a practical viewpoint, the subordinate acceptance approach is not extensively used in the management of a nursing facility. It is difficult to imagine that a subordinate or department head has the choice of accepting authority; very little choice is left if the only alternative to not accepting the authority is to be dismissed. It should be noted that the subordinate's power to disobey under this theory cannot deprive the superior of his or her authority. A number of management theorists believe that when the behaviorist school of subordinate acceptance discusses authority, it really means a form of leadership and not authority.

### Authority by Law

Under this theory, the rightful power is granted by law. It gives an office holder that power necessary to perform his or her job. Some examples of authority given by law are justices of the U.S. Supreme Court or circuit or magistrate courts, governors, mayors and other elected federal, state or municipal officers.

### Authority by Personal Qualities or Technical Competence

Under this theory, authority remains with an individual; it cannot be delegated or assigned. A person who is a recognized expert in a particular field is often referred to as an authority on certain problems. In this instance, the person has authority by virtue of what he or she knows. The decision is accepted because of knowledge—not because of the position in the organization. An example of this kind of authority in a nursing facility is when the nurse aides and orderlies go to a staff RN to assist them when making decisions rather than go to the director of nurses. Under the formal authority theory, the director of nurses would be the one who has authority to make decisions. However, in this case, the staff RN has the necessary special competence, and the aides and orderlies go to him or her and thus circumvent the director of nurses.

### Limitations on Authority

The concept of authority has specific express and implied limits. These limitations may be internal or external.

Some of the internal limitations are:

- **Articles of Incorporation and Bylaws**—These documents are necessary to form a profit or non-profit corporation. It is not unusual to delineate limitations or constraints on the authority of the administrator in these documents in the areas of budget, staffing, purchasing and others of important decision making.
- **Policies and Procedures of the Facility**—In many nursing facilities, the administrator's authority is outlined or limited in a formal document known as the policy and procedure manual.
- **Tapering Concept of Authority**—In the typical nursing facility, each manager in a particular position is subject to specific authority limitations spelled out in the assignment of duties and delegation of authority. The administrator may have the authority to make capital expenditures up to $10,000,

whereas the department head may not exceed the capital expenditures of $1,500. The general rule is that more limitations are placed on the scope of authority as one goes down the managerial hierarchy—hence, the term *tapering concept of authority*. The lower down the managerial hierarchy, the more restrictions on authority; the higher up in the managerial hierarchy, the less limitations and the broader the scope of authority. An inverted triangle is used to illustrate this principle (see Figure 3–1).

Some of the external limitations on authority are:

- **Codes and Laws**—All active administrators in the health care field are familiar with the mountains of rules, regulations, standards, codes and laws that are thrust upon them and restrict or modify the authority in the facility. Department of health rules and regulations, licensing rules, conditions of participation for Medicare and Medicaid, Occupational Safety and Health Administration (OSHA), resident's bill of rights, and the standards for the handicapped and disabled are but a few examples of external constraints put on the facility.
- **Political, Ethical and Economic Considerations**—The concept of what is politically acceptable, mor-

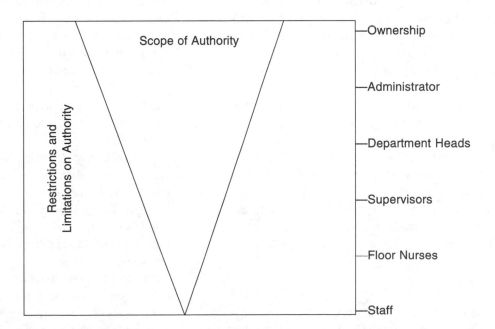

**Figure 3–1** Tapering Concept of Authority

ally right and financially feasible for the elderly influences many social laws that directly affect the operation of a nursing facility.

- **Labor Unions and Collective Bargaining**—The manner in which the administrator may manage a facility is directly affected if the facility has a collective bargaining agreement or is directly involved with a labor union. The administrator no longer has the last say on decision making, but may have to work with the labor leader or union representatives in the areas of benefits, discipline, hiring and firing.

## Delegation of Authority

Delegation of authority is essential to the effective operation of a health care facility. To delegate means to grant or confer. Delegation means conferring authority from one executive or organizational unit to a subordinate for the purpose of carrying out a particular assignment or assignments. By so doing, the administrator expands his or her scope of management. Although the executive gives up some control over work performance, delegation of authority does not mean surrender of authority. An administrator delegating authority always retains overall authority for assigned tasks given to a subordinate. For example, in approving vacations or pay raises, the authority of the administrator may be delegated to a department head who in turn may delegate to a supervisor, but the ultimate responsibility for implementation of wages and salary administration remains with the administrator.

A chain of authority is established following the formal organizational structure. Authority is delegated only to the extent required to perform an assigned task in a satisfactory manner. Delegation may be downward, upward or lateral. Downward delegation is illustrated by an administrator delegating to the assistant administrator or to department heads, upward delegation by state government to federal government, and lateral delegation by certain departments delegating to other departments on the same organizational level.

### Reasons for Delegation

Delegation of authority is important for more efficient and effective operation of a nursing facility because it establishes the formal organizational relationships among the departments of the facility, gives the facility managerial depth that is a resource of managers able to carry on if the need arises, and develops subordinates by permitting them to make decisions and apply their knowledge gained from backgrounds, meetings and training.

### How to Delegate

The process of delegation is important. It consists of three aspects:

- **Assignment of Duties**—The administrator or department head is the one who decides how the work is to be divided among the subordinates. By reviewing his or her own functions and duties, he or she will be able to determine the functions to be delegated. Three groups of functions the administrator or department head may wish to review are: routine functions that are time consuming, functions requiring a certain degree of skill, and functions that cannot be delegated and must be performed by the administrator.
- **Granting of Authority**—The second part in the process of delegation is the granting of authority to make decisions, use resources and take action to perform the allocated duties. Duties are assigned and authority is delegated to positions within the facility—not to individual people. However, because positions are filled by people, one commonly speaks of delegation of authority to subordinates. Once the duty or function is delegated, commensurate authority to perform the duty is granted. The scope of authority is necessarily related to the duty to be performed. It should not be larger than necessary to perform the assigned duty or function.

  The authority granted may be specific or general. It is much better to be precise and clear than to require the subordinate to guess how far authority may go. The authority granted should be in writing, if feasible. Charts, manuals and job descriptions will be a valuable assistance in determining the scope of authority.
- **Unity of Command**—This concept states that the delegation of authority and issuance of orders or commands comes only from a single supervisor to a single subordinate, and each subordinate reports only to one supervisor. Simply stated, "A servant

cannot serve two masters." One subordinate with several supervisors results in divided loyalties and possible conflicting orders that are bound to lead to unsatisfactory performance by the subordinate and result in a confusion of authority. If a subordinate has two bosses, he or she does not know which of the two superiors has the authority that will contribute toward his or her success in the organization. Having only one superior to which to report eliminates fragmenting accountability and the resulting conflicts.

## Span of Management

The span of management concept states that a manager can effectively supervise (direct and control) only a certain number of subordinates. This theory is sometimes referred to as span of control. The number of employees a manager can effectively supervise depends on:

- **Training of the Administrator or Chief Executive**—The educational background, experience and work knowledge of the administrator helps determine how many subordinates he or she can supervise.
- **Type of Organization**—Whether the organization is a factory or a nursing facility will influence the span of management of the chief executive. Generally, if the organization requires many judgmental evaluations, the span will be fewer personnel. On the other hand, if the nature of the work is repetitious and simple, the span of management is usually greater in number.
- **Capacity and Make-up of the Subordinate**—The greater the self-direction of the subordinate, the broader the span of management for the supervisor. Those who possess technical skills and are highly trained do not require the same degree of supervision as those who are untrained.
- **Communication**—The manager who communicates effectively broadens his or her span of management. Thus there is usually a direct relationship between the effect of communication and the span of management.

In a nursing facility, a supervisor can supervise between 8 and 12 persons due to the frequency of contact required to carry out resident care and related duties properly.

## Responsibility

Another major aspect of delegating authority is the creation of an obligation on the part of the subordinate to the superior for the satisfactory performance of assigned duties. The acceptance of this obligation by the subordinate creates a responsibility. Responsibility results from a contractual agreement in which the subordinate agrees to perform assigned duties with commensurate authority in return for recognition.

The authority to perform and accomplish the specific job flows from the superior to the subordinate, and the responsibility is the obligation that is exacted from the subordinate to accomplish these duties. Responsibility may be a continuous function or it may be terminated by the accomplishment of a single act. The relationship between the administrator and the department heads is an example of a continuing obligation; if the administrator arranges for someone outside the facility to do a study on salary structure, the responsibility is discharged with the completion of the study.

### Delegation of Responsibility

Quite often one hears a manager talk about delegating responsibility. Responsibility cannot be delegated or shifted to the subordinate. An executive can delegate the authority to perform a specific job to a subordinate, but in doing so he or she does not delegate the responsibility in the sense that once duties are assigned, the delegator is relieved of all responsibility for them. The delegator retains the overall responsibility in the matter. Although out of necessity the administrator may delegate certain tasks to department heads and the department heads may in turn delegate to supervisors, neither of them delegates his or her responsibility. Because responsibility is an obligation to carry out a task, it cannot be shifted or reduced.

For example, an administrator learned that someone had broken into the business office and emptied the wooden drawer of cash and safekeeping valuables. When the claim was turned over to the insurance company for collection of money for the valuables, the facility was informed that it was not covered because the valuables were not kept in a safe. A wooden drawer is not safekeeping said the company, and the claim was denied. The business office manager was delegated the authority to implement a safekeeping procedure. It was assumed that the manager removed the valuables from the drawer each evening. After the incident was completed, the board of directors held the administrator responsible even though the authority to run the business office was delegated to the business office manager.

One of the most widely accepted principles of management is that authority and responsibility should be equal. This means that the subordinate must have been delegated enough authority to undertake all the duties assigned to him or her for which he or she has accepted responsibility. Inequality between delegated authority and responsibility produces undesirable results. If authority exceeds responsibility, a misuse of authority can result. Conversely, the executive who accepts responsibility without adequate authority is likely to be in a frustrating situation.

## MANAGEMENT THEORY

Several theories exist concerning what managers assume about human nature in relation to work accomplishment. These assumptions will affect their approach to leadership. Some of the principal theorists and their approaches are as follows.

**Henri Fayol**—Management Process School. Fayol's contribution was the insistence that management principles can be identified, isolated and used. He stated that management is a separate and unique function and that a valid theory of management could be applied to all forms of organized human cooperation.

**Frederick Winslow Taylor**—Management Process and Human Behavioral School. Taylor is considered the "Father of Scientific Management" and contributed two basic principles of management theory: (1) that both worker and management must take their eyes off the division of surplus (profit) as the all important matter and together must turn their attention toward increasing the size of the surplus; and (2) that both managers and workers must recognize as essential the substitution of exact scientific investigation and knowledge for the old individual judgment or opinion of the worker or manager in all matters relating to the work to be done.

Taylor asserted that management is partly a matter of mechanics (creating and controlling the physical environment of the worker) and partly a matter of dynamics (inspiring and energizing the group of people who work within this framework). Unfortunately, people using his method often have emphasized the mechanical aspects of his teachings and have completely ignored the people-oriented side.

**George Elton Mayo**—Human Behavioral and Social Systems. Mayo emphasized the importance of human factors and, particularly, social factors in industrial situations. He stressed the need to study social behavior in the organization as a means for determining how to improve the productivity of the organization.

Together with others, he was responsible for the "Hawthorne Studies" (1927–1933) that suggested that economical factors are less important than the emotional and nonlogical attitudes and sentiments of the workers, that the work enviornment is a social environment and that the workers respond to attention. These studies give rise to the idea that by giving workers lots of attention, a manager can get greater production.

**Kurt Lewin**—Decision Theory. Lewin suggested that workers would do better if they could participate more in the affairs of their organization, if they could help with decision making and if they were treated more democratically with respect to decisions about matters affecting their employment.

**A.H. Maslow**—Human Behavioral and Social Systems. Maslow felt that there is a hierarchy of needs in workers. From the highest to the lowest, these needs are:

1. **Self-actualization**—Realizing one's own potentialities fully.
2. **Self-esteem**—Respect and recognition by others for real achievement, status, power and capacity.
3. **Social acceptance**—Being loved and accepted by others, and belonging.
4. **Safety and security**—Being safe from physical harm.
5. **Physiological needs**—Adequate food and shelter.

He argued that a worker is dominated by efforts to meet needs at each level starting with the lowest. When the lowest need is satisfied, one becomes strongly interested in meeting the next higher level of need, and the lower level need drops out of the picture. Maslow pointed out that the hierarchy may function in a different order of ascendancy for some individuals but follows the order he identified for most people.

He suggested that most workers in the United States have had the bottom three needs largely satisfied and are concerned primarily with meeting the self-esteem and self-actualization needs. Just before his death, Maslow identified two kinds of self-actualization equating the highest with mankind's highest aspirations where man reaches fulfillment and contributes to mankind. He called these people transcenders, citing as examples: Aldous Huxley, Albert Schweitzer, Martin Buber and Albert Einstein. He suggested that regular self-actualizers are individuals who reach the expectations of McGregor's Theory Y (see later in this chapter) and transcenders come under Theory Z, commonly called participative management where employees have input into decisions on work performance, thus utilizing their knowledge as well as their efforts and skills.

**Clayton P. Alderfer**—Human Behavioral School. Alderfer suggested there are three needs in man. He developed the "ERG" theory of need:

1. **E**xistence needs including both material and psychological desires such as: pay, satisfactory working conditions, food and shelter.
2. **R**elationship needs with family, fellow employees, supervisors, friends and other people.
3. **G**rowth needs which motivate productive and/or creative influence of a person on him- or herself or on his or her environment.

**Frederick Herzberg**—Human Behavioral School. Herzberg suggested that individuals have two kinds of needs that operate in the job environment on two separate continuums:

1. One type he called hygiene factors that grow out of the worker's job environment and that management can control. He argued that these factors are important only in that they can cause dissatisfaction in the worker. Such areas (termed dissatisfiers) call for preventive action and include: physical working conditions, supervisory policies and activity, climate of labor and management relationships, pay and incentive pay, fringe benefits and money rewards, and security. Meeting worker needs and desires in these areas removes sources of dissatisfaction but does not sustain worker motivation. Like with eating and hunger, a pay raise, for example, may satisfy the worker today, but he or she will soon become dissatisfied later wanting more pay.
2. The second type of need he called motivation factors (satisfiers) and argued that they grow out of what the worker does or the nature of his or her job. These are harder for management to effect but do serve as incentives by producing satisfaction and motivating workers to produce better. Under this category are such factors as: feelings of accomplishment, feelings of growth in skills and professions, recognition and increased responsibility. One of Herzberg's recommended means for increasing motivation is job enrichment—a deliberate enlargement of responsibility, scope and challenge.

**Saul Gellerman**—Human Behavioral School. Gellerman defined behavioral science as a systematic measurement of worker attitudes—actions and factors in the environment that can affect them by using the findings in psychology, sociology, anthropology and many of the specialized branches of these disciplines (such as social psychology or industrial anthropology).

He stated that behavioral science has been moving in recent years to identify the techniques used by successful managers who get more productive and profitable operations and to see if these techniques can be applied successfully in different settings, situations, industries and occupations. Research is showing a variety of factors, some of which are listed below.

1. Workers are almost never used at more than their minimum capacities.
2. Workers today are better educated, more in demand and more independent than they were a generation ago.
3. The threat of losing a job or the attraction of getting more money do not motivate them effectively.
4. The environment of managers is seen by managers as being full of challenge and opportunity; the same environment is seen by workers as being rather dull and unstimulating.
5. People are motivated not so much by what someone else wants them to do as by their own desire to get along as best they can in their environment as they see it.
6. The manager, to workers, is just a part of their work environment, to be adjusted to in whatever

way will best realize the attainment of what the workers value most.

7. The process of managing and motivating people is very complex. A manager must analyze specific situations and try to deal with them creatively.

8. Some approaches that work in some situations to get better motivation are:

   - **Stretching**—Deliberately assigning duties to an employee that are more difficult but which the manager thinks the employee can handle. The experience of successful achievement can encourage the employee to develop a desire for doing more difficult things.

   - **Management by Objectives**—Giving the employee rather broad discretion in how he or she handles the details of his or her work, provided the employee reaches defined targets and stays within cost and time boundaries. Here goals are identified, plans are determined, time limits set and progress continually measured.

   - **Participation**—The general strategy of getting employee comments, suggestions and discussion before something significant affecting them is decided. Even if their suggestions are not accepted, they will usually be less likely to misinterpret what is being done and why.

**Douglas McGregor**—Decision, Empirical and Human Behavioral School. McGregor suggested that a manager's style of managing reflects his or her assumptions about people. He identified two basic styles:

- **Theory X**—If a manager exercises very tight control over the workers, supervises very closely, gets satisfactory performance by ordering and forbidding, uses authority and coercion to control and motivate them, and is generally autocratic and rewards successes and punishes mistakes, the manager is acting on the assumption that workers:
  1. Are basically lazy and lack integrity.
  2. Want security and to work as little as possible.
  3. Avoid responsibility and decision making and prefer to be directed by others.
  4. Work only to get money, are indifferent to organization needs and are not interested in achievement.
  5. Are incapable of directing their own behavior.
  6. Are not very bright.

McGregor emphasized that whether a supervisor is tough on workers (hard-nosed, autocratic), is soft (bribes to get people to work, being permissive, catering to worker demands) or is firm and fair (teaching, inspiring, judging, rewarding, punishing), he or she is practicing Theory X and trying to control the workers. Under this theory, the manager relies completely on external control of the behavior of the workers, assuming that they are children and treating them accordingly.

- **Theory Y**—If a manager lets workers participate in setting objectives and work standards, gives them freedom to direct and control their own work, expects some mistakes, considers them a part of their own growth and learning, and provides them with advice and support, he or she is acting on the assumption that workers:
  1. Are not lazy and have integrity.
  2. Like responsibility and are willing to assume it.
  3. Take pride in their work and like to achieve.
  4. Can direct their own behavior and like to do so.
  5. Want their organization to succeed.
  6. Are willing to make decisions.
  7. Are not stupid.

   Under this theory, the manager relies heavily on the workers' self-direction, self-control and commitment to organizational objectives. It is assumed that they are mature adults and are treated as such.

McGregor adopted Maslow's hierarchy of needs as descriptive of what people seek and argued that Theory X type of management fails because the workers' physiological and safety needs already are met, and they are trying to satisfy their social, self-esteem and self-fulfillment needs. He suggested that when the latter needs are not met on the job, the workers do become disinterested, passive and unwilling to follow their demagogue leader to meet what they feel are unreasonable demands just for economic benefits. In effect they become less productive. He argues that Theory Y management does not mean abdication of managerial leadership or a lowering of standards. By providing the opportunity for workers to meet their higher wants on the job, they are motivated to meet even higher standards, expanding the effectiveness of leadership by producing even better results.

**Rensis Likert**—Human Behavioral School. Likert stated that most organizations can be rated on a four-system scale that indicates their prevailing management system.

- **System 1** is exploitive authoritative (arbitrary, coercive, highly authoritarian, little concern for the needs of humans) management that developed in the 19th century. Although it is seldom found in pure form today, it still lingers as the dominant style of some managers.
- **System 2** refers to benevolent authoritative (paternalistic, more interest in workers' welfare, more benefits) management that grew up after studies showed that workers respond to attention—a sort of System 1 with a pleasant veneer.
- **System 3** is consultative (employees given a chance to be heard and to participate although management keeps the right to accept or reject ideas) leadership that evolved as managers learned that workers support better what they have helped create.
- **System 4** involves participative management. With the influence of talent and competence rather than authority permeating the organization, workers are given access to information and trusted to use their creativity and initiative in setting goals and solving problems. Mutual confidence and trust and genuine teamwork characterize all relationships. This management harnesses the power of human resources by relying on three basic principles:
  1. Use of supportive relationships and dealing with people in ways that maintain and enhance their feelings of self-worth.
  2. Creation of an organization of tightly knit, highly motivated work groups strongly committed to achieving the objective of the organization and knitting the groups together by having persons with memberships in more than one group.
  3. Setting high-performance goals for the whole organization.

Likert has said that research shows the closer an organization gets to System 4, the more likely it is to have sustained high productivity, good labor relations and high profitability. Converting an organization toward this system is not easy; it requires massive re-education of all those involved. However, even small shifts toward the system will get improved performance in these areas.

**Chris Argyris**—Human Behavioral School. Argyris's views are based on extensive studies of behavior in actual business organizations and have the underlying assumption: "People, if left free to develop, will naturally grow more mature. Most adults are motivated basically to be responsible, self-reliant and independent." He suggests that if a manager treats people like children, they will act like children; if the manager treats them like adults, they will act like adults.

Many of the key element in the working environment create frustration and unhappiness in the worker. For example:

1. In task specialization, the individual uses only a few abilities—suppressing individuality and causing frustration and unhappiness.
2. In the chain of command, individuals become subordinate to and dependent on leaders.
3. Unity of direction of the organization comes when leaders set the goals, thus preventing workers from setting and pursuing their own goals, and eventually becoming frustrated.

As a result, workers tend to reduce their interest in the job, treating it with indifference and even contempt as a necessary defensive maneuver that allows them to preserve self-respect. Argyris suggests that workers are apt to be in conflict with and antagonistic to an organization and the achievement of its goals because their own needs are unmet. He feels productivity would be enhanced if satisfaction of the individual's needs and the attainment of the organization's goal could be integrated so that the same behavior of workers would accomplish both.

He argues that job security, pay and fringe benefits are necessary but do not motivate workers because workers want their jobs to be stimulating, dignifying and a source of pride and accomplishment. He is not advocating making workers happy, but creating conditions where the workers will derive a greater sense of personal value and significance from their work. Their jobs become more the central focus of their efforts and ambitions because it is where they experience many of their major satisfactions.

**B.F. Skinner**—Human Behavioral School. Skinner stated that behavior that goes unobserved and unrewarded will tend to extinguish itself. Employees want to know that they are doing a good job and that their efforts are appreciated. Positive reinforcement (i.e., longevity pins, commendations, congratulations), praise and recognition—as long as these are based in fact and earned—may motivate better effort and higher morale as workers feel their efforts contribute to the facility's goals.

Although none of these theories are all inclusive or thoroughly supported by evidence, they do affect the field of management and are worth considering as managers seek to motivate employees to take an interest in their work and the organizational goals, to cooperate with others and to do their fair share of the workload. The major techniques, functions and skills of directing are discussed later in this chapter.

## TEAM MANAGEMENT

A team is two or more people who interact and coordinate their efforts for the accomplishment of a specific obligation. Teams may be as small as two or as large as 100 persons; for the most part, teams average about 15 people. There must be interaction as a team and a common objective or goals. Teams will achieve greatest potential when they enhance problem solving through increased member efforts, personal member satisfaction, merger or diverse abilities and skills, and organizational flexibility.

### Types of Teams

A **formal team** is one created by the formal organizational structure.

A formal **vertical team** in a nursing facility is composed of the administrator and the department heads according to the formal chain of command (see Figure 3–2).

A formal vertical team also may be composed of a department head or supervisor and his or her subordinates in the organizational structure (see Figure 3–3).

A **horizontal team** (sometimes called a task force) is a formal team composed of employees from about the same hierarchical position on the organizational chart in different areas of expertise (see Figure 3–4).

A **special purpose team** is created outside of the formal organizational structure to undertake a special project. For example, the administrator of a skilled nursing facility appoints a special team to determine the feasibility of creating a home health outreach to the community. Another form is where the administrator appoints several individuals within the same department to help improve quality and efficiency in their work environment.

A **self-managing team** consists of 5 to 20 semi-skilled workers who rotate their jobs to perform a major organizational task. The team may be empowered to make decisions within their work realm. They work with minimum supervision and may elect one of their own as supervisor.

### Team Development

The **forming stage** is a period of orientation and getting acquainted. The team members test one another for friendship possibilities, task orientation and which behaviors are acceptable to others. During this stage, members are concerned with: "Will I fit in?", "What is expected of me?" and "What is acceptable?" During the forming stage, the team leader helps members to get acquainted and encourages informal social discussion.

During the **storming stage**, individual personalities and roles emerge. People become assertive in claiming roles and expectations of them. This stage may be marked by conflict and disagreement. During this stage, the team leader should encourage participation by each team member to talk about their ideas, disagree with one another, and work through conflicting perceptions about team norms and values.

In the **norming stage**, conflicts are resolved, and the team becomes adhesive. Generally, there is consensus

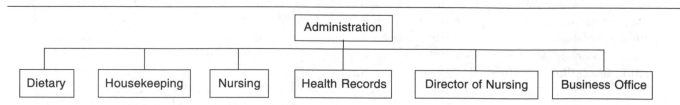

**Figure 3–2** Formal Vertical Team

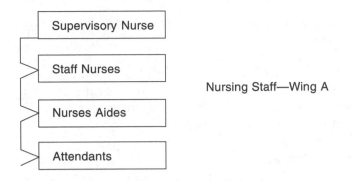

Nursing Staff—Wing A

**Figure 3–3** Formal Vertical Team

as to members' roles, who has the power and who is the leader. This stage is of short duration. The team leader emphasizes unity and clarifies the team's roles, norms and values.

In the **performing stage**, the major emphasis is on problem solving and accomplishing the assigned tasks. The members should be considerate to each other and handle conflicts in a mature way. The leader should get high task performance as team members interact frequently to achieve team goals.

The **adjourning stage** occurs on committees, task forces and teams that have limited tasks to perform. Emphasis, therefore, is on gearing-up, gearing-down and disbanding.

### Managing Team Conflict

Conflict is an antagonistic interaction in which one party attempts to thwart the intentions or goals of another. Teams develop action types for dealing with any conflict based on the desire to satisfy personal concerns versus another's concerns. The following styles of handling conflict may be used to fit a specific situation.

1. The **competing style** reflects being assertive to get one's own way. This style is used to resolve an important issue or an unpopular action in an emergency or crisis situation.

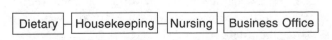

**Figure 3–4** Horizontal Team

2. The **avoiding style** is used when there is a need to delay action to gather more information or when a disruption could be very costly.
3. The **compromising style** reflects assertiveness and competitiveness. This style is used when both sides have equal powers as both sides work to split the difference or when management has to arrive at an expedient solution because of time constraint.
4. The **accommodating style** reflects a maximum degree of cooperativeness. This is used when maintaining harmony is especially important.
5. The **collaborating style** reflects a high degree of assertiveness and cooperativeness, enabling both parties to be winners, although it may require substantial bargaining and negotiation. This style is used when ideas of several parties need to be merged into a common solution.

## MANAGERIAL FUNCTIONS

Everything a manager does falls into one or several of the functions of planning, organizing, directing or controlling.

### Planning

Present day administrators operate in a dynamic economy where change is the rule rather than the exception. Planning helps the manager to master change. The planner is the one with the greatest opportunity to bring together all the resources of the enterprise into a more effective business entity.

Planning is the intellectual aspect of future growth, requiring imagination and foresight. Planning is the foundation of management. No manager can manage successfully over a period of time unless he or she has planned.

Planning is the function that determines the objectives or goals of the business and the course of action (policies, procedures, rules or budgets) to be followed in the attainment of those end results. It consists of selecting and relating facts and the making and using of assumptions regarding the future in formulating proposed activities necessary to achieve desired results. It is looking ahead and preparing for the future. The work of the manager, relative to planning, involves general activities such as clarifying, amplifying and determining objectives of the facility—deciding how, when and who will do the various tasks.

Adequate planning should take place before acting. Every manager has a planning function to perform. Top managers (board of directors, administrators and department heads) are primarily involved with broad policy setting and short- (a few days to one or two years) and long- (three years or more) range goals. As a person assumes the role of middle management and staff, the planning activities become more restrictive.

Planning exists in all health care facilities regardless of their size. In larger facilities, its presence is more apparent due to top level managers giving all or a good portion of their time to planning efforts. In contrast, in a facility of under 100 beds, planning is usually done somewhat informally, and the administrator does most of it.

The planning effort is continuous. All plans are tentative and subject to revisions and amendment as new facts become known and as the variables are reevaluated.

The scope of planning is related directly to the position in the organizational hierarchy. Planning at the very top level is broad and far reaching. The chairman of the board or president is concerned with the total picture. Major plans are formulated by the governing body to implement objectives. This determines the general form of the organization, its functions and activities. Each department head then formulates departmental policies that are directed toward carrying out the major goals of the facility.

### Types of Plans

The use and integration of plans within an organization is a primary tool of management. Each plan used must in effect support every other plan and contribute to the major goals of the health care facility. Within a given facility, plans are interdependent. The policies followed are in keeping with the objectives. The long-range plans must be compatible with the operational plans and the growth plans with the user plans. Plans tend to beget plans. The human tendency is to add or modify existing plans. This means that current plans serve as guidelines in developing new plans. The need for continuous updating and integration of plans or programming is a permanent consideration in planning.

Because planning is applied to all types of activities, there are many classifications of plans. Some plans deal with small areas; some with narrow ones; some concern space; others emphasize performance, costs, quality or other major attributes.

- **Strategies**—These are general plans of action focusing on long-range goals of the facility such as accommodating future community needs and funding facility and service changes.
- **Policy**—A policy is a broad guide to thinking that starts to tell how the goals are to be reached. The distinguishing attribute of a policy is that it sets overall boundaries for activities; policies are broad, general, comprehensive and usually established by the ownership. They often express the business philosophy. Because policies are broad, they allow flexible decision making by the departments of the health care facility who, regardless of their function, must formulate department policies to help carry out those established by the ownership. Policies developed by the administrators, department heads and supervisors must be approved by the governing body. Various types of policies are:
  1. **Originated Policy**—A policy, which is originated by the ownership and follows the lines of organizational structure starting at the top of the organization and flowing downward, is called an originated policy. Occasionally, an originated policy will start at the lower levels of the organizational structure and be adopted by top management. These policies flow from the bottom to the top of the organization.
  2. **Appealed Policy**—This is a policy established to cope with an unusual or exceptional operating problem. A department head, for example, appeals to the administrator for a quick decision because of his or her inability to handle the present situation. Appealed policies are made to solve current problems on a short-term basis.
  3. **Express Policy**—An express policy is one that is recorded in an official document of the business enterprise. These would include bylaws, the constitution or operating rules and regulations. Express policies are always written or recorded.

4. **Implied Policy**—An implied policy is one that exists within an organization, but is not recorded in the business records. Implied policies are sometimes defined as customary practices. For example, a firm refuses to hire applicants over the age of 40. There is no express policy to this effect, but it is a customary practice because there are no new employees in the organization over 40 years of age. This would then be an implied policy.

5. **Internally Imposed Policy**—A policy which is established and enforced by the ownership from within the business organization itself is an internally imposed policy. Examples are bylaws and operating rules and regulations.

6. **Externally Imposed Policy**—These policies are imposed upon the enterprise by outside influences such as federal, state and local governments, and unions and civil rights groups to achieve compliance with laws and regulations. Examples include the Medicare and Medicaid laws. Labor policies may be imposed by labor laws and by the terms of a collective bargaining agreement.

7. **Written or Oral Policies**—Policies in a business organization may be oral or in writing. Policies that are orally communicated are implied policies. The more feasible way of promulgating policies is to have them in writing. The process of writing will compel top management to review and discover any discrepancies. The written policies may be used in supervisory training and orientation programs because they are recorded and provide management with a specific reference. It can be a disadvantage if these policies get into the hands of individuals who may not understand their purpose or need due to flexibility in interpretation. Also, when policies are written, management is often reluctant to change them. However, the advantages of written policies far outweigh the disadvantages.

• **Programs**—A program is a comprehensive type of plan that brings together a group of varied plans. It may include long- or short-range plans, orientational plans, operational plans, objectives, policies and procedures. It usually involves large segments of a facility summing up the means to accomplish basic goals. A major program will involve several departments or the entire facility, whereas a minor program will be effective within a department.

• **Procedures**—A procedure is a plan that provides a sequence of tasks in proper order to perform certain designated work. It points out the specific task, when it is to take place and by whom it is to be performed. Procedures are used a great deal in repetitive tasks and are more numerous and exacting at lower organizational levels. Procedures assist primarily in acting rather than in thinking. A written Standard Operating Procedure (SOP) is followed in a given situation but allows some discretion. Procedures show how to implement policies.

Procedures are prepared by supervisors, submitted to the administrator and approved by the governing body. Quite often, procedures tend to remain longer than they are useful. For this reason, it is important to review procedures on a regular basis with the view toward eliminating obsolete procedures and updating those that are necessary.

• **Methods**—A method is a plan for action. It is more limited in scope than a procedure and describes a specific course of action in showing how the work is to be done. Time and motion studies currently used by methods engineers are based upon methods analysis and work simplification principles and used to improve work output.

• **Rules**—Rules are an authoritative guide to specific action. Rules make no allowance for decision making or discretion, have no time sequence and are reinforced by some form of discipline depending on the severity of the breach. These should be developed with some input from the administrator and other employees to help make them operational and enforceable.

• **Standard**—A plan that points out norms or an expectancy used in management is a standard or a guideline. Standards include the goals, policies and plans that guide work performance and employee behavior. For an administrator to evaluate performance, a reference point or a norm must be available so that a meaningful comparison can be made between what is accomplished and what is expected. However, a standard should not represent perfection. Standards are vital to that function of management termed controlling.

## Organizing

Organizing is a basic function of management. Organizing assembles and arranges all the required resources to achieve an objective. The work of the administrator relative to organizing is the breakdown of work in operative duties defining position requirements, delegation of authority and provision of facilities and personnel. The goal of organizing is to assist people in working together to carry out the plans and meet the business goals effectively and without friction. An administrator must know which activities to manage, who provides help, the channels of communication, the relationships among individual employees and the general makeup of a work group.

Organizing becomes necessary when the work to be done is too much for one person to handle. There must be a coordination of efforts to accomplish the defined work and to provide work satisfaction. The administrator strives for **synergism**, which is the simultaneous action of separate but related parts to produce a sum greater than its separate components. The term organizing comes from the word *organism*, which means to create a structure with the parts so integrated that their relation to each other is governed by their relationship to the whole. Organizing consists of parts (the grouping of each activity) and relationships (the activities in the facility to accomplish its necessary objectives). Thus, it involves determination and assignment of duties to employees and the establishment and maintenance of authority relationships. It is a structural framework in which individual efforts are coordinated, and it takes place at all levels of management.

### *Department Functions*

In a typical nursing facility, activities are grouped into separate departments or work units of assigned activities. The departments vary according to the size of the institution, but the functions of the nursing facility regarding its organization remain the same. There are three main divisions of functions:

1. **Professional Care of the Resident**—Under the category of resident care, functions include the nursing department, health records, dietary department, admissions and discharge, pharmacy, medical services, occupational therapy and physical therapy.

2. **Supporting or Paramedical Services**—These services support the professional and resident care departments and serve the entire nursing facility. They include the business office (accounting, bookkeeping, accounts receivable, accounts payable, payroll, switch board, information office and general clerical staff), the procurement or purchasing department and the personnel department. Volunteer services, public relations department and social and rehabilitative services are included in some of the larger institutions.

3. **Upkeep and Maintenance**—The materials management division include the housekeeping department, the maintenance department and linen department.

Each department has a department head responsible for the performance of the department, and authority relationships are well-defined. This process is called departmentalization. Within the department, the department head finds the right person to place in a specific job. This process (termed staffing) involves recruiting and selecting the proper employees and subsequently the training, analysis of work performance, discipline and promotion of these employees.

### *Theories of Organizing*

There are several theories that are meaningful and offer helpful knowledge about organizing. Some of the more important are:

- The **systems theory** views organizing as a system of mutually dependent variables that include the individual, the formal arrangement of functions, the informal arrangement of functions, the behavioral patterns of the employees, and the physical environment. This theory considers all of these factors existing within the system—reacting and shaping the environment as a unit. The manager must keep these variables moving together toward the business goal.

- In the **quantitative theory**, measurable factors that affect organizing are related and processes so as to derive the best organization. Two of the factors measured are the number of decisions made by the administrator and the span of management or number of employees reporting to the administrator. This theory strives to increase preciseness.

- The **fusion theory** points out that a person uses an organization to achieve his or her own goals, and in turn the organization uses the individual to pursue its goals. By a personalization process, the individual seeks freedom of decision and optimum performance; by a socializing process, the organization requests completion of work assignments and gives rewards and penalties. The personalizing and socializing processes are fused by means of organizing.

- The **neoclassical theory** emphasizes work accomplishment. Maximum work achievement is sought through maintaining a balanced arrangement of functions necessary to the business. Division of labor is followed, and jobs are defined. This theory also recognizes the impact of human relations on the structure and considers environment and social values that are woven into an overall pattern of interdependency of these values on the organization.

### Tangible Parts of Organizing

Four tangible parts of organizing exist:

- **Employees**—Each person is assigned a specific portion of the total work. The assignment takes into consideration the employee's interest, experience, skill and behavior. The assignment may consist of a part of the work of an organizational work unit or all the work of that unit.

- **Work**—The functions to be performed come from the stated objectives. The functions form the essential work of the department. In a nursing facility, clusters of similar work are grouped together and formed into departments such as nursing, dietary, business office, management and maintenance.

- **Environment**—The physical means and the general climate within which the employees are to perform their work is called the work environment. The nurses station, location of nursing units and desks, general morale and attitudes all make up the nursing facility environment.

- **Relationships**—This involves the relationship of an employee to his or her work, the interaction of one employee with another and the interaction of one work unit or department to another within the organizational structure. Interdepartmental relationships are very important to the smooth function of a facility.

### Organizational Structure

An organizational structure shows the flow of interactions within a facility. The interaction pattern is set by the work, and the employee is assigned to it. Two forms of behavior are considered within the organizational structure:

- **Formal** behavior results from using prescribed communication channels, standard methods for performing tasks, work-oriented attitudes, clearly defined jobs and stated lines of command among employee work units. Quite often desirable social conduct is spelled out, and the employees are encouraged to conform with accepted norms of behavior to develop a sense of duty. Pay increases and promotions depend on such conformity.

- **Informal** behavior is neither prescribed nor included in the formal organizational structure. The fact that it is not a part of a formal organization does not mean that it is undesirable. Informal behavior may be advantageous. Some of the influences leading to informal behavior are cultural likes and dislikes, individual values and socializing on the job.

### Organizational Chart

An organizational chart is drawn to help visualize the formal organization that has been approved by the governing body. This chart shows what activities are performed by whom, the work grouping of the activities and their relationships to each other. Chart lines joining the organization's work-employee units indicate the formal flow of communication and decision making.

Most organizational charts place those with the greatest decision making at the top of the chart and those with the least at the bottom. A solid line indicates a line authority decision-making position; a broken line indicates staff authority. Figure 3–5 shows an example of a typical nursing facility organizational chart.

Within the organizational chart, different types of authority relationships exist. A discussion of authority and its relationships follows.

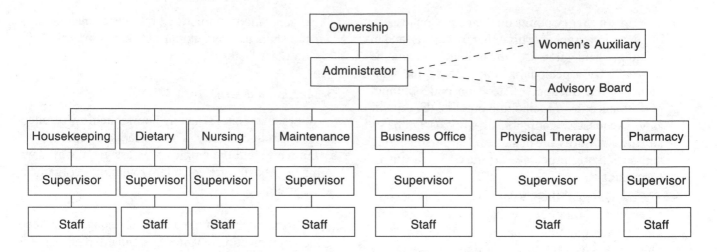

**Figure 3–5** Organizational Chart

*Line Authority.* Line authority (or the scalar chain) is a relationship in which the supervisor exercises direct command over one or several subordinates. A person with line authority has charge of and is responsible for the work of his or her department and its contribution toward the goals of the facility. Line authority is sometimes referred to as direct operative authority. Under this arrangement, decision making is expedited because each member of the management team has authority over a complete department and need only consult his or her immediate supervisor when necessary.

Such a relationship is characterized by vertical growth showing a superior-subordinate relationship where the superior delegates authority to the subordinate who in turn delegates authority to another subordinate and so on, forming a vertical line from top to bottom. Thus, the line formed gives rise to the term vertical line authority: each member in the organization knows from whom orders are received and to whom one reports. Figure 3–6 shows an example of vertical line organization.

A straight-line authority organization is where a facility uses a pattern of employing only individuals who have line authority. There are no advisory or staff specialists in a line organization. Each department head in the facility is concerned directly with his or her own department. For example, in the dietary department, the chief dietitian is responsible for hiring, firing, scheduling of work, planning of work, promoting and reprimanding. The straight-line organizational structure is commonly used in nursing facilities with fewer than 100 beds.

Some advantages of this type of organization are quick decision making, elimination of buck passing, understandable work authority relationships, and simplification of discipline problems. Some disadvantages are: the facility tends to rely too heavily on the administrator, the growth of the facility may place too much burden on top executives, and no place is made for specialists or advisers. See Figure 3–7 for an example of straight-line authority.

*Centralized Authority.* The centralized concept of authority means the concentration of authority in one individual or in one department. Under this theory, the autocratic technique of directing is used primarily. All department heads in the facility report directly to the administrator, who makes all the major decisions, and there are no staff department in the organization. Essentially very little delegation of authority is made to department heads.

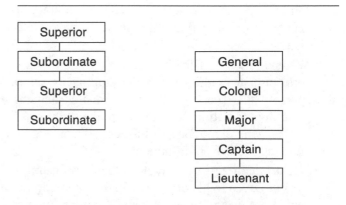

**Figure 3–6** Vertical Line Organization

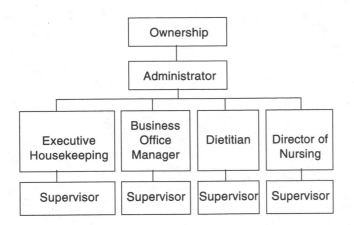

**Figure 3–7** Straight-Line Authority Organization

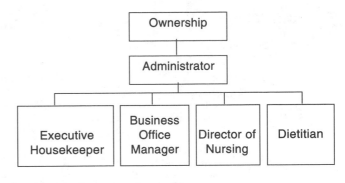

**Figure 3–8** Centralized Authority Structure

Advocates of centralized authority list the following advantages: duplication of functions is avoided, uniform policies and practices are promoted, and prestige and full utilization of the administration is won. Figure 3–8 shows an example of a centralized authority structure.

*Staff Authority.* In addition to the line authority relationship, the modern nursing facility uses the concept of staff authority. The word staff historically means a stick carried in the hand for support. Hence, staff authority supports or assists line authority. It is the function of staff authority personnel to advise, counsel, guide and assist the persons in line authority positions. A staff authority person does not make management decisions for the organization. Within a specific department in the nursing facility, the department head is the line authority figure who participates in the decision making and retains the decision-making authority whether or not the organizational structure is straight-line or line-staff.

A staff authority relationship is always designated on the organizational chart as a broken line. In most nursing facilities, the personnel department is a good example of staff authority. The function of this department is to provide advice to all department heads. The personnel manager has expertise, and the department will be involved in recruiting and screening job applicants and administering the wage and salary program.

A staff authority relationship is like the relationship between a general practitioner and a consultant. The general practitioner may use the services of a specialist in cardiology, hematology or radiology, but the control and legal responsibility for the resident ultimately rests with the general practitioner. The advice of the consultant may be accepted or rejected.

Quite often, friction exists between line and staff authority persons. This may be because the concept of line and staff authority is not clear; the administrator should explain the function of each clearly to the employees. A good staff authority employee is a person who is satisfied to work behind the scenes giving advice to the department heads, needs not be in the limelight and is not too sensitive to complaints or rejection. It is important for the administrator and department heads to have open lines of communication with staff authority personnel. Department heads should be encouraged to use staff authority personnel.

*Decentralized Authority.* The decentralized concept of authority means disbursing the authority throughout the organization to key department heads and supervisors. Under this theory, the consultive and free rein techniques of directing are used extensively. Department heads throughout the facility are delegated authority to help manage the facility. A great deal of input is received from department heads and employees under this system.

Advocates of decentralized authority list the following advantages: effective human relations are encouraged, greater opportunity to develop and to manage is provided, teamwork and self-sustaining organization are promoted, and risk of losses of personnel and facilities are spread out. Figure 3–9 depicts a decentralized authority structure.

*Functional Authority.* Functional authority is a relationship where one person, usually a specialist, has control over a specific function and supervises all personnel working in that area of specialty. This specialist can advise how the task is to be done but cannot

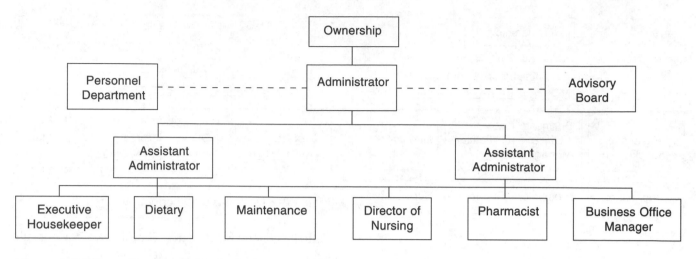

**Figure 3–9** Decentralized Authority Structure

correct errors or discipline. The personnel director in a nursing facility would have this type of relationship where he or she has line authority within departmental boundaries, although the entire department acts in a staff capacity in relationship to other departments in the facility; he or she reports to and is supervised by higher management levels. Consultants often have functional authority and report directly to the administrator. Functional authority requires assignment to well-defined work areas to avoid overlapping authority and dividing responsibility. It is conceivable that several lines of authority could be placed over one worker leading to several bosses and confusion of responsibility.

### Directing

Directing is the integration by communication of the efforts of all employees so that by accomplishing their assigned tasks, they will meet the individual and group objectives. It includes ordering, teaching, supervising, guiding and coordinating. While planning, organizing and staffing are preparatory managerial functions, directing is the managerial function that starts the organized action and is performed by all managers at all levels within the organizational structure. A technical definition of directing is to issue directives to get a job done. It involves explaining of objectives, guiding subordinates, developing employees to their full capacity, using praise and reprimands, and providing recognition by monetary and non-monetary rewards for outstanding performance.

An important tool of directing is the order. This can stop, start or modify an activity. It is used at all levels of management. An order is given in the nature of a command requiring a subordinate to act in a certain manner in a given circumstance. An order is not given by a subordinate to the supervisor; it follows the chain of command and organizational structure. Characteristically, a good order must be:

1. Reasonable so that compliance can be expected.
2. Compatible with the objectives of the organization and the subordinate's job duties.
3. Intelligible to the subordinate. It must be stated clearly, simply and precisely.
4. Conveyed in an objective and business-like manner.

### *Techniques of Directing*

Three major techniques or styles of directing are discussed below.

*Autocratic (or dictatorial).* This approach is also referred to as management by edict or fiat. The manager or administrator using this approach gives direct, clear and concise orders to subordinates. He or she explicitly gives instructions as to what is to be done, and how the work is to be accomplished. The executive who uses this method of directing exclusively believes that employees are paid to follow orders and not to exercise independent thinking. The focus is on task not human relations.

The advantages of the autocratic approach are: quick decision making, firm guidance to subordinates, and use in chaotic situations to bring order.

Some disadvantages include: does not give the subordinate an opportunity to participate in management decisions, kills initiative, and does not help develop management skills of the employee.

*Consultive (or democratic).* The administrator consults with his or her department heads or subordinates and receives input from them regarding the problem or decision to be made. The executive will consider the input, but retains decision-making authority, issuing a directive or making the final decision. The individual or group consulted does not have decision-making authority. The consultative technique of directing is a powerful management tool. It emphasizes the human relations aspect of management. An executive who uses this technique should be genuinely interested in the viewpoints of the employees. This approach does not weaken the executive's formal authority position because the final decision making rests with the administrator. When using consultive directing, a free interchange of ideas and discussion of alternative solutions should be used.

Some of the factors to consider in using the consultative approach are:

1. Consultative directing is time-consuming. If the problem is one that must have an immediate solution, consultative directing may not be feasible.
2. Subordinates' capacity and willingness to offer ideas is recognized. If the department head or supervisor is not willing or capable of recommending ideas to solve the problem, there is no need to receive input.
3. Not all department heads are going to be interested in all specific or specialized problems.
4. Directive conflicts with the interest of the employee may result. For example, a decision to close down a nursing unit may be in conflict with the jobs of the nurses working on that unit.

The advantages of the consultative approach are:

1. A directive issued as a result of consultation may not blatantly appear as an order but more as a solution in which the subordinate participated.

2. Normally, the morale of the employee is better if the individual is asked to participate in decision making.
3. Consultation gives management personnel an opportunity to use their management skills and communicate their ideas.
4. Communication is improved. The executive and the subordinate understand each other more clearly.

The disadvantages of the consultative approach are:

1. It may give the subordinate the notion that the executive cannot make a decision.
2. It may lead to confusion if the solution is not summarized by the executive.
3. The subordinate may feel he or she has a right to be consulted in all operative decisions if this approach is used exclusively.

### Free Rein (or laissez-faire)

The administrator or executive encourages the subordinate to use initiative and ideas to solve a problem. The executive assigns a task, outlines the problem and requests that the subordinate find the solution. In using this technique, the executive must delegate authority and decision making to the subordinate. The final decision is made by the subordinate, not the executive. The executive may be available for assistance, but the final decision rests with the subordinate.

This technique is used in those situations in which the subordinate has specialized knowledge or skill that the executive does not have. A typical situation in a nursing facility using this technique is when an administrator seeks a solution to a medical problem from a physician. Although some say that 80% to 85% of employees work effectively under this technique, it should not be used unless the executive feels he or she is working with a subordinate who has the ability and the willingness to handle the problem. This technique can cause many problems for an administrator if used indiscriminately.

A skilled administrator of a health care facility will not use any of these techniques exclusively. Depending upon the situation and employees, they may be used independently or simultaneously. A combined use of these techniques appears to be the most feasible.

## Controlling

An administrator wants to get stated or planned results. In order to do this one must use the management tool of controlling. Controlling is the process of evaluating performance against initial objectives and, if necessary, taking corrective action to assure the attainment of planned goals. Controlling is like a checkup to make sure what is done is what is intended. It is objective oriented. It is a means to an end and is designed to get the employees to do what must be done to accomplish the goals of the facility. Controlling is practiced at all levels of management by all managers. There are three basic steps in controlling: setting the standard, checking on performance, and taking corrective action. These steps must be followed in sequential order.

### Setting the Standard

Standards are criteria against which results are judged. The overall goals of a nursing facility are broken down into various objectives for each department, and within these departments, these objectives are further broken down into such areas as quality, schedules or budgets.

In setting standards, the department head usually has working knowledge of how much time it takes to perform a particular task, how much material is required and what constitutes a conforming or nonconforming job. Policies, procedures and rules are established, and the staff is oriented to them. Goals that are verifiable by qualitative or quantitative terms are considered the best standards. In hospitals and the nursing facilities, methods analysts assist in setting acceptable standards. The specialized area of work simplification uses such techniques as work distribution charts, motion and analysis, and flow process charts.

Standards may be tangible or intangible. A **tangible** standard is one that is capable of being objectively measured. For example, the standard of a clean resident room is capable of objective evaluation. On the other hand, some **intangible** standards found in a nursing facility are reputation in the community, high morale among employees and high quality resident care. With so many subjective evaluations involved in these standards, they are difficult to measure precisely.

### Checking on Performance

The second step in controlling is to check on performance. After standards have been established, the su-

pervisor compares actual performance with the standard. Several means for the determination of performance are observation, reports and statistical data.

Observation means directly looking at the work done. Direct observation provides an intimate picture of the performance. For example, an inspection of resident room is a good way for the executive housekeeper to check on the quality of cleaning in the rooms. Direct observation may be used to evaluate both quality and quantity of work, methods involved and general work environment. However, because of the time-consuming aspect of direct observation, the administrator or department head may find it impractical to make personal observations of all his or her subordinates' work.

The more removed a supervisor is from the actual work site, the more reports will have to be relied upon. Reports are of two types: written and oral. A report should be brief, clear and complete.

- **Oral reports** may be a face-to-face communication on an individual or group basis. In a nursing facility where the nursing department is operational 24 hours a day, the process of reporting becomes very vital to its operation. After each eight-hour shift, it is customary practice for nurses to report to the oncoming shift the status of each resident. The use of monthly department head meetings, individual conferences with department heads and supervisors, and training and orientation sessions are all considered oral reports.

  An oral report is satisfactory for situations having very wide coverage or where opportunity for questions is needed to clear up any misunderstanding or to secure additional information. In oral reporting, the administrator or executive should pay special attention to significant deviations from established standards.

- **Written reports** are those that are recorded in some manner. They may be descriptive or contain statistical information and are best when comprehensive detailed information needs to be conveyed. A permanent record of the reports is kept in the event they are needed later. The format of a written report should be designed so that it is easy to read. Some commonly used written reports used in a nursing facility are those prepared by the administrator and presented to the ownership at a board meeting, reports of various advisory and operational committees, accident reports, budgetary and other statistical reports, and the many reports required from federal, state, county and city officials in the daily operation of the facility. Written reports should be reviewed periodically to establish the continued need for them.

### *Taking Corrective Action*

The third step in controlling is taking corrective action. When a difference is found between the established standard and the performance, judgment is needed to assess the significance of the differential. In some cases, a slight deviation may be serious; in others, it is not. The comparison between standard and performance should be made as near to the time of performance as possible. Special attention should be given to those comparisons showing deviations greater than normal expectancy. An administrator concentrates his or her controlling efforts on these situations.

Taking corrective action also consists of seeing to it that the operations are adjusted to get results consistent with the standards or objective in a particular department. Modifications in any one or all of the managerial activities may be required. Sometimes a method must be changed, a goal clarified or altered, an authority line of communication cleared up, or better motivation scheduled. An analysis of the reasons for significant deviation is especially important. It is advisable to hold the department head responsible for implementing any required corrective actions that must take place within the department.

In dealing with correcting an employee's behavior, several guidelines are recommended to help prevent defensiveness and misunderstandings:

1. Bring the first error to the employee's attention as soon as possible and in private.
2. Deal with the issue and not the personality; be specific and factual concerning the error.
3. Be business-like; listen to the employee's response— focusing on the issue and ensuring mutual understanding of the expectations of performance.

Program Evaluation and Review Technique (PERT) is a planning and control technique used to monitor how the parts of a program fit together in event and time. A flowchart is developed, indicating an event or goal and a plan with a target completion date. This forces all levels of management to plan on the event for which they are responsible and to concentrate on crucial activities needing correction, allowing for any necessary action at the right time and place. This technique is limited when routine recurring events are planned without an existing responsible estimated time schedule. PERT is time-oriented and requires specific training for use in nursing facility management.

## MANAGEMENT SKILLS

Management is an integrated system where the previously mentioned functions will overlap and enforce each other. An administrator needs to develop other skills in order to achieve a well-run organization.

### Coordination and Cooperation

All the functions of management in one way or another use the concept of coordination. The administrator must have department heads and supervisors coordinate their efforts of planning, organizing, directing and controlling so that the objectives and goals of the nursing facility will be accomplished.

**Coordination** is the orderly synchronization of the varying interests and efforts of workers leading to the stated objective. It is not a separate function but a process by which the manager gets unity of action toward the accomplishment of a goal. Coordination is more difficult at the higher levels of management because more levels of supervisors exist where activities must be coordinated. The manager must reconcile different approaches, efforts, interests and goals to bring them into common action toward the organizational purpose. It is an exercise in futility to order an employee to coordinate. Coordination is a byproduct coming into existence as a result of actions and special efforts.

**Cooperation** is the collective action of individuals in pursuing the objective. It indicates the willingness of an individual or employee to help out.

For example, consider the efforts of a football team. Obviously the players on the team are willing and eager to cooperate with each other; they want to win the football game and they are aware of their common purpose. At this point in time, they are cooperating. Next the proper signal is given and the play starts. The ball is passed from the center, and at that split second each man carries out his preplanned role during the play—one man blocks, another feints to the left, and another runs and stops to the right. The quarterback hurls a successful pass to the end, and a touchdown is scored. This is coordination. Each effort had to have a proper act, the exact timing and synchronization so that the team could score a touchdown.

## Leadership

Organizations exist that create positions and roles for managers. Leadership, although similar to management, involves the creation of a willingness in people to follow those whom they believe will provide the means of achieving their own personal goals. The leader must have a fundamental understanding of people, their motivations and their needs; he or she must be able to create and administer ways to satisfy these needs and to get the desired response to achieve the business purpose and goals. The management theories discussed earlier involve management and leadership.

Leadership skills have been found to involve a minimum of four major ingredients: the authority of the leader, understanding that an individual's motivation will vary with different situations, ability to develop motivation and style of the leader.

## Decision Making

The ability to make sound decisions is one of the most important qualities of an effective administrator. Decision making is at the base of planning. To achieve the goals and objectives of the facility, the administrator must continuously decide what actions are necessary and how they can be carried out.

Decision making takes place at all levels of management in every department of the facility. It is the rational selection of an alternative from two or more choices to determine the most desirable course of action and involves thought, feeling and knowledge. The decision maker also is dealing with future values; therefore, a certain amount of uncertainty is present. Although decisions quite often include just two alternatives (yes or no), for each the possible outcome is predicted and evaluated. The decision also is influenced by one's values and subsequent conflicts in values. The resolution of the conflicts is sought because decision making means coming to a conclusion.

### Factors Involved in Decision Making

The basis for making viable decisions and evaluating alternatives are plentiful. The factors usually relate to the administrator's background and knowledge. The following are considered important.

*Subjective Factors.* These are factors relating to the makeup of the decision maker.

- **Intelligence**—Intelligence of the decision maker is important but is often overrated. Generally speaking, those individuals with higher intelligence will produce more meaningful decisions if the problem is so complex that intellectual resources are necessary. Poor decisions are not caused by a lack of intelligence alone, but by other factors that interfere with the proper use of intelligence. Individuals who have a high IQ may still make poor decisions because they lack practical judgment or "common sense," which is often quite uncommon.
- **Self-Confidence**—Self-confidence of the decision maker is directly related to effective decision making. When a manager or supervisor makes a decision, he or she is taking a risk. Very seldom are the alternatives black or white. Even after the accumulation of evidence and the weighing of alternatives, a wrong decision could still be made. A manager must be willing to take that chance. To decide is to act and to act requires courage as well as judgment. To be an effective decision maker, the administrator or executive must have the confidence to fail.
- **Intuition**—Some decision makers act on impulse or intuition: The decision is based upon an inner feeling of the decider. It may be a sixth sense or an unexplainable insight into a certain state of affairs. Normally the impulse decision maker does not take the time to gather facts. He or she is characterized by been quick tempered, loose tongued and lacking self-control. This process of decision making is highly irrational and follows no set pattern. Intuition is most likely present to some degree in most decision making. It does not always give satisfactory results, but it quickly supplies a decision.

- **Psychological Values**—Many problems an administrator must decide are not economic or measurable. Decisions concerning the size of a department head's office, personal satisfaction of one's ego, adherence to an established set of traditions or a desire to become big in itself are some psychological values that may be determinative in a decision.

- **Experience**—The experience of the decision maker directly affects the decisions made. Intimacy with and the understanding of problems requires experience. Experience supplies guidelines, and helps to separate the important from the unimportant and to take advantage of past situations. Some management theorists maintain that reliance upon experience may be an important factor in decision making but should not be used exclusively.

*Objective Factors.* Objective factors are those factors that may be used by executives that are not directly related to the makeup or personality of the decision maker. They may be used by a variety of manager "types."

- **Use of Facts and Statistics**—Research and the fact gathering is indispensable in making an effective decision. Studies, research papers, market analyses, study of legislation in the long-term care field, and statistics from similar-sized facilities on rates, incomes, expenses and attitudes are all related to decision making. The administrator or executive must be familiar with the professional literature, methods and procedures, and motivations and needs of employees.

- **Experimentation**—Trying out the alternative and seeing what happens is one method used in decision making. This is a common technique used in scientific inquiry. Experimentation is expensive and is based upon the assumption that the future will duplicate the past.

- **Analysis**—What decision to make can be aided by breaking down a problem into its component parts and then studying each part in relation to the whole. By critical analysis, the way decision-making causal relationships affect the objectives are identified. This approach narrows the essential facts to the most important specifics.

*Effective Timing.* The timing of a decision may be a critical factor in its success or failure. On occasion, immediate decisions are necessary. Emergency staffing, disciplining an employee and immediate need for certain supplies are examples of such decisions. At other times, making a quick decision is to lose the advantage of valuable information. There are even times when the best decision is not to make any now. It is imperative that the time factor be considered in making decisions. Set target dates for deciding important issues and conform to those times. Do not put off decisions unless a tangible reason exists to do so. Probably one of the biggest complaints that employees have about their supervisors is that they put off making decisions.

*Intangible Factors.* Some of the intangible factors an administrator must contend with are changing rules and regulations of the state health and social service agencies, changes in Medicare and Medicaid, quality of care, employee morale. These are normally quite difficult to evaluate. They must be recognized, ranked in terms of their importance and compared with respect to their probable effect upon the ultimate results.

*Tangible Factors.* These include such factors as net income over expenses, man hours, utilization of equipment, per diem costs and other quantitative data. These factors are interrelated. Proper use of expensive equipment, realistic staffing and cost containment all contribute to the profit factor. When many tangible factors and a few intangible factors are available, the selection of an alternative is relatively simple.

*Steps in Decision Making.* Generally, the steps in making a decision will include:

1. Determining the basic problem behind any symptoms, identifying causes, collecting related facts and figures.
2. Identifying alternative and possible solutions.
3. Evaluating each alternative in terms of the goal sought.
4. Choosing the alternative or making the decision. (Determine how this will be implemented and monitored for effectiveness.)

Decisions may be made on an individual or group basis:

- **Individual decision making** is common when the decision to be made is simple and all of the alternatives are easily understood. Emergency decisions often are made on an individual basis. Whether or not to defer to an emergency decision is determined by the consequence of not deciding.
- The most common mechanism for making group decisions is through a committee. By using the process of **group decision making**, those who will be affected will be given the opportunity to participate in the decision. It also makes it possible to include judgment of specialists and technicians who have specialized knowledge concerning the issues being decided. The contribution of individuals in the group will vary; some will say very little and others will speak a great deal.

In the last analysis, decision making is essentially a lonesome task. Even when using the committee, the final action must be taken by the individual decision maker.

## Communication

A major skill required of the administrator of a health care facility is the ability to communicate effectively. Gaining the acceptance of policies, seeing that instructions are understood and improving performance all depend upon effective communicating. The administrator who is unable to get his or her department heads and supervisors to understand what is wanted will not succeed in getting them to do it. Therefore, all the functions of management are facilitated by communication, management is not communication alone, but an essential part of it.

Such a thing exists as an illusion of communication. This happens when an executive believes that mutual understanding has taken place because one person has spoken to another or because what was written by one has been read by another. What is expressed is not always what is understood.

It has been estimated that 90% of an administrator's or an executive's time is expended in sending or receiving information. Communication is the process of passing on information from one person or group to another with mutual understanding ensured through feedback. All communication is two way—when one speaks, the other listens; when one writes, the other reads. The speaking and the listening or the writing and the reading are essentially ingredients of communication. Exchange of ideas opens the way for effectively transmitting information and gaining understanding.

### Types of Communication

Communication is classified in the following manner:

*Downward Communication.* This is when communication flows from the top to the bottom managerial levels of a facility. Downward communication is most frequently used in a nursing facility. It helps to coordinate the different departments and the levels of management. It is used to communicate to subordinates orders, instructions and memos, as well as objectives, policies and procedures. It follows the organizational structure.

*Upward Communication.* This communication flows from subordinates to supervisors. This form of communication may or may not follow the organizational structure and chain of command. It is used to communicate suggestions, grievances and reports to management.

*Formal Communication.* Formal communication is established by the organizational structure following the chain of command and lines of authority. This generally takes the form of specific orders. Examples of formal communications are monthly department head meetings, monthly meetings with the board of directors, telephone conferences, posters and direct mailings to employees.

*Informal Communication.* This communication exists because of personal and group interests of people. Unofficial or informal lines of communication exist, called the grapevine. Personnel on all levels want to be "in the know." The grapevine is said to be direct, fast and flexible. It is based on hearsay and rumor and is in most cases inaccurate. Even though it does not have access to official information sources, the believability of the information by the employees is high. The grapevine is used by personnel to vent their anxieties and apprehension about their job situations. It can create an informal organization where a key group of people communicate without the administrator and can have influence on line decision making. An administrator and executive should acknowledge the existence of the grapevine and try to use it to their advantage.

*Oral Communication.* Oral communication represents all types of nonwritten communication. It may take the form of speaking or gestures. It is imperative that an administrator or executive is capable of clearly expressing himself or herself when speaking. Oral communication is said to be one of the most effective means of communicating. It is usually face to face and provides opportunity for immediate reaction or feedback. It can be changed immediately if not understood.

It has been said that actions speak louder than words and will color communication. Many books of popular interest have been written on nonverbal communication. Gestures include actions of the body, a facial expression or the way one uses his or her hands, arms or legs. Thus slamming of an office door by the administrator needs no verbal explanation to inform the employee or bystander of the frame of mind of the administrator.

Department head, supervisory and staff meetings have been commonplace as formal ways to use oral communication. Encouraging group participation, the popularity of participative management and keeping employees informed are some reasons why formal meetings are popular. To be of greatest value, a meeting should be:

1. **Planned**—Each member attending should be given the purpose, program and time.
2. **Specific**—Discussion and presentation should be kept relative to the issues.
3. **Illustrated visually**—Illustrations should be used especially if complicated concepts are involved or statistics are used.
4. **Recorded**—This should supply a record of what was covered and decided.

*Written Communications.* All communications that are reduced to writing are said to be written communications. The ability to write clearly is mandatory for an executive who wants to effectively communicate. Written communications may take the form of reports, memos or letters. Written communications should be complete, clear, concise and correct.

### Roadblocks or Barriers to Communication

Many roadblocks to communication can arise that administrators must be aware of in order to develop better communication skills. Some are as follows:

- **Individual Differences**—Employees are individuals who have a singular personality of their own. The way a communication is interpreted very often will depend upon the background, cultural and social status, and the experience of the receiver. Because human personality and behavior is so personal, the message attempted to be communicated must take into consideration those differences.

- **Language Barriers**—If employees are from a different country or even from different parts of the United States, a real language barrier may occur. This is especially true with minority groups who are employed in routine, custodial and maintenance jobs. Background will influence the receiver's interpretation of the information.

- **Defensiveness**—When an employee receives a message from the supervisor, several reactions occur. There is an evaluation of the message in relationship to the background and education of the receiver. A subordinate is eager to appear favorable in the eyes of the supervisor and, therefore, any feedback he or she may give would tend to be what he or she feels the boss wants to hear.

- **Resistance to Change**—Most employees prefer the status quo and do not welcome change with open arms. Any communication that tends to upset the status quo, therefore, is greeted with suspicion, and the receiver's mind becomes like a filter, rejecting new ideas if they conflict with the present manner of doing things. Changes are perceived as threats to the status, ego and self-image of the employee.

- **Lack of Feedback**—One of the most common roadblocks to effective communication is lack of feedback or failure to follow up if a communication problem exists. Oral face-to-face communication is highly desirable because the sender gets an immediate feedback or reaction from the receiver and can act accordingly. Written communications, however, do not have the same feedback. If an employee or receiver of a written communication does not understand it, there is no way that this message is brought to the attention of the sender unless the receiver makes a special effort to do so, or unless the sender follows through and seeks feedback or reaction to the message.

- **Distractions**—Nothing is more disturbing than to listen to oral communication and be distracted by a variety of noises, sounds and activities. A distraction may be: the physical setup of a room, a color scheme, lack of a public address system, or the arrangement of chairs and tables in the meeting room. A distraction also may be in timing. Certainly a communication should not be given if waiters and waitresses are busy picking up dishes, silverware or trays.

- **Ineffective listening**—The definition of communicating includes the understanding of a message that is being related. To be physically in a room while a speech is being delivered does not guarantee that the message is getting across. Some people can be physically present in a room, but their minds are wandering. In order to get the most out of an oral communication, individuals must listen attentively to what is being said.
- **Poor Retention**—Depending on a variety of the previously mentioned and other factors, individuals retain only a part of the information given to them and must be reminded at regular intervals.

### 10 Commandments of Communication

Consideration of the following 10 commandments of communication will help improve effectiveness in conveying information.

1. **Seek to clarify ideas before communicating**. The information to be sent to the receiver and the problems to be resolved must be carefully organized. The sender must have a resource of information to answer unexpected questions or expand on any associated or relevant topics.
2. **Use direct and simple language.** One of the most common barriers to effective communication is the use of technical, complicated and garbled language. Whether the communication is verbal or written, it is necessary to use as simple language as possible to relay the idea to be communicated. Don't beat around the bush; make sure the message is clear and direct.
3. **Do not confuse by over- or undercommunication**. One of the greatest challenges in communication is to avoid talking or writing too little or too much. Giving too much information is very common. It results from too great an eagerness to fully use available resource material and communication channels. Some employees cannot digest a mountain of communication, particularly if it is not essential to their work. The other extreme is the failure to give enough information to perform the work or achieve desired results. This also can be devastating. To avoid both extremes and communicate adequately, the sender must be sensitive to feedback and use past experience as a guide.
4. **Make sure the information communicated is meaningful to the receiver**. Under ideal conditions, the information communicated is what the receiver wants to know and what the sender believes the receiver should now. Employees like to be informed about promotion possibilities, working conditions, facility policies, employee benefits and the general condition of the facility.
5. **Realize that communication may be altered in transmission**. Change in communication may take place as it is interpreted by each in a line of receivers. The change may be either favorable or unfavorable. Most people dislike passing on facts about unfavorable results and tend to sweeten the communication; this happens more often in upward communication where an employee reports to a supervisor.
6. **Use proper symbols, gestures and visual materials**. All communication employs symbols to represent persons or things. Symbols may include signs, colors, words, gestures and characters. They stand for something meaningful. The use of appropriate pictures, charts or diagrams help the human mind to comprehend complex material that may be confusing if described by words alone.
7. **Seek not only to be understood, but to understand**. Very often the sender is so involved with the information that he or she is trying to communicate, the receiver does not get the message. Don't automatically shut off conflicting positions on the issue being presented; give the receiver an opportunity to relate to the sender's stand. The sender should try to understand the feelings and attitudes of the receiver.
8. **Follow-up communication; seek feedback**. One of the most valuable ways to determine if face-to-face oral communication is effectively communicated is to seek immediate feedback. Give the audience an opportunity to ask questions or make comments or suggestions. By the same token, if a memo or written communication is conveyed to

employees, give them the opportunity to comment or make suggestions (constructive or otherwise) about the communication. Too often administrators assume their communication is crystal clear and do not seek any feedback. This can be disastrous if the communication is not written clearly or is ambiguous in its intent.

9. **Be sure actions support the communication**. Administrators or executives have many opportunities to back up words by appropriate action. It is important when communicating certain ideas that actions are fitting or consistent with the materials presented. Imagine the reaction of employees if—when attempting to convey the importance of tidiness, cleanliness and orderliness—the speaker appears disorganized, disheveled and dirty at the meeting. Sometimes actions do speak louder than words.

10. **Be consistent, redundant and responsive**. As a communicator, it is necessary to present information to employees in a consistent manner. A good communicator will repeat the message several times during the communication by using different words or symbols to emphasize important points in the material. An effective executive also will be responsive to the feelings, attitudes and expectations of the employees being addressed.

### Managing Conflict

The administrator is constantly faced with conflict in the daily operation of a nursing facility; thus, conflict resolution becomes important. These conflicts often may occur between employees or department heads in the facility and within professional organizations. When a person or thing does not measure up to expectations of another person or plan, a conflict results.

It does not make sense to deny the existence of conflict in an organization. Acknowledgment of the existence of a conflict is the first step in approaching conflict resolution and creating a positive feeling that is proactive rather than reactive. In the multifaceted relationships within a nursing facility, three basic approaches to consider in conflict resolution are:

1. **Lose-Lose**—Both parties in a conflict lose as a result of the final resolution. This takes place when a compromise is reached between the par-

ties but neither party is satisfied. This is not an effective way of conflict resolution.

2. **Win-Lose**—One of the parties appears to win, and the other party appears to lose. This occurs when a disagreement between parties is resolved by a third party to the benefit of one and to the detriment of the other.

3. **Win-Win**—When this strategy is correctly applied, each party in the conflict agrees that the best solution has been reached. This is the preferred strategy to use as neither party is a winner nor a loser.

### COMPUTER INFORMATION COLLECTION PROCEDURES

A managed information system is an organized method for providing past, present and projected information relating to internal operation of the facility. It is a means of organizing the large quantities of information so that the information is usable. It is believed that complex care management and documentation are better managed under a uniform computerized system where the information and records are reproducible and easy to update.

With the introduction of computers in the business world, the modern nursing facility administrator is using them to provide easily accessible information for decision making by both the administrator and department heads. The growth of managed and subacute care has brought increasing complexity to the delivery of quality care and requires the ability to track individualized patient needs, medical outcomes and cost analysis. Information in such areas as accounting (payroll, billing), personnel, census records, survey findings, resident assessment (MDS, care plans, RAI), medicinal (pharmacy) and dietary needs to be readily stored and accessible. To deliver these services and maintain costs effectively, analyses pairing the outcomes of treatment from admissions to discharge and the value, time and cost of services needs to be accomplished. Because regulatory agencies require a vast amount of information, it is essential to coordinate, integrate and translate such data into useful information.

Computerization can supply an organized method of obtaining integrated data, ranging from financial billing to resident care plans, quickly and efficiently. The administrator and top management make the choice to computerize and must include commitment to a computer system that connects the various functions and departments of the entire facility and becomes an integral part of both the management and treatment teams. The system must meet the facility's particular needs and those of the nursing staff. Resources need to be identified, and coordination of the vendors, management and users have to be planned. Factors to consider are staff acceptance and training (scope, cost, hours), scope of the system (resident care planning, menus, financial), software (cost of tailoring, additional informational needs, revision), and physical location (wiring, telecommunications needs). Communication needs to be established among the the various users within the facility. Capital expense is required to provide and install the equipment and to train relevant staff to run the system. Generally, computers have been introduced to the facility in the business office, followed by word processing for secretaries and clerks, and then into resident assessment and care plans. Computer software packages are available for nursing, dietary, housekeeping and maintenance.

## MARKETING AND PUBLIC RELATIONS

Marketing is basic to the success of a business endeavor. Whether product- or service-oriented, any business will be unlikely to succeed, grow and survive without effective and innovative marketing to potential customers. Hand in hand with supporting marketing efforts is public relations, which seeks positive image and key public support. Marketing involves selling the particular facility and its services to targeted audiences, whereas public relations is the building of the image of the long-term care industry as a whole.

The nursing facility administrator needs to be aware of the roles of marketing and public relations in a service-oriented industry that is facing critical challenge from poor image, elderly care alternatives and predicted increasing demands in the near and distant future. The administrator should understand management's objectives and the long-term care market. In spite of high occupancy rates, little public trust is found in long-term care facilities. Awareness by the general public of alternatives, such as life and continuing care communities, home health care, HMO expansion and specialized elderly housing, can increase family decisions for non-nursing facility choices. Although

most people in nursing facilities rate their facility favorably, the public as a whole continues to view long-term care facilities as a last resort that warehouses the dying; the public needs to know that facilities, resident care and administrative professionalism have been and continue to be upgraded.

### Marketing

A provider's present and future success depends on its ability to meet the needs and expectations of elders and their families. Thus, the administrator must integrate a planned program of marketing into management and public relations. Marketing involves interaction with customers, all organizational levels providing service and other providers to assure that the marketing messages developed are met with and support the customer's expectations. The administrator may formulate and carry out marketing plans with the assistance of outside expertise, public relations training and/or utilization surveys and reports.

Generally, the administrator will need to utilize a systematic approach to develop a marketing strategy. It has been determined that a marketing opportunity analysis (MOA) implemented before and throughout planning will help provide the identification of desires, needs and locations of the elderly, the nature of the competition, and information for developing and communicating the facility's services in accordance with current and predicted trends in the health care market. To assist in awareness of the marketplace, MOA examines five general characteristics:

- **The nature of the demand** of the nursing facility users is the basis for the provision of service. This would include developments and concerns in social/cultural, economic, technological, political/legal and/or ecological environments. What are special needs in the area the facility serves? How and who meets these needs? Can the facility feasibly fill any gaps in the market?
- **The diversity in the immediate market** helps identify and helps pinpoint what unique type of service is needed, in what combinations, by whom, where, at what age and at what income level. This assists the administrator in tailoring services to the ongoing present and future needs of the facility's area.

- **The trend and developments within the nursing facility industry as a whole** indicate what alternative care providers are meeting the market areas. This also helps identify areas of potential growth and industry trends.
- **The level and nature of the competition** will help clarify the nature of immediate competing facilities and hospitals with swing beds and long-term care units. What positive unique services are offered? Where does the competition fail? Answers to such questions also will provide a basis for comparison to evaluate the facility's existing services.
- **The effectiveness of distribution of the facility's service** (referent analysis) considers intermediaries or those referring people in need of nursing care such as physicians, social workers, fraternal groups, churches, hospitals or skilled nursing facilities. This focuses on identification of the intermediaries and establishment of relationships of mutual services.

The "three Ms" of marketing (measuring, molding and monitoring) present broader guidelines for formulation of an effective and sound program:

- **Measuring** is a feasibility study to target the audience or customers and to determine the present and future needs and services. This can be achieved by looking at factors such as supply (service, quality, cost, percentage of occupancy) by competitors, demographics (where qualifying age and income groups reside), and results of surveys and interviews from focus groups. They will help provide direction for the next two steps.
- **Molding** formulates the strongest preferences identified by the measuring process into a simple, clear and concise marketing message for the targeted audience. At least one service (quality of care, atmosphere, location, physical environment, activities) offered should be unique—setting the facility apart in the marketplace. It should meet a real need while reinforcing any other services available. Ad copy, radio spots and other communications should be consistent with the original image and message conveyed. The marketing plan with budget estimates and rationale for each step of the overall program should be drawn up.

- **Monitoring** checks for effectiveness of the marketing program and involves attention to three elements:
  1. The marketing components to determine the number and characteristics of responses.
  2. The training, policies and effectiveness of the sales staff.
  3. Information regarding age, location, income level and needs of those reached by various types of advertising.

In marketing, the administrator must consider the facility from the customer's perception. Customers include residents, families, faculty staff, consulting and attending physicians, hospitals, community organizations and the government. Each has varying demands and expectations. Families and potential residents want assurance that when they can no longer care for themselves, qualified facilities and staff will provide professional care with an attitude of respect and compassion. They expect caring attentive nurses, good activities programs, cleanliness and nutritious, attractive meals. Generally, our society is demanding a safe hospitable environment from community, organizations and/or institutions for the many members growing older each year. The family makes the majority of admission decisions and is a primary marketing target. This requires that the facility be aware of their expectations, satisfactions and dissatisfactions and respond to these aspects (using family, staff and physicians surveys; resident meetings; admissions policies; opinion cards; open door to the administrator; and routine follow-up). Various other individuals with whom the facility works in delivering services to residents interact with the facility and each other and are "ambassadors" to external audiences.

## Public Relations

Because a long-term care facility's customers buy directly from the facility (supplier) and not from dealers or specialized distributing organizations, public relations is a primary marketing tool. This is a process of developing and maintaining positive relationships with key support groups. Customer relations are founded on perceptions that come from knowledge about and/or experience with the facility and/or the administrator. Personal experience is the strongest influence on the overall perception of the nursing facility. In day-to-day contact, both internal and external customers are witness to the care and concern given by management and staff and can feel cared for and valued or ignored, abused and undervalued. Public relations concerns internal and external activities of the facility reaching internal and external audiences and reflecting on the facility's image as a whole.

Internally, the health care facility staff plays a significant public relations role in daily interaction with residents, the administrators, families and visitors and among themselves. Focusing on employee selection and satisfaction, opening communication channels to employee needs and feelings, and increasing the staff's awareness of its role and value in customer relations and in the provision of quality service and care can increase customer satisfaction and contribute positively to the facility's image. Similarly residents, their families and the medical staff need to be kept informed, considered and treated as significant to the operation and success of the facility.

Several means exist of establishing good marketing and public relations with the internal audiences. These methods can contribute to a positive image of a quality, caring facility:

- For employees, notice of employee meetings, awards programs and newsletters focused on staff concerns.
- For residents, newsletters concerning day-to-day activities, resident works such as stories, poems or reminiscences, and admissions packets giving detail of the facility services, policies and activities.
- For families, special meetings, individualized notes (thank you notes upon admission of a relative, periodic reports on resident's care and progress), open houses and tours.
- For physicians, a personal visit from the administrator concerning related resident(s) condition and care, marketing/informational packets.

Externally, community relations is an important factor to consider in the facility's marketing strategy. Most referrals are from the community and its medical care and service providers. Thus, good community outreach and service programs can benefit the facility in terms of visibility, positive image, higher employee morale, recognition and resident referrals.

Daily contacts are basic considerations to the public's image of the facility. Good telephone procedures—how calls are answered and how the inquiries are handled—have a great deal to do with the initial perception. Each individual (whether a potential resident, family member, serviceperson or vendor) should be treated with respect and courtesy. Literature, packets and brochures concerning the facility and the rules and regulations; its nursing, dietary, office, pharmacy and other services; the available activities; complaint procedures; and costs will inform the public, potential residents and their families on the kind of care the facility can furnish. Well-organized discharge planning enhances communication with other community organizations and presents an image of a rehabilitative facility working to help residents back into the community.

### Marketing and Public Relations Program

Several steps dovetailing with the marketing guidelines are recommended in formulating an effective public/community relations program. The plan should be practical and individualized to the facility and meet the needs in both the target market area and the facility. Major areas to consider cover:

- **Deciding what is to be accomplished and establishing objectives** that will bring results within the facility's own objectives. Specific facility goals might include increasing resident referrals or facility name recognition. Consider the facility and its services from the customer's view; address and remedy problem areas. Take into account the immediate competition such as hospitals and nursing facilities, life care centers, acute care units, and any marketing efforts and results they may use.
- **Identifying the target audience** by researching the population (density, vital statistics such as age and income) and profile (traits and abilities as determined by ratings and surveys). Geographic areas with health care providers, agencies and individuals providing referrals to the facility will help define the present and potential market area.
- **Establishing programs and tasks, developing focused messages and selecting the method and media** best suited to the audience's preferences and the facility's goals. Such public relations tools might include:

1. Inviting the public to the facility (special events such as a 75th anniversary of the facility, food service tours, facility tours to individuals, agencies, social service groups and community leaders).
2. Distributing facility newsletters and/or brochures and regular contact with medical providers (social workers, hospital discharge planners, physicians), direct mail, newspapers, and radio and television presenting information on professional quality long-term care.
3. Providing public services such as nutrition education to residents, families and the public, and provision of meals with the cooperation of various community organizations to the elderly and needy; health fairs and blood pressure checkups; employee-volunteers to medical clinics, hospice, meals on wheels; volunteers and programs involving community organizations such as Green Thumb; media use for human interest, health care issues; and information on insurance and health care legislation.

- **Implementing the public relations program** considers schedules, budgets and personnel. One designee should oversee such implementation. Notes and impressions of effective programs can be recorded to supplement review and revisions of the entire strategy.

As one marketing official has said, "Marketing is a function of the entire organization and that clients' perceptions and expectations evolve with each interaction with your organization." Thus, public relations must be planned and fully integrated into management. It must be supported by time, diligence, a well-organized and well-run facility offering quality services meeting special needs, a positive internal audience and community involvement. The resulting good image will evolve and be communicated to present and potential customers.

## NURSING FACILITY ADMINISTRATION

The **mission statement** of a nursing facility points out what the purposes of the facility are and why it is doing what it is doing. This operational philosophy serves as a guideline for the overall management and operation of the facility and assists all its employees in integrating the values and ethics of the leadership to carry out the philosophy of the organization.

## Administration
### *42 CFR, Sec. 483.75, Chap. IV (10-1-98)*

For the facility to participate in Medicare (Title XVIII) and/or Medicaid (Title XIX) and receive funding for long-term care, it must comply with the Code of Federal Regulations (CFR). Under these requirements, "facility" means a skilled nursing facility (SNF) or a nursing facility (NF) meeting these requirements. It may be all of or a distinct part of a larger institution, but may not be an institution for the mentally retarded or other mental diseases (Sec. 483.5).

### *Achieving Compliance*

A facility must be administered in a manner that enables it to use its resources effectively and efficiently to attain or maintain the highest practicable physical, mental and psychological well-being of each resident.

*Licensure.* A skilled facility must be licensed in accordance with state or local law if that law requires it.

*Compliance with Federal, State and Local Laws and Professional Standards.* The facility must operate and provide services in compliance with all applicable federal, state and local laws, regulations and codes and with accepted professional standards and principles that apply to professionals providing services to such a facility.

*Relationship to Other HHS Regulations.* In addition to compliance with the regulations set forth in this subpart, facilities are obliged to meet the applicable provisions of other HHS regulations, including but not limited to those pertaining to: nondiscrimination on the basis of race, color or national origin (45 CFR Part 80); nondiscrimination on the basis of handicap (45 CFR Part 84); nondiscrimination on the basis of age (45 CFR Part 91); protection of human subjects of research (45 CFR Part 46); and fraud and abuse. Although these regulations are not in themselves considered requirements under this part, their violation may result in the termination of, suspension of, or the refusal to grant or continue payment with federal funds.

*Governing Body.* The facility must have a governing body, or designated persons functioning as a governing body, that is legally responsible for establishing and implementing policies regarding the management and operation of the facility.

The governing body appoints the administrator who is:

1. Licensed by the state (where licensing is required).
2. Responsible for management of the facility.

*Staff Qualifications.* The facility must employ on a full-time, part-time or consultant basis those professionals necessary to carry out the provisions of these requirements. Professional staff must be licensed, certified or registered in accordance with applicable state laws.

*Use of Outside Resources.* If the facility does not employ a qualified professional person to furnish a specific service to be provided by the facility, the facility must have that service furnished to residents by a person or agency outside the facility under an agreement.

Arrangements or agreements pertaining to services furnished by outside resources must specify in writing that the facility assumes responsibility for:

1. Obtaining services that meet professional standards and principles that apply to professionals providing services in such a facility.
2. The timeliness of the services.

*Disclosure of Ownership.* The facility must provide written notice to the state agency responsible for licensing the facility at the time of change, if such change occurs, in:

1. Persons with an ownership or controlling interest who:
   a. Have direct or indirect ownership interest, or a combination of direct and indirect ownership interest, totaling 5% or more in the facility.
   b. Own interest of 5% or more in mortgages, deed of trust, note or other obligation secured by the facility (if the interest totals 5% or more of the assets of the facility).
   c. Are officers or directors of a corporate facility.
   d. Are partners in a partnership facility.

2. The officers, directors, agents or managing employees.
3. The corporation, association or other company responsible for the management of the facility.
4. The facility's administrator or director of nursing.

The notice must include the identity of each new individual or company.

## ORGANIZATION OF THE GOVERNING BODY

The governing body is the individual, group or corporation that has the ultimate authority and responsibility for the operation of the long-term care facility. In some instances, the administrator and governing body may be the same individual. The operation of the facility includes satisfactory compliance with all related laws, rules and regulations. Attending physicians are responsible for the medical care of the residents. The governing body must work with physicians to ensure the welfare of the residents and provide sufficient and adequate equipment, supplies and personnel for effective practice in a proper environment. The legal duties of the governing body should be written.

Generally speaking, the size of the governing board or body should be adequate to meet the needs of a community. The size will differ depending upon the type of institution—whether a hospital or nursing facility, or a proprietary or nonprofit corporation. Some SNFs have large boards in order to obtain a broad contact with the community. However, with a large board, it may be difficult to be able to make decisions and to find qualified individuals to serve. The number on governing boards varies from 3 to 30 persons with the average numbering about 15. This number has been found to constitute a more manageable board. Some organizations have decided to add advisory boards for community reaction, but this could prove dangerous and promote duplication unless the role and the functions of the advisory board are clearly and concisely defined.

### Qualifications for Members of the Governing Body

If possible a broad representation of disciplines should be on the board. Lawyers, physicians, educators, labor, business and consumers are the types of community leaders desired. At one time it was almost heresy to allow a physician on a board, but today it is customary practice to have a medical representative. It is also customary to involve consumers of long-term care on the board. A nonprofit facility usually will appoint the members of the first board for a specific term of years (i.e., one third of the members for 3 years, one third for 2 years, and one third for 1 year). Other facilities may appoint board members for 1-year terms subject to reappointments every year.

In selecting a board, the members—whether they be professional, business or labor representatives—should be chosen on the basis of proven leadership qualities in the community, not as patronage for a favor done for the nursing facility. A businessman who is a leader in the community might have certain organizational abilities. A lawyer may or may not be the attorney for the health care facility (if retained by the health care facility, he or she should not be asked to give formal legal opinions at board meetings, but can be used as a guide regarding legal implications involved in setting policy in the health care facility). A physician on the board should represent the feelings of the physicians in the community—not those of colleagues with an axe to grind with administration or with fellow colleagues. This selection should be based on individual qualities, not merely because of the medical profession. The labor leader can be of valuable assistance in determining policy regarding the benefits the health care facility wishes to offer its employees. Some boards appoint a certified accountant or a financial analyst to assist in general financial problems that may arise.

It is quite important to select a board member who is successful in his or her respective field. If the individual is a failure in his or her own profession or business, the chances are he or she will not be of much assistance on the governing body. A member of the board must be honest and above reproach and free from political influence. If he or she is a controversial politician in the community, decisions on policy matters might be based upon what is politically expedient instead of upon what will benefit the health care facility. Finally, the board member should not have a personality that is too aggressive and will not allow the chief executive officer to manage the facility. On the other hand, he or she should not be a rubber stamp or avoid participation in the necessary board decisions.

He or she must be prepared to devote a great deal of time to the affairs of the facility.

## Duties and Responsibilities of the Governing Body

Members of the governing body must act in good faith and for the best interests of the health care facility. They must use due and reasonable care, exercise diligence and act within the scope of authority conferred upon them. Board members are expected to keep themselves informed as to the long-term care industry generally and their facility's activities specifically. It is their duty to see to it that their health facility obeys the law and maintains its activities within its powers.

Board members are treated as **fiduciaries** with respect to the business. Their relationship to the health care facility involves responsibility and accountability. It is their duty to administer the business affairs for the common benefit of all owners and exercise their best care, skill and judgment in its management.

Three general duties defined by cases handed down by the courts are:

1. A duty of **obedience,** meaning that the board members are to perform their activities within the powers conferred upon the business by its bylaws and/or articles of incorporation. The courts have pointed out that the willful violation of this duty may make the board member liable to the business.
2. A duty of **diligence,** meaning that board members should exercise that degree of care that the reasonably prudent individual would exercise under the same or similar circumstances as to the general management of the business.
3. A duty of **loyalty,** meaning that a board member must refrain from engaging in personal activities in any manner that could injure or take advantage of the health facility. That is, the board member may not make secret or private profits out of his or her official position and must give the business the benefit of any advantages gained due to this relationship of trust with the facility.

Specific duties of the governing body include to:

1. Establish the overall policies of the health care facility by taking into consideration the health

needs of the community with a view toward elimination of duplicating efforts.

2. Provide adequate equipment necessary to fulfill the objectives and purposes of the health care facility.

3. Ensure that professional standards of health personnel employed in the institution meet the minimal requirements of the federal, state and municipal regulatory agencies.

4. Receive reports from the administrator that keep them advised of financial, professional and administrative aspects of the operation of the health care facility.

5. Approve a budget submitted by the administrator to ensure the solvency of the health care facility.

6. Ensure that all rules, regulations and ordinances of federal, state and municipal agencies are complied with and to receive adequate records regarding such compliance.

7. Receive reports from the administrator regarding activities of the several departments within the facility.

Because the governing body is the ultimate authority in the facility, procedures must be established to:

1. Make sure board members are aware of any statutory requirements regarding the incorporation or establishment of the health care facility.

2. Provide reports from the administrator to keep members informed in a general way of all activities taking place in the organization.

3. Remind board members to avoid self-dealing in any matter relating to the business.

4. Make sure any member's dissent in disagreement with a board action is properly identified and in the board minutes.

5. Remind members to attend the board meetings on a regular basis.

6. Make sure that members know the duties and responsibilities, rules and regulations, and bylaws of the health care facility.

### Committees of the Governing Body

Committees of the board fall into two broad categories: standing and ad hoc committees. Standing committees are of a permanent nature and are designed to carry out in a general way the statutory responsibilities of the governing body. Ad hoc committees are special committees usually established to carry out a specific purpose, and they cease to exist when that purpose is complete. Ad hoc committees may be a nominating committee, a special fund-raising committee, and a surveys and study committee.

Standing committees include the following.

- The **executive committee** usually consists of the officers of the governing body and several members at large. Some organizations include the immediate past president as a member of this committee. When the governing body is large, this committee may serve as the authority to whom the administration must report. On decisions of a major nature, such as the dissolution of the business, major building programs, or capital financing efforts, this committee's actions should be ratified and approved by the full board. When the board meets on a quarterly basis or less often, it is important that the executive committee meets on a monthly basis to carry out the business activities of the facility. If the board is a small group meeting on a monthly basis, the functions of the executive committee become less vital; they would deliberate only on matters of an emergency nature.

- The **ethics committee** is appointed to establish and write ethics policy and to promote ethics education in the facility. The governing body of a nursing facility, whether it is a corporation, partnership or sole proprietorship, is confronted with complex ethical decisions involving the operations of the facility. The size and composition of the ethics committee in a facility varies; some use their professional employees and community members (clergy, lawyers, physicians and social workers). Their task is to help recommend policies on such moral ethical issues as advance directives, withholding or withdrawing treatment, use of restraint and other dilemmas brought on by serious illness and aging. (See Chapter 7, Resident Care.)

- The **finance committee** should be composed of three to five members. Ideally, these members have a background in business, law and accounting. This committee recommends the monetary policy and ensures financial stability by remaining up to date with both the short- and long-range financial status of the facility. Major functions are to review the annual budget, which is prepared and submitted to the governing body by the administrator, and to submit related recommendations to the full board. This committee also reviews with the administrator, the facility's salary and wage program or may take the necessary steps if the facility is planning to borrow money for expansion of its services or major plant repairs.

- The **public relations committee** may consist of three to five members with backgrounds of journalism or psychology and/or a basic knowledge of human relations. This committee becomes very important in the small long-term care facility which does not generally retain a full-time public relations director or have in place a systematic approach to this essential function. The public image of the health care facility is an important factor in attracting and maintaining community support. For too many years, nursing facilities have had a poor public image because the community receives insufficient information regarding their activities and functions. The committee should regularly prepare news releases, covering human interest stories, an innovation or interesting procedure, new equipment, and resident activities.

- The **building committee** may be composed of two to three members who assist the administration with maintenance, remodeling or renovation, or when building plans are being projected. Individuals active in the community in building and real estate might serve as members of this committee.

- The **fund-raising** committee assists in any continuing fund-raising projects and with special projects undertaken by the health care facility.

- The **joint conference committee** is very important in nursing facilities. Its members consist of several officers of the governing body, the administrator of the facility, and physician representatives such as medical director or attending physician. It serves as an excellent method of communication to the board members regarding activities of a medico-administrative nature. It is a committee that is required by the Joint Commission on Accreditation of Healthcare Organizations, the Public Health Service and other regulatory agencies.

Ad hoc committees include two types:

- The **nominating committee** is usually appointed by the president of the governing body and is concerned with the nomination of new officers and board members of a health care facility.

- The **survey and study committee** would undertake special studies or projects before possible implementation. A study of the facility's community image or community needs might be a function of this committee.

## Meetings of the Governing Body

Meetings of the governing body include regular, special and annual meetings. The governing body ideally should meet on a monthly basis to carry on the general management of the facility. The meetings are general in nature and are customarily set up in the following order:

- Call to order.
- Reading of minutes of previous meeting.
- Old business.
- Communications.
- New business.
- Reports of officers and committees.
- Adjournment.

Special meetings may be called by the officers or by a designated member of the board as provided for in the bylaws of the health care facility. For example, some bylaws provide that the president may call a special meeting if adequate notice is given. The time considered adequate may be anywhere from 3 to 30 days. Usually the bylaws provide that the reason for a special meeting be indicated in the notice sent out to the board members. Generally, only the business of the special meeting is heard.

The annual meeting is called for the purpose of electing new officers and to receive reports from the administrator regarding the operation of the facility. The annual report should outline by department the activities in the health care facility during the past year. This fiscal report is then discussed, and the financial operation of the health care facility is reviewed accordingly. The annual budget, including salary budget, supplies and expense budget, and equipment budget, also may be discussed.

## ADMINISTRATOR'S DUTIES

A nursing facility administrator is a licensed professional specifically trained for this position. Administrators are held to the standards of professional competence in the same manner as a nurse, pharmacist or other professional paramedical licensed personnel who are hired to provide a direct service.

The administrator is hired to manage the facility and must meet certain standards of professional conduct. He or she is the chief executive officer and legally has the responsibility for all activities in the health care facility but often delegates some of this authority. The administrator is responsible for a broad spectrum of activities involving not only the internal operation of the facility but external activities in the community. The ownership or corporate board of directors of the facility retains the ultimate legal responsibility. If the administrator fails to meet the duties and obligations within standards of professional conduct, any resulting liability could be imputed to him or her personally or to the facility.

### Code of Ethics

High standards of integrity and ethical principles are an essential part of the professional responsibilities of long-term health care administration. The American College of Health Care Administrators (ACHCA) promulgated the following fundamental rules as basic to carrying out this responsibility.

The welfare of persons for whom care is provided is predominant. In support of this, the administrator needs to:

1. Provide the highest quality of appropriate services possible in light of available resources.
2. Comply with laws, regulations and standards of recognized practice in the operation of the facility.
3. Protect each resident's confidentiality of information.
4. Conduct administrative duties with personal integrity, earning confidence, trust and respect in the community.
5. Avoid any illegal discriminatory actions that are not related to the bona fide requirements of quality care.
6. Not disclose professional or personal information regarding residents to unauthorized personnel un-

less required by law or to protect the public welfare.

The administrator must maintain high standards of professional competence and must:

1. Possess and maintain the competencies that are necessary to effectively carry out his or her responsibilities.
2. Practice administration in accordance with his or her capabilities and seek counsel from other qualified persons when appropriate.
3. Obtain continuing education and professional development actively.
4. Present truthfully qualifications, education, experience or affiliations.
5. Provide other services than those for which he or she is prepared and qualified.

In the practice of long-term care administration, each administrator must strive to maintain professionalism, placing the interest of the facility and its residents first and shall:

1. Avoid partisanship, providing a forum for the fair resolution of disputes involving the management of the facility or delivery of services.
2. Disclose to the governing body or other appropriate authorities any circumstances concerning him or her that might create conflict of interest or have a substantial adverse impact on the facility or its residents.
3. Refuse to participate in any activity that might create a conflict of interest or have a substantial adverse impact on the facility or its residents.

Long-term care administrators also honor their responsibilities to the public, their profession and the relationships with colleagues and members of related professions. In this area, they:

1. Foster increased knowledge and support research efforts within their profession.
2. Participate in community planning to provide a full range of health care services.
3. Share their expertise with colleagues, students and the public to promote understanding of long-term health care.

4. Inform the ACHCA Standards and Ethics Committee of violations of its code of ethics and cooperate with related sanctioned inquiries.
5. Do not defend or support any unethical conduct of colleagues, peers or students.

## Administrator and Governing Body

The relationship of the administrator to the governing body or ownership is one of employer-employee and principal-agent. As an employee, the administrator holds the same legal relationship to the employer as other employees do. His or her immediate supervisor, however, is not one person but the total board of directors. The principal-agent relationship is contractual based on mutual consent (employment contract) between the administrator and the governing board, whereby the administrator represents the governing body in dealings with third parties (insurance, contractors) to manage affairs or perform some service.

The board has the ultimate legal responsibility for the management of the health care facility and, therefore, must establish policies and be kept informed of activities within the facility. The board may guide the administrator in a general way, but being successful businessmen, businesswomen and leaders in the community does not necessarily qualify them as experts in the health care field; the administrator must be the expert. It is very important that the administrator be given the proper authority to carry out his or her legal responsibility of operating the facility. Although the governing body must delegate authority to the administrator, he or she remains accountable to them. The administrator is not the business manager but is the overall supervisor of all functions both administrative and medico-administrative.

Recent legal cases demonstrate that the business activities of a health care facility are interrelated with the quality of care being offered in the facility. The administrator should assist the board in establishing general policy. The administrator then has the responsibility to implement the policy once it has been established by ratification of the board. He or she should attend all meetings of the governing board and its committees.

A general trend exists today to put the administrator on the same level as other board members. In private corporations, the president of the corporation is a member of the board but not necessarily the chairman of the board. The administrator as a board member should not vote on any matter that concerns him or her personally (such as employment contracts or fringe benefits) because courts may hold that this is a conflict of interest.

## Reports by the Administrator

Communications between the governing body and the administrator are very important. One way in which the administrator may communicate effectively with the board is to present reports to them on a monthly basis. An agenda for board meetings should be prepared by the administrator and distributed to the members before the meeting. When several items require statistical documentation, enough time should be provided to study the material and prepare any questions in time for the meeting. Monthly profit and loss statements are prepared and discussed at the meetings. The business manager may prepare the report, but the administrator presents the reports to the board.

Some health care facilities invite the business manager to attend the meetings of the board to answer any details about the preparation of the report. However, the responsibility for reporting remains with the administrator. The administrator should study any problems, do the detail groundwork in gathering statistics to present, and make an appropriate recommendation to the board about who may or may not accept the recommendation.

## Administrator's Duties within the Facility

The administrator is the liaison officer between the governing body, the organized medical staff (if there is one) and the department heads in the health facility. He or she must communicate policy to the members of the general staff. The number of organized departments varies with the size of the facility, but the functions that must be performed do not vary. Whether the facility is large or small, functions, including those in the following areas, must be performed: bookkeeping and accounting, personnel, dietary, housekeeping, laundry, pharmacy, and resident care.

### Relative to Personnel

The selection of all department heads should be made by the administrator. Because these individuals are the key to the successful operation of the health care facility, the administrator must have a good working relationship with them. All department heads must report to the administrator. In large facilities, very often an assistant administrator coordinates the activities of some of the departments and then reports to the administrator.

The administrator is responsible for the training of personnel concerning the mission, rules and regulations of the facility and for keeping employee morale high. In the small health care facility, he or she may be responsible for establishing and implementing personnel practices. In the larger institution, a personnel manager may assist the administrator in carrying out this function.

### Relative to Quality of Care

The landmark case of *Darling v. Charlestown Community Hospital* (211 NE 2d 253 [1965]) established a duty upon the administrator to be involved in the quality of care being rendered in the facility. OBRA 1987 mandates that the facility have an operational quality assessment and assurance program and a committee to monitor the quality of services in all areas. All providers must meet the provisions of a quality assurance program that stresses health outcomes and provides data to measure outcomes and other indicators of quality.

The nursing facility administrator coordinates resident care management and must be able to plan, implement and evaluate the care program. He or she requires a broad knowledge in the areas of the needs of those coming into the facility for care, the roles and standards of the personnel (including nurses, aides, dietitians and social workers) caring for the residents, and all applicable standards, rules, regulations and new legislation to make sure that the facility is in compliance. A breach of federal or state standards would be an important consideration in determining what standard of care should apply in negligence actions.

### Relative to the Medical Director

Most nursing facilities do not have a formal organized medical staff. However, the governing body through its medical director, must monitor physicians to see to full compliance with all regulations regarding physicians with patients in a nursing facility. The medico-

administrative decisions regarding these regulations are part of the responsibility of the administrator.

The medical director of a nursing facility is usually a full- or part-time physician. Some of his or her duties are to implement and enforce the policies relative to medical care in the facility as required by Federal and State law. The Code of Federal Regulations, Part 42, 430 to end, 10-1-98, requires nursing facilities to ensure that:

1. a physician must personally approve in writing a recommendation for an individual to be admitted to a facility,
2. each resident is under the care of a physician,
3. another physician supervises the medical care of a resident when the attending physician is unavailable.

In most cases, the legal status of an attending physician in a nursing facility is one of independent contractor. This means that any negligence caused by the attending physician would not be imputed to the nursing facility under Respondeat Superior, because the medical director is not an employee of the facility relative to medical care. (However, some large corporate facilities do employ a physician as medical director.)

The administrator should be involved in, and supervise, contractual agreements between the medical director and the facility regarding their duties, responsibilities and compensation. The administrator should also ensure that the rules are adhered to regarding physician visits, frequency of physician visits, availability of physicians for emergency care and proper physician delegation of tasks to be performed by a nurse practioner, clinical nurse specialist or physician's assistant, who is not an employee of the facility but who is working in collaboration with the physician.

### Relative to the Nursing Service

The primary role of the nursing department in the facility is the proper care of the resident. The administrator is responsible for the selection of the director of nursing with authority to both employ and discharge her or him. Because of the importance of this position in the facility, it would probably be judicious for the administrator to consult with the board and/or medical director before such action is taken.

The administrator delegates some of his or her authority to the director of nursing to operate the nursing department. Because the administrator retains the legal responsibility for the operation of the entire facility, mechanisms for receiving reports and communications from the director of nursing should be established.

### Relative to the Dietary Department

The food service of a facility is an important factor in therapy and quality of life to the resident and in maintaining good public relations with the community. The resident judges the quality of the health care facility by the type of nursing service rendered, the cleanliness of the facility, and the food served. If the food is therapeutically good for the resident, is hot when received by the resident and is attractively served, the image regarding food service should be good.

A qualified dietitian should be on the dietary staff on a full-time or on a consulting basis. The administrator is responsible for retaining the dietitian who will report directly to him or her. The purchasing of food for a health care facility is very often done by the dietitian.

### Relative to Fiscal Solvency

The administrator is responsible for the fiscal solvency of the institution. To carry out this responsibility he or she should prepare, or have prepared, an annual budget for submission to the governing body for approval. This budget includes salary projections, supply and expense projections, and equipment projections. A personnel department may assist the administrator in obtaining information for the establishment of a wage and salary program, and the administrator should be empowered to fix all salaries within the limits of the budget.

If the facility has a comptroller or a business manager, he or she should be given the responsibility of doing the actual detail work on the budget to be reviewed and approved by the administrator before he or she submits it to the board for approval. Once the budget is approved, the administrator operates the health care facility within its guidelines.

### Relative to Risk Management

Risk management is a program to anticipate possible legal problems and to manage or reduce these occur-

rences. Identification of the risks is a first step in such a program. Generally, risk may fall into:

1. **Physical risks**—This includes such physical plant concerns as: fire safety, disaster, emergency procedures and all of the different standards (Life Safety Code, ANSI, ADA) that the facility must meet in order to be licensed, certified or accredited.
2. **Resident care risks**—This includes poor policies and procedures relating to the resident care, such as poor record keeping, ignoring residents' rights, improper use of restraints, poor medication procedures, and negligence in keeping records of incidents that take place in the facility. Lack of preemployment tests for screening new employees also falls into this category.

Some steps that can be taken to reduce occurrences that may lead to legal liability are:

1. Adequate insurance coverage to cover the risks that may be incurred (see Chapter 5).
2. Documentation of all incidents and accidents that occur in the facility.
3. Good inservice training for employees (see Chapter 4).
4. Active quality assessment and insurance committee (see Chapter 7).

### Relative to the Business Office

The lifeblood of any health care facility, whether profit or nonprofit, is the ability to generate income and keep the operation solvent. The administrator must work closely with the office manager regarding the fiscal operations. With the advent of third-party payers, most health facilities are financed primarily by insurance policies (such as private insurance companies, Blue Cross and Blue Shield, Medicare and Medicaid) held by residents either on a group or an individual basis. The administrator, therefore, must be familiar with the prospective payment system, the legislative requirements of Medicare and Medicaid, and the total insurance process as it relates to the facility. Unless he or she has special training in this area, the administrator is not expected to do the accounting for the facility. However, he or she should be familiar with accounting statements in order to properly interpret and analyze profit and loss statements and balance sheets, and be conversant with procedures relating to accounts payable and accounts receivable within the organization.

### Relative to the Purchasing Function

The administrator has certain responsibilities as an agent for the facility to make sure proper purchasing procedures are established. One responsibility is to protect the assets of the corporation; in order to do so adequately, good procedures must be established and implemented. Larger facilities will have a purchasing agent who does all the ordering for the facility, with the exception of food, in coordination with the administrator and department heads. In smaller facilities, this is combined with another function. It is sometimes feasible to form consortiums with other health care providers in the area to achieve greater economy in the provisions of services and supplies.

### Relative to the Physical Environment

The administrator needs to have a broad knowledge of the state and federal regulations applicable to the physical environment (NFPA, ADA/ANSI, OSHA) to ensure the facility's compliance for the protection of its residents and others coming into the facility. An infection control committee must be operational to prevent, control and monitor contagious disease and infections, and to ensure the use of universal precaution measures. Equipment used by residents must meet their needs and be on a preventive maintenance program. Disaster and fire preparedness programs must be established and operational.

Generally, the housekeeper is responsible for the cleanliness of the facility, and the maintenance engineer is responsible for all other physical aspects of the operation. These department heads a report to the administrator and keep him or her informed of any related problems of a significant nature. Because of possible negligence on the part of the facility, the administrator must be informed immediately about any defects in operating equipment either on the grounds or in the building.

### Administrator's Duties Outside the Facility

### Relative to the Health Field

The duties of the administrator are not limited to activities within the four walls of the building. Nursing facilities are an integral part of the community. From the view of health care planning, it is very important that all health care providers and hospitals work together and cooperate with each other when possible. The administrator of a health care facility should be active in local, state and national health organizations such as the local nursing facility council, state association, the American Health Care Association and ACHCA. By keeping active in the health field, he or she will keep abreast of the many changes that are taking place in a very dynamic area of management.

### Relative to the Community

The administrator is considered a leader in the community and his or her actions are often interpreted as representative of the health care facility. The administrator may be active in the community, joining a service club or participating on the boards of credible organizations if requested to do so. As part of the public and community relations program, he or she may tell the story of the facility to the community by presenting talks to various service clubs.

The public image of health care facilities historically has been poor. Part of this poor image is due to lack of disclosure of information such as the finances of the institution, the adequacy of the accommodations, and approval by accrediting agencies. Therefore, it is imperative that the administrator have a good working relationship with the press because of the help it can give in presenting favorable information (i.e., new personnel employed, new techniques or new equipment used, special resident activities) to the community.

### Sample Job Description of an Administrator

The administrator has a number of responsibilities including:

- Exercising general management of the nursing facility.
- Providing for implementation of policies, directives and resolutions promulgated by the governing body.
- Overseeing that rules and regulations of the state board of health and other state and federal regulatory agencies are complied with regarding the operation of the health care facility.

- Developing, maintaining and administering a sound plan of organization.
- Being responsible for maintaining high standards of resident care.
- Maintaining the nursing facility in a solvent condition and making such recommendations to the governing board as necessary to the attainment of this objective. The administrator is responsible for the supervision and preparation of the annual budget.
- Reporting regularly to the governing body and submitting an annual report on the operation of the health care facility.

In addition, in regard to capital expenditures, the administrator is granted the authority to present for approval of the governing board requests for new and replacement of existing equipment not included in the annual budget in amounts over $1,500.

The approval of the governing body is necessary for plans and procedures involving major structural changes of the physical plant; for major personnel policies and wage and salary programs; for plans and procedures to introduce, expand or delete health services; for major changes in rates and charges for services and raising additional income from sources outside operating income; for initial contractual agreements regarding third-party payers; and for creation of new positions, new departments and new educational programs.

The administrator shall arrange a contract agreement with the medical director regarding the duties, responsibilities and compensation of this position. He or she will supervise medico-administrative decisions in relation to federal and state regulations and facility policies concerning physician and medical director responsibilities in the facility and will ensure their implementation.

In regard to relations with other health care facilities, the administrator shall develop a working relationship with third-party payers and negotiate contractual agreements, subject to approval of the governing body; cooperate with other health care agencies so that the health needs of the community are coordinated; and develop and maintain a favorable image of the health care facility by keeping the public informed through cooperation with the news media.

The duties of the administrator at any time may be assigned by the governing body.

## Administrator's Traits

According to one of the leaders of the health care field, the administrator needs to:

1. Have tact and diplomacy. The administrator is constantly working with many types of people. He or she may be working with a sick resident or with a doctor, planning a project with the auxiliary or discussing the institution with a lawyer or businessperson.
2. Be firm and be able to make a decision when it is required. The most ineffective administrator is one who sits on the fence on all issues and refuses to make a decision for fear he or she may upset someone. When a decision must be made, it is up to the administrator to make it.
3. Spend a great deal of time organizing the facility as chief executive officer of the health care facility. It is impossible to have an efficient operating facility unless departments are properly organized and lines of communication are established within the organizational structure.
4. Be a leader in the health care facility and in the community. The administrator should know how to work with people and develop confidence in them. Leadership must be shown by the administrator's actions on a daily basis.
5. Maintain high principles and be impartial in working with physicians, personnel and other individuals in the health care field. The administrator must have the administrative courage to adhere to his or her principles.
6. Like the work. The administrator is technically on the job 24 hours a day and should take a personal interest in the work.
7. Process administrative ability to coordinate the activities of others. In the larger facility, he or she will delegate much of the administrative authority to highly qualified department heads. In the smaller facility, the administrator may be performing the functions of many job titles.
8. Appear neat and tidy. The administrator should set a good example for others in the health care facility.
9. Have the ability to communicate both verbally and in writing. Therefore, a command of the English language is important.

10. Be able to analyze fact situations, to separate the unnecessary verbiage, and to present ideas in a concrete form.

11. Like to read and keep up with the current trends in the industry.

12. Be imaginative and innovative in the health care field.

13. Have empathy and like to work with older people.

## BIBLIOGRAPHY

*Black's Law Dictionary*. 1990. St. Paul, MN: West Publishing.

Brandt, M.E., and S. Allen. 1986. Marketing the image inside and out. *Provider*.

American College of Health Care Administrators. 1989. *Code of ethics*. Alexandria, VA.

Code of Federal Regulations, Title 42, Parts 430 to end.

*Darling vs. Charlestown Community Hsopital*, 211 NE 2d 253 (1965).

Davis, W. 1994. *Introduction to health care administration*, 4th ed. Bossier City, LA: Publicare Press.

Giordano, L. 1987. Computerizing the facility creates better management. *Provider*.

Hoerr, J. 1989. The payoff from teamwork. *Business Week*, July 10, 1989.

Koontz, H., C. O'Donnell, and H. Weihrich. 1988. *Management*. New York, NY: McGraw-Hill Book Co.

Lambert, N., and J. Thanopoulous. 1985. A dynamic planning framework for nursing homes. *Nursing Homes*.

Miller, D.B. 1982. *Long-term administration desk manual*. Greenvale, NY: Panel Publishers.

National Association of Boards of Examiners—NHA. 1997. *NAB study guide*, 3rd ed. Washington, DC.

Owens, T. 1991. The self-managing work team. *Small Business Reports*.

Pincus, J.D. 1986. Public relations: prescription for an ailing public image. *Provider*.

Seip, D.E. 1987. The three M's of marketing. *Contemporary LTC*, March 1987.

Shonk, J.H. 1992. *Team-based organizations*. Homewood, IL: Business One.

Sullivan, W. 1994. High tech. *Provider*, March, 1994.

Sundstrom, E., K. Demeuse, and D. Futrell. 1990. Work teams. *American Psychologist*, February, 1990.

# Appendix 3-A

## Glossary

### MANAGEMENT TERMS

**Administrator**—The chief executive officer of a nursing facility. Sometimes referred to as the executive vice president or president, this person is duly licensed by a state to practice as a nursing facility administrator.

**Advisory Board**—A board consisting of members who advise the decision makers in the facility. However, this board does not have decision-making authority.

**Authority**—The power or right to act, command or exact action from others.

**Case Mix**—A procedure in which the functioning levels of the residents are based on the resident's ability to perform the activities of daily living (ADLs) and the cost of providing the level of care.

**Chart of Organization**—A diagram that shows the various levels of management and the lines of authority and communication within the facility.

**Communication**—The passing of information from one person to another with mutual understanding of what has been conveyed.

**Compensation**—This term includes salary and wages, incentive pay and employee benefits.

**Competition**—An organization or entity that has similar or the same goals and objectives as another nursing facility.

**Controlling**—The process of evaluating performance against initial objectives and, if necessary, taking corrective action to assure the attainment of the planned goals.

**Corporation**—A legal entity that may conduct a business, sue or be sued. A corporation is created by the state and has limited liability.

**Coordination**—Getting personnel to work together to accomplish a common goal.

**Decentralized Authority**—Disbursing authority throughout the organization so that department heads are delegated authority to help manage the facility.

**Delegation of Authority**—Giving a part of one's authority to a subordinate to accomplish a specific goal of the organization.

**Departmentalization**—Setting up separate units of activities of a similar nature (i.e., nursing, dietary, housekeeping).

**Directing**—A management function involving the methods and communications a supervisor uses to complete tasks and efforts of the organization. It includes ordering, teaching, supervising, guiding and coordinating.

**Economy of Action**—A management principle stating that any time a higher paid employee makes a decision that a lower paid employee can make as well or better, the facility is wasting resources and money.

**Feedback**—When a sender of information receives knowledge that his or her message has been received and understood.

**Formal Organization**—The organizational structure approved by the governing body of a facility.

**Functional Authority**—A relationship in which one person has control over a function but not over the people who carry it out. He or she can instruct how a task is to be done but cannot correct errors or discipline. Individuals who are experts in a certain area (i.e., legal counsel, labor relations consultant) have this type of authority.

**Goal or Objectives**—The end result toward which all the organization activities are directed.

**Governing Body**—An individual or group of people who assume legal responsibility for establishing and implementing policies in the nursing facility. In a sole proprietorship, the governing body is the individual; in a partnership, it is the partners; and in a corporation, it is the board of directors.

**Grapevine**—An informal informative method of communication outside of the established formal structure of the organization.

**Guidelines**—A term referring to a plan of operations or standard.

**Hierarchy**—A theory of human motivation expounded by A.H. Maslow, which indicates that all workers have certain needs, ranging from psychological needs to self-actualization.

**Human Resource Planning**—A process by which a facility assesses its future needs and the ability of the staff to meet these needs.

**Informal Organization**—Loosely organized unofficial groups (such as a grapevine or a clique) that operate outside the formal structure.

**Levels of Management**—A facility's levels of management that are comprised of top, middle and line management.

**Line Authority**—An authority relationship in which a manager exercises decision-making supervision over subordinates.

**Management**—The process of achieving the goals of an organization through the work of its employees. It involves all personnel working together with the least amount of friction to accomplish the facility's goals.

**Management Information System** (MIS)—An organized way of providing the past, present and future information relating to the operation of the facility and the external environment in which it functions.

**Management by Objectives** (MBO)—A form of management in which objectives are clearly stated, planned and monitored toward attainment by the manager.

**Mission Statement**—A statement of the purpose and the objectives of a nursing facility.

**Motivation**—Encouragement for inducement to an employee to carry out the job tasks in the desired manner.

**Open Door Policy**—A policy whereby a supervisor allows any employee at any organizational level to come to him or her directly with problems.

**Organizing**—The grouping of people and activities to achieve goals or objectives. This function establishes the formal activities of an entity and defines formal lines of communication.

**Participative Management**—A management style in which employees take an active role in the decision making by giving input to the decision makers.

**Partnership**—An association between two or more persons to carry on as co-workers of a business for profit.

**Payer Mix**—A procedure by which the residents are categorized by source of payment (such as Medicare, Medicaid, private pay).

**PERT**—A program evaluation and review technique to monitor how the parts of a program fit together in event and time.

**Planning**—A basic function of management that determines the objectives and the course of action to attain these goals.

**Policy**—A broad guide to thinking and decision making.

**Positive Reinforcement Problem Solving**—The reinforcement of positive behavior by rewards (such as praise or recognition) or approval to promote and build employee morale.

**Procedure**—A plan that provides a series of tasks in the necessary order to perform specific designated work.

**Principle of Exception**—A management principle that states that recurring decisions should be made at the lowest level of the organization. Only the unusual or exceptional decisions are brought to the attention of higher level management.

**Program**—A comprehensive type of plan that brings together a group of varied plans.

**Public Relations Function**—The process of communicating a positive image of the facility internally among employees and externally among the community and other health care providers.

**Responsibility**—The creation of an obligation on the part of a subordinate to the supervisor for the satisfactory performance of assigned duties.

**Rule**—A specific demand for action that has no exceptions.

**Risk Management**—A program established by administration as a means of anticipating problems and protecting the facility by insurance or other preventive measures.

**Scalar Chain**—A type of organizing that shows different levels of management from the top echelon to line workers.

**Span of Management**—The number of employees the manager can effectively supervise.

**Staff Authority**—A person with expertise in a specific area gives advice and recommendations to the decision makers but cannot enforce decisions or discipline employees.

**Staffing**—The function of management concerned with recruiting, selecting, training, orienting, promoting and demoting. Its purpose is to fill the different positions in the facility with qualified individuals.

**Standards**—The goals, policies or procedures to use as a guideline for employee performance and behavior.

**Strategic Planning**—A process used to reevaluate the facility's mission, identify long-term goals and select the strategies to carry out these goals.

**Tactical or Operating Planning**—The process of selecting and evaluating short-term goals (less than one year).

**Theory X and Y**—Human behavioral theories developed by Douglas McGregor. They state that a manager's style reflects his or her assumptions about people. Theory X is autocratic and assumes that work is distasteful and unsatisfactory. Theory Y assumes that workers enjoy their work and are self-directed to a great extent.

**Theory Z**—This theory was developed by William Ouchi and is based on the assumption that trust, long-term goals and incentives will encourage employees to cooperate with each other.

**Total Quality Management** (TQM)—A relatively new participative management method aiming toward continuous quality improvement which is based on mutual respect and open communication among employees and management. This concept is to build employee interrelationships through work teams.

**Two Factory Theory**—A theory developed by F. Herzberg based on dissatisfying (hygiene) factors and satisfying (motivating) factors. It states that people who are dissatisfied with their work associate the negative feelings with their work environment, and that people who are satisfied with their work associate the positive feelings with the nature of their work.

**Unity of Command**—An employee has one superior to whom he or she reports for direction.

## LEGAL TERMS

**Abuse**—In regard to resident abuse, this term refers to ill treatment by coarse, insulting words or harmful acts.

**Advanced Directive**—A written instrument (such as any living will or durable power of attorney for health care) given by a competent adult to his or her agent to become operative in the event of incapacity or incompetency.

**Affidavit**—A written or printed declaration or statement of facts made voluntarily and confirmed by oath or affirmation of the party making it, usually before a notary public.

**Agent**—A person authorized by another to act for him or her.

**Aggrieved**—A person who has suffered a loss or injury.

**Assault**—An intentional tort threatening bodily injury and creating fear or apprehension to another.

**Assignment**—Transfer of rights of real or personal property to another person.

**Battery**—An unlawful touching of another without that person's consent.

**Cause of Action**—A personal action suing another usually for liquidated damages or money.

**Civil Law**—That law dealing with actions between private parties where a government subdivision is not a party.

**Claimant**—One who claims or asserts a right, demand or claim.

**Code of Federal Regulations** (CFR)—A publication containing codified laws, rules and regulations of federal agencies. Title 42 CFR Part 430 to end, for example, concerns Medicare and Medicaid requirements for long-term care facilities.

**Competent**—One who is legally fit and has mental capacity to understand the nature of his or her act.

**Complainant**—One who signed a complaint in a criminal lawsuit.

**Common Law**—That body of law which derives its authority from usages and decrees of the courts.

**Contract**—An agreement between two or more persons.

**Corporate Negligence**—A breach of duty owed to a person by a business entity.

**Criminal Charge**—Concerns violation of a criminal statute.

**Criminal Law**—That body of law in which the parties to an action involve the violation of a criminal statute.

**DNI**—Do not intubate.

**DNR**—Do not resuscitate.

**Damages**—A money compensation recovered in the courts by any person who has suffered loss or injury. Liquidated damages are the amount of damages as determined by a judgment or a specific sum of money agreed to by the parties. Punitive damages are those relating to the punishment of a defendant for a willful, malicious or intentionally fraudulent act, or for outrageous conduct.

**Decedent**—One who has passed away; used in law of wills and estates.

**Deed**—A written conveyance of title, duly notarized, from one person to another.

**Defamation**—Libel or slander; an untrue statement injuring the character or reputation of another.

**Deposition**—Testimony of a witness under oath; for use in legal proceedings.

**Durable Power of Attorney**—A written instrument authorizing another to act as one's agent on his or her behalf, which becomes effective when he or she becomes disabled.

**Durable Power of Attorney for Health Care**—A legal document where the principal appoints an agent to make all types of health care decisions if and when the principal becomes incapable of making them. A health care proxy is used in states where there are no laws covering durable power of attorney for health care.

**Estate**—All real or personal property in which one has an interest of ownership.

**Executor**—A male person appointed under a will to administer an estate of the decedent.

**Executrix**—A female person appointed under a will to administer an estate of the decedent.

**Felony**—A crime punishable by a prison term of one year or more.

**Fraud**—An intentional false representation to deceive another so that he or she shall act upon it to his or her legal injury.

**Holographic Will**—A will that is handwritten, dated and signed by the one making the will.

**Incompetency**—Lack of legal ability to understand the nature of one's act.

**Independent Contractor**—One who is personally liable for his or her negligent acts.

**Informed Consent**—An agreement allowing something to happen (i.e., medical treatments, medical procedures or surgery) based on full disclosure of facts, risks or alternatives.

**Intestate**—One who dies without a will.

**Invasion of Privacy**—An intentional tort violating the right of privacy.

**Law**—A set of rules and principles established by a governing body.

**Legal Guardian**—A person appointed by a court to handle the affairs of one who is incompetent.

**Legacy**—A disposition of personal property under a will.

**Liable**—Having the responsibility to compensate a legal wrong to another.

**Libel**—A written form of defamation.

**Lien**—An encumbrance upon personal or real property.

**Living Will**—A document that gives precise instructions directly to one's physician, directing the life sustaining treatment to be received or not be received in the event of a terminal illness or condition and inability to participate in medical decisions.

**Malpractice**—A negligent act by a professional.

**Misappropriation of Property**—Term used in OBRA 1987 relative to the stealing of resident's personal property. There must be specific intent to steal, not the mere negligence of handling the property.

**Misdemeanor**—A lesser criminal act usually punishable by one year or less in a county prison.

**Negligence**—Omitting to do an act that a reasonable prudent individual would do under the same conditions and circumstances.

**Negotiation**—An act settling or arranging terms of a transaction.

**Notary Public**—A public officer who administers oaths.

**Personal Representative**—A person appointed by a testator to carry out the directions and requests in his or her will and to dispose of the property accordingly.

**Plaintiff**—One who brings an action at law.

**Power of Attorney**—A written instrument authorizing another to act as one's agent.

**Privileged Communication**—A communication that is privileged or confidential such as between physician and patient, husband and wife, lawyer and client, clergy and penitent.

**Probate Law**—Law that deals with wills and estates.

**Public Law**—Law involving a government subdivision such as criminal, administrative or constitutional law.

**Respondeat Superior**—A form of vicarious liability, meaning "Let the master respond for the acts of his or her agents."

**Seizure**—To forcibly take possession of property.

**Slander**—A form of oral defamation.

**Statute of Limitations**—The time period in which an action must be started.

**Subpoena**—An order from a court directing a person to appear before the court in a legal proceeding.

**Subpoena Duces Tecum**—An order from a court directing a person to produce documents in his or her possession.

**Subrogation**—Substituting one person for another with reference to a lawful claim, demand or right.

**Summons and Complaint**—The initial documents required to start a lawsuit.

**Theft**—Taking of property without owner's consent. Popular name for larceny.

**Testator**—One who makes a will.

**Tort**—A private or civil wrong or injury.

**Trespass**—An unlawful entry upon the property of another.

**Uniform Anatomical Act**—An act concerned with the giving of one's organs at the time of death.

**Vicarious Liability**—Holding a person or entity liable in monetary damages for the negligence of another.

**Noncupative Will**—An oral will declared by the testator in his or her last sickness before a sufficient number of witnesses and later reduced to writing.

**Probated Will**—A will that has been admitted to probate by a court.

**Reciprocal Will**—One in which two or more persons make mutual provisions in favor of each other.

**Self-Proved Will**—Self-proved by affidavit of attesting witnesses, eliminating the need for the witnesses to appear in court.

## MARKETING & PUBLIC RELATIONS TERMS

**Competition**—Rivalry between similar/same businesses seeking to sell products and/or services.

**External Audience**—Refers to those people (physicians, social workers, clergy, families, hospital discharge planners) having contact or potential contact with the facility.

**Internal Audience**—Refers to those people within the facility (i.e., residents, employees, medical staff, consultants).

**Market**—A geographical area of demand for services or products.

**Market Diversity**—Refers to the various needs or groups of needs within a given market.

**Market Opportunity Analysis** (MOA)—An organized system for identifying and assessing the market for a particular product or service.

**Market Segmentation**—Recognizes and pinpoints the various groups and their unique needs within the market.

**Marketing/To Market**—The selling of goods or services by the producer to the consumer.

**Marketing Research**—Basically involves formation of questions regarding a potential market, collecting relative facts, analyzing these facts and proposing a plan of marketing.

**Measuring**—A study to determine present and future needs of a potential market.

**Molding**—Formulation of a concise marketing message.

**Monitoring**—Checking the effectiveness of the marketing program.

**Public Image**—Reputation or general view or impression held by the public relative to areas such as function, quality or costs of a particular business or industry.

**Public Relations** (PR)—Developing reciprocal understanding and goodwill between the facility and the public.

**Referent Analysis**—Examines the role of intermediaries (such as physicians, social workers, hospitals) referring people to the long-term care facility.

**Strategy**—A careful plan or method to accomplish specific goals.

# CHAPTER 4

# Personnel Management

## PERSONNEL DEPARTMENT

The personnel function in the nursing facility exists whether the facility has 20 beds or 200 beds. A basic decision the administrator must make is if this department will be a full-time or a part-time function. If the facility is over 150 beds, it is probably advantageous to set up a full-time personnel department. In a smaller facility, the personnel function may be combined with another staff (rather than line) authority position. Some may use the administrator's secretary as a personnel assistant because of the open communications in this instance. Other possible combinations include: personnel director–purchasing agent, personnel director–office manager, personnel director–public relations.

### Role and Function of the Personnel Department

The general functions of the personnel department include the interpretation of policies established by the governing body and implemented by the administrator; employee recruitment and training; and the administration of a wage and salary program. It should be clearly understood that the relationship of the personnel function to the department heads is advisory. The personnel director can do much of the preliminary screening and recommend applicants to the appropriate department head, but he or she does not make the final decision to hire.

### Qualifications of the Personnel Director or Assistant

An important consideration is that this person enjoys working on a staff level behind the scenes. Usually a person who desires the limelight and wants credit for innovation is better qualified for a line position. The person for this job must have tact and salesmanship, enabling him or her to gain the confidence of the line department heads by pointing out that he or she functions on a staff level to assist them and not to run their departments.

As a major communications link between the employees and the administration, the personnel director or assistant needs to be familiar with basic human relations elements. Personnel problems are important because 65% to 70% of a health care facility's cost is reflected in personnel. The personnel director must be interested in people, have a good sense of humor after a tough day, and have the confidence and respect of the employees at every level of the organizational structure. Previous experience in the health care field is not an absolute prerequisite, but it is helpful because the organizational structure of a health care facility is quite different from other corporate structures.

## PERSONNEL POLICIES

Every health care facility must have written personnel policies established and ratified by the ownership or board of directors (in a corporation) to be implemented by the administrator. A good set of such policies has a positive effect upon human relations, deters union activity, and protects the facility from unjustified unemployment compensation claims by employees. A copy of the personnel policies should be distributed to each employee in the facility and used extensively throughout the organization.

### Federal and Case Law Requirements for Personnel Policy Procedure

The Code of the Federal Regulations (42 CFR Part 430 to end 10/1/98) spells out the following as to personnel policies and procedures. The facility must have written policies and procedures that support sound resident care and personnel practices and address:

1. Control of communicable diseases.
2. Review of employee incidents and accidents to identify health and safety hazards.
3. A safe and sanitary environment.
4. Personnel records that are current, available to each employee and contain sufficient information to support placement in the position to which assigned.
5. Referral or provision for periodic health examinations to ensure freedom from communicable diseases.

Generally, no documentation of information concerning religion, politics or arrests and convictions should be made when the latter are related to an individual's job. Some states, however, now are requiring a criminal record check before employment.

Personnel records must be kept confidential. An employee handling these records cannot discuss their contents with anyone except as authorized by the administrator. These records need to be kept under lock and key, and made available only to authorized staff (such as personnel record clerk, supervisor, individual employee or administrator).

Personnel records are an objective source of data for making decisions on personnel matters. They may be checked by Occupational Safety and Health Administration (OSHA), Equal Employment Opportunity Commission (EEOC), wage and hour divisions of state and federal departments of labor, state licensing and certifi-

cation agencies and other appropriate authorities requiring that certain data be kept in personnel files.

### Items in Personnel Policies

Some basic items to be included in a good set of personnel policies are:

1. Definitions of terms used in the policies.
2. Wage and salary administration.
3. Vacations.
4. Leaves of absence (see below).
5. Sick leave.
6. Death in the family.
7. Military absence.
8. Jury duty.
9. Employee selection, preference to present employees.
10. Grievance procedures.
11. Rights of probationary and temporary employees.
12. General policy as to training with or without pay.
13. Policy regarding review for pay increases.
14. Lay-offs and unemployment compensation (see below).
15. Termination, nature of termination and terminal pay.
16. Discrimination.
17. Employee benefits (see below).
18. Employee health services, pre-employment and annual physicals.
19. Relationship between employee health status and job performance (see below).

### Family Medical Leave Act of 1993

The act provides that the employer must grant up to 12 weeks of leave a year to eligible employees:

1. for the birth, adoption or foster care of a child
2. to care for a spouse, child or parent with serious health conditions
3. for a serious illness, preventing performance of job functions

The leave is without pay, but the employee does not lose time or benefits and must be reinstated to his or her job upon return. To be eligible for family medical leave, the employee must have worked at least 1,250 hours during the past 12 months. This includes any part-time worker employed as much as 60% of the time. This leave may run concurrently with a worker's compensation leave.

### Unemployment Compensation

All employees who participate in the Social Security Act are eligible for unemployment compensation when laid off by the employer. Normally, unemployment compensation is available for up to 26 weeks through the state employment agency if the worker agrees to accept any suitable comparable work offered through the agency. Unemployment compensation is funded by the Federal Unemployment Tax (FUTA) and paid totally by the employer in most states. This tax is based upon the wage of each employee. A separate record is kept for each employee. Once the nursing facility has paid the required revenue, its rate of taxation is reduced. Employers with the fewest unemployment claims will have the best rates. It is important that the nursing facility documents discharge of employees accurately and follows prescribed disciplinary procedures in order to successfully refute unemployment compensation claims.

### Workers' Compensation

Workers' compensation helps pay for injuries to a worker who is hurt on the job. In most states the workers are paid a percentage of their wages while recovering from injuries. The cost of hospitalization and medical care are covered under this law. Employers with good safety records pay less than those with large claims.

### Employee Health Status and Job Performance

A facility that maintains programs implementing employees' health will be more successful in having good job performance by the employees. Close compliance with OSHA (see Chapter 2) will go far in ensuring adequate performance by employees. The administrator and department heads must pay careful attention to the laws concerning the health status of its employees and make sure these laws are properly implemented in the facility.

### Establishing Personnel Policies

Who makes personnel policies? The establishment of personnel policies is a board or ownership function. However, a great deal of work is accomplished usually by the administrator before these policies are ready to present to the governing body. The personnel director may advise the administrator and department heads concerning the policies. However, neither the personnel director nor other department heads should write the policies. The administrator and other key individuals have the total picture in mind; individual department heads tend to take into consideration their particular departments only. Personnel policies can be compiled several ways:

- The **administrator writes the policies** and submits them to the governing body for approval. This procedure for writing the personnel policies would be used by an administrator who is autocratic and management policies. He or she is the kind of administrator who centralizes most of the decision making with himself or herself and, therefore, feels impelled to make the policies on the basis of what he or she feels is best for the organization before submitting them to the governing body. In a small facility, this type of procedure may be used extensively. However, it is not considered a good one from the human relations or psychological viewpoint of dealing with employees.

- The **administrator appoints a committee** composed of the personnel director (if one is employed), the comptroller and other department heads to write policies and to submit them to him or her for review. The administrator then presents the policies to the governing body for final approval. This involves committee meetings by two or three of the key personnel given the responsibility of writing the personnel policies. One of the problems with this procedure is that other employees in the organization may feel that they are being slighted when not asked to participate in such an important aspect of the operation of the nursing facility. Personnel policies should be written with all personnel in mind and with what is best for those personnel. Therefore, this procedure is not recommended; those not involved may perceive that the administrator shows favoritism toward certain key personnel and is not interested in obtaining the ideas of other employees in the organization.

- The **administrator asks the department heads and other key personnel to submit ideas with regard to personnel policies**. In this procedure, the ideas are recorded and discussed to get participation of as many employees as possible at a series of meetings of department heads, supervisors and staff personnel. The ideas then are incorporated into a final set of personnel policies. This procedure is recommended because it involves participation of all personnel in the organization. The actual writing of the policies can be accomplished by a committee appointed by the administrator or by the administrator personally. After they are completely written and have been reviewed by all interested personnel in the organization, the administrator then will present the policies to the board of directors or the ownership for approval and ratification.

To remain effective, personnel policies must be reviewed constantly to reflect changes in employee requirements and federal and/or state statutes and regulations.

### Publicizing Personnel Policies

Good personnel policies are a vital part of the operation of the nursing facility. Once written, it is important that they be communicated to employees and other interested persons. Some ways the personnel policies may be publicized are:

- **Personnel Handbook**—These may be handed out to personnel when hired and/or during orientation to the facility and its policies. Questions can be answered at once and possible misunderstandings cleared up before becoming future problems.
- **Use of a House Organ or Internal Publication**—If the facility publishes a monthly or quarterly newspaper that is distributed to employees and other interested persons, the new policies or changes in personnel policies may be featured in a news article. Some nursing facilities publish a small leaflet as a means of keeping employees, physicians and others informed on what is happening.
- **Memorandums**—Memorandums clearly and precisely written are excellent mechanisms for publi-

cizing new or revised personnel policy changes. These memorandums may be distributed to department heads to hand out to employees or may be placed in with the employees' paychecks. The latter method may be used where department heads either misplace or do not remember to distribute the memos—particularly to the employees on the night shifts.
- **Meetings with Department Heads, Key Personnel and Staff**—Personnel policies may be publicized by holding meetings with department heads, key personnel and staff. Any questions regarding the new or changed policies can be discussed and clarified immediately.
- **Women's Auxiliary**—Personnel policy changes may be publicized by informing the auxiliary of the changes. Some of the members of the women's auxiliary are active in the community and communication of such policies may enhance public relations.

## SAMPLE PERSONNEL POLICIES OF PRAIRIEWEED NURSING FACILITY

### History of Nursing Facility

A history of the development of the nursing facility, how it came about, what physical facilities it has, and a mission statement concerning the purposes and objectives of the facility are covered in this section.

### Welcome

(This paragraph may include a message to the personnel indicating their importance to the operation of the nursing facility.)

Many positions in a nursing facility do not involve direct resident contact; however, it is only through the satisfactory performance of each employee, regardless of his or her particular duties, that we can achieve our goal of efficient quality care for all residents. Regardless of what you do in the facility, your job is important. You are the Prairieweed Nursing Facility to our residents and their visitors. The impressions you create in dealing with the residents and the people with whom you work establish the reputation of our facility.

Prairieweed Nursing Facility believes in the policy of nondiscrimination regarding race, color, creed, national origin, sex and political affiliation.

You will want to know what the Prairieweed Nursing Facility offers you as an employee and what the facility will expect of you in return. It is for this reason that this handbook has been prepared. We look forward to a constructive and harmonious working relationship with you.

## Terms Used in Personnel Policies

**Administrator**—The chief executive officer of the nursing facility. He or she is responsible to the governing body for the coordination of all activities in the facility.

**Department Head**—An individual who is in charge of an official department of the nursing facility.

**Permanent Part-Time Employee**—An employee who regularly works 20 hours or more per week.

**Permanent Employee**—An employee who has been appointed to a position, and who has successfully completed the probationary period.

**Probationary Employee**—An employee who is serving the probationary period of six months, or one who is put on probation by reasons of disciplinary action.

**Reinstated Employee**—An employee who is returned to active employment following an authorized leave of absence. Such an employee will retain his or her rate of pay, seniority and all employee benefits that he or she had accrued prior to a leave of absence.

**Rehired Employee**—An employee who was formerly employed and who did not take a leave of absence but is reemployed as a new employee subject to all rules and policies of a new employee.

**Seniority**—Refers to a period of continuous employment.

**Supervisor**—An individual who is given administrative responsibility within the organization.

**Temporary Employee**—An employee who is appointed for a limited period of time. The duration of employment is fixed in advance and in no instance may exceed six months.

## Administration

(In this section it may be wise to outline the role and function of administration. Following is a sample paragraph to be used as a guideline.)

The administrative offices are established and maintained to be of service to the employee. Its aim, a simple one, is the satisfaction of mutual needs—the individual needs as an employee and the needs of the nursing facility.

The personnel office or the person handling personnel functions is a part of the administrative office and its functions include conducting initial interviews, reference verification and, in some instances, testing. The personnel office does not hire or fire. These decisions are in the hands of the department heads with the approval of administration. This office has the necessary forms to organize and maintain a system of centralized personnel files able to give ready analysis of personnel records, wage increases, promotions, transfers or terminations.

Through the administrative offices, the uniform employment policies, regulations and practices established by the Prairieweed Nursing Facility will be related and interpreted to facility employees. The administrative staff will work to keep the employees informed about nursing facility activities, policies and regulations through the use of handbooks, bulletins and the facility newsletter.

## Outline for Grievance Procedure

Employees should feel free to discuss any problem with their immediate supervisors. Supervisors are encouraged to refer an employee to a department head whenever they feel they have not satisfactorily helped with the problem. In any event, employees should feel free to directly approach the next highest level of management whenever they fail to achieve the satisfaction with their immediate supervisor. The administration has final and complete responsibility for the overall operation of the nursing facility; their decisions are binding. The employee can be assured of fair and impartial consideration.

## Benefits at Prairieweed Nursing Facility

(The employee benefits given have a real dollar cost to the facility and a real dollar value to the employee. Typical benefit programs may run from 18% to more than 65% of the payroll costs.)

### Health Program

Continued good health is the concern of all co-workers and each resident who enters the Prairieweed Nursing Facility. A preemployment physical examination is required. The laboratory tests and the chest X-rays will be done at the expense of the facility. To aid in a positive health program, complete annual physical examinations are required within three months of each employee's birthday. A physical examination form is sent prior to the birth month.

### Workers' Compensation

Employees are covered by insurance for injuries incurred while at work. In order to benefit from this insurance, a written report of the incident must be made by the employee and given to the supervisor or delegate within 24 hours. (If the nursing facility has a health nurse, a statement should be made here that any employee needing treatment during the day should report to the health nurse.)

### Cafeteria

The cafeteria service schedule is posted in the cafeteria where attractive meals are served to all employees. Employees bringing their lunches may eat in the cafeteria.

### Rest Period

Two 15-minute work-rest periods (one in the morning and one in the afternoon) are provided during an 8-hour work period.

### Sick Leave

One day per month with pay is allowed for illness effective after 6 months continuous employment. The nursing facility reserves the right to require medical verification of illness. Payment will be withheld for ill days taken during the last month of employment that is not substantiated by a physician's statement. If an abnormal amount of absenteeism is incurred by an employee, he or she may be asked to have a complete physical examination; the advice of the physician will be sought with regard to further employment. Indis-

criminate use of sick leave has a decided effect on personnel consideration for promotion.

(If the nursing facility has a policy with regard to accumulation of sick leave, this may be put into this paragraph, indicating what that policy is and whether or not sick leave may be accumulated. The customary practice is to allow a liberal amount of accumulated sick days.)

### Leave of Absence

After one full year of employment, a leave of absence not to exceed six months may be granted without loss of accrued benefits. Types of leaves of absence are illness, maternity, education or special. During any leave of absence, benefits will not accrue. Upon returning from leave, the employee may be offered a position for which he or she is qualified and will be given an opportunity to return to his or her former position if and when the position is open.

Leave of absence is also granted for up to 12 weeks to those eligible under the Family Medical Leave Act.

### Absence Due to Death in the Family

In case of death in the employee's immediate family (father, mother, sister, brother, husband, child, father-in-law or mother-in-law), the department head or his or her delegate should be notified immediately. The department head or delegate must notify the personnel office in writing of such a situation. Absence of 3 days with pay will be granted to the bereaved employee. This benefit is effective after six months of full-time employment.

### Absence Without Pay

Absence without pay may be approved by the department head for up to 10 days leave granted for urgent personal business. The department head or immediate supervisor must be notified prior to the absence. Three consecutive days of absence without proper notification or previous planning will result in automatic dismissal. Additional time may be granted upon approval of administration.

### Paid Vacations

(The length of paid vacations is contingent upon the customary practice in the community or particular part of the state. The vacations outlined in this policy are prevalent in the area in which this nursing facility is located.)

After 6 months full-time employment, an employee will be eligible for 1 week of vacation with pay; and after a full year of employment, 2 weeks with pay. Vacations are earned in accordance with the following schedule:

1. 2 weeks (10 working days) after 1 year of regular full-time service.
2. 3 weeks (15 working days) after 5 years of regular full-time service.*
3. 4 weeks (20 working days) after 10 years of regular full-time service.*

*Vacations in excess of 10 days will be arranged at the discretion of the department head.

### Terminal Vacation

Upon termination, with required notice, those who have been in the service of the nursing facility for at least 6 months will receive vacation pay earned. Terminal vacation is that which is earned from the last anniversary date. It will be added to the final earnings check, except in case of failure of an employee to give proper notice of termination or of dismissal for cause.

### Holiday Pay

Seven holidays with pay, or a day in lieu of each, are granted to full-time employees who have completed 6 months of regular service. These are: New Year's Day, Memorial Day, Independence Day, Labor Day, Veteran's Day, Thanksgiving Day and Christmas Day. Absenteeism before or following a holiday must have prior approval of the department head.

### Continuing Education (In-service Education)

Ongoing programs are being developed for all departments. The planned orientation for each new employee is to help meet job requirements. An in-service training program is conducted for ward clerks, aides and orderlies. Each employee is reimbursed for meeting time if off duty when the class is held.

### Employee Health Insurance

The nursing facility encourages all full-time and permanent part-time employees to enroll in the facility insurance plan unless covered by their own insurance. The insurance coverage for employees may be with Blue Cross or commercial insurance companies. If an employee wishes to take a family plan, that single benefit cost is paid by the nursing facility and the difference between the single benefit plan and the family plan is paid by the employee. Under OBRA, a terminated employee may continue with the facility's insurance carrier for up to 18 months, if the employee pays the premium.

(A decision should be made by administration as to whether the full premium of insurance will be paid for the employee or whether a part of the premium will be paid. A customary practice is to pay the full single benefit of insurance premium.)

### Jury Duty

If called for jury duty, an employee must notify the department head as soon as possible. Time will be granted for this service. If the jury pay is less than the salary at the nursing facility, the difference will be paid by the facility. The employee is asked to bring the check for jury duty to the payroll office and arrangements will be made for reimbursements.

## Also at Prairieweed Nursing Facility

### Solicitation Protection

To protect the employee from solicitation, raffles, charity drives and so on, employees are strictly prohibited from soliciting other employees, residents or visitors without the approval of the administrator on any matter while on nursing facility business. Violation of this policy will subject an employee to possible dismissal.

### Service Awards

Service award pins are presented to employees during the year. The length of service is determined by using the last date of hire as of January 1 of each year. Pins are awarded for 5, 10, 15, 20, 25, 30 and 35 years of continuous service.

### Chapel

A chapel is on the premises. Clergymen of the various faiths are frequent visitors. Religious services are conducted in the chapel regularly. The time of services is posted at the chapel entrance. Employees desiring to take advantage of these services should make their requests known to their immediate supervisors. Whenever possible, employees will be privileged to participate in such services on their own time. The chapel is open and available to employees, visitors and residents.

### Suggestion Box

The purpose of the suggestion box is to provide a systematic means for employees to communicate to management their constructive ideas to decrease costs, save time, improve the operating efficiency and quality of the nursing facility, and provide a way for these ideas to be evaluated and publicly recognized for their worth. All employees are eligible to submit suggestions. A cash prize, letter of recognition and certificate will be presented to the employee submitting an outstanding suggestion. All suggestions must be signed by the employee submitting the idea.

### Wage and Salary Policy

Basic salaries are based on job classification and wage scales within the state. Minimum and maximum pay scales are developed for each classification. Six months after the date of employment, each employee will be reviewed by his or her department head and a recommendation made concerning a pay increase (based on job performance and/or cost of living). Thereafter, subsequent job review and pay increases will be considered annually and may be given during the month of February of each subsequent year.

### Pay Day

Employees are paid for actual hours on a weekly [or biweekly or monthly] basis. Pay day is every Friday. To allow for sufficient time to prepare the payroll, any hours worked in the week prior to pay day are not included in that paycheck but will be included in the following paycheck.

The withholding tax, Social Security and health insurance premium payments will be deducted from the first check issued during the given month. Withholding tax, Social Security and any group life insurance will be deducted from the second check. An employee with a question concerning his or her paycheck should consult the department head or payroll office.

### Overtime

Time and a half is paid for overtime after 8 hours in one day or 40 hours in a 1-week period. All overtime must be authorized by the department head and approved by administration.

## Employee Rules and Regulations

### General Appearance and Deportment

All employees are required to be neat, clean, proper in appearance, courteous and orderly at all times while on the premises. The use of intoxicating beverages while on duty is absolutely forbidden and will be grounds for immediate dismissal.

### Smoking

Smoking is permitted only in designated areas. All other areas are smoke-free.

### Confidential Information

The release of confidential information by an employee to anyone concerning the diagnosis, treatment or care of a resident or another employee without authorized consent will be considered a cause for dismissal.

### Parking

Parking facilities are provided, and employees are urged to use the area designated for them.

### Wage Garnishments

Wage garnishments are costly to the nursing facility. Any frequency of wage garnishments may be taken into consideration at the time of the evaluation of the employee.

## *Tardiness*

Habitual tardiness will be cause for termination of employment.

## *Absenteeism*

Employees may be interviewed upon return to work. Any employee who is absent for three consecutive days without the proper notice to his or her department head is considered to have quit without notice, and employment is terminated.

## *Signing In and Out*

Each employee is responsible for accurately punching his or her own time card in and out on the cards provided. The nursing facility will pay wages only for time shown on the time card. An employee signing in or punching a time card of another employee will be considered to have breached the rules and regulations of the facility and may be subject to dismissal.

## *Political Activities*

The nursing facility does not endorse political activities on the premises.

## *Identification*

Identification badges are issued to all employees by the personnel department. Employees are required to wear their badges in plain view at all times while on duty. A charge will be made for the replacement of lost identification badges. The loss of a badge must be reported immediately by the employee to the personnel department.

## *Accidents and Safety*

In the interest of protecting residents, visitors and employees from injury due to accidents, prescribed safety rules and common safety practices shall be observed by employees at all times. All accidents, no matter how minor, must be reported to the supervisor immediately. An incident report must be filed and signed within 24 hours and submitted to the administrator's office.

## *Bulletin Boards*

Bulletin boards are provided for the purpose of passing on information to all employees. In order that erroneous or otherwise undesirable information not be posted, only official nursing facility notices may be routinely posted on them. Other notices or material must be approved by administration prior to posting.

## *Theft and Destruction of Property*

Of necessity, the nursing facility is open 24 hours a day. Employees, therefore, are urged to be alert for the entry of unauthorized persons. If anyone is seen who does not appear to be an employee, or who may be outside his or her regular working area, he or she should be offered assistance in reaching his or her destination. Employees shall refrain from abuse, theft, deliberate destruction of or tampering with the property and equipment of the facility, fellow employees, residents and visitors. Violations must be reported to the supervisor immediately.

## *Uniform*

Uniforms are to be worn only during an employee's tour of duty.

## *Moonlighting*

Because outside remunerative operations might affect health or quality of work at the nursing facility, employees must have the approval of the department head.

## *Discipline or Employee Performance Standards*

(It is of primary importance that the facility have a clear and concise statement on how it will suspend or discharge an employee for violations of the policies, procedures and/or rules of conduct.)

Some of the common reasons for discipline in a health care facility are tardiness (most common), excessive absences, disorderly conduct, abusive language, use of alcohol or drugs during work, fighting, possession of firearms, theft or breach of confidentiality of resident records. Disciplinary action may be taken when an employee disregards a procedure or rule or fails to respond to repeated corrections of errors. Such discipline is geared to change or modify employee behavior from unacceptable to acceptable. Employees will be reprimanded in private and praised in public. Forms of discipline include:

- **Oral Reprimand**—A verbal warning given to an employee to modify or terminate certain forbidden behavior.
- **Written Reprimand**—Conducting a formal conference with the employee. The meeting and results are documented, dated and signed by the immediate supervisor and the employee. It is kept as part of the employee's personnel record.
- **Docking Pay**—A reduction of the 8-hour work personnel pay by the number of moments or hours the employee has failed to work.
- **Suspension**—The employee is forbidden to work for a specified period of time (days or weeks) possibly without pay.

### Termination of Employees

An employee who intends to resign from his or her position is required to give adequate advance written notice to the department head. Adequate notice is considered to be two weeks for staff personnel and one month for department heads.

On termination of employment, all benefits are automatically discontinued and cannot be applied in the case of rehiring. An employee, who has one full year of service and whose employment record has been satisfactory, may at the discretion of the department head be rehired within six months at the salary on record at the time of termination. A terminal interview will be requested of all employees.

### Dismissal or Termination for Cause

The nursing facility reserves the right to dismiss an employee for a violation of professional conduct. Violation of the policies, rules and regulations may result in firing an employee from his or her job on a permanent basis. If an employee's work is unsatisfactory, he or she will be informed of this by the department head or delegate and encouraged to improve.

(It is of primary importance that the employer apply discipline without discrimination. Discipline must be applied equitably and without any partiality on the part of the supervisor, department head or administrator.

Employment security officials and EEOC prohibit discrimination.)

The use of progressive discipline where a verbal warning is followed by a written warning is highly recommended. Many employers lose lawsuits relating to unemployment compensation for fired employees because of failure to adequately document progressive discipline in the personnel file of the employee involved. A record should be made documenting that each employee received a copy of the personnel handbook explaining the policies and rules of the facility; each employee should sign a statement and indicate the date that he or she received a copy of these policies.

### Telephone Calls

Telephones within the nursing facility must be kept free for the facility business. Public telephones for use of residents and visitors are at various locations throughout the premises. If it is necessary to make a call while on duty, ask the supervisor for permission to do so. Personal calls are discouraged while at work, except in instances of real necessity.

## WORK ENVIRONMENT

Human relations among employers and employees is an important consideration in accomplishing the goals of both the facility and the employees. Good communications among the administrator, supervisors and staff will help create a positive work environment and good relationships.

## Promoting Communication

Communication has a direct bearing on the quality of resident care by enhancing morale, quality of work, productivity and well-being of employees. The attitude and behavior of both the administrator and personnel director are important to maintaining the self-esteem and motivation of the staff. Employees need to know the employer is interested in their concerns, as well as those of management. Each seeks to contribute important services and work accomplishment, to receive recognition and reward for effective efforts and time, to be involved in decision making and to part respect from peers.

### Supervisor-Employee Relationships

The following are guidelines for creating a positive work environment and facilitating the process of communication between all staff and the business management:

- **Keep Employees Informed**—If a change in policy or procedure occurs, the changes should be communicated to directly affected employees as soon as possible.

- **Provide Job Recognition**—This is one of the most important non-financial incentives. The recognition of the job an employee is doing and of his or her accomplishment will contribute to a positive feeling on the part of the worker.

- **Listen to the Employee**—Every worker wants to know that he or she is being listened to. Employees enjoy expressing themselves, especially when superiors take the time and effort to listen attentively.

- **Maintain Accessibility and Availability of the Supervisor**—Maintaining a schedule of employee meetings and conferences with an attempt to receive input from the employees is very helpful in enhancing employer-employee relationships, allowing the employees to air problems and express opinions.

- **Create a Relationship of Trust**—The relationship between supervisor and employee should be premised upon the basis of trust. Mutual obligations should be created when promises are made. Fair treatment and respect for the human dignity of the employee are parts of this trust relationship.

- **Promote Based Upon Quality of Work**—When considering a promotion for an employee, take into consideration not only the length of employment but also the special skills and attitude of the individual and relate these to the quality of work. This sends a message that quality work is rewarded.

- **Provide the Best Wages and Working Conditions Possible**—This topic is covered extensively in the review of personnel policies in this chapter. Good wages and environment encourage employees to stay on the job.

- **Sponsor Facility Social Events**—Establishing events such as a bowling team, golf team or other sports activities and facility-sponsored picnics or outings with participation by management, staff and their families may give the employer and employee a chance to associate with each other in a new atmosphere.

### Newsletters

Another important communication tool that the administrator may use is an informative newsletter. Usually the facility publishes a newsletter on a monthly basis to report interesting activities concerning the residents and the facility and to recognize the accomplishments of its employees, staff and volunteers. Well-written and properly constructed, a newsletter can help promote public relations with both the employees and community.

### Employee and Facility Goals

Part of maintaining a positive atmosphere in a facility is the resolution of possible conflicts between the goals of the facility and the goals of the employee. The overall goals of the facility should be clearly stated in the mission statement and general policies, outlining the broad functions and purposes of the organization. Each departmental policy should then carry out its specific goals and relate them to the overall organizational goals.

Each employee has certain personal goals he or she wishes to achieve. These goals often are reflected in work attitude. Employees with positive personal goals generally will perform a better job. A.H. Maslow pointed out the goals of a typical employee:

1. Satisfaction of physical needs (food, clothing or shelter).
2. Safety and security (from physical harm or tyranny).
3. Social acceptance (love and acceptance by others).
4. Self-esteem (respect and recognition by peers).
5. Self-actualization (realizing one's full potential).

### Counseling

Some of the larger facilities employ specially trained persons to counsel employees regarding personal growth and job performance. Career counseling is geared to help an employee reach his or her optimum level of performance and competence.

### Grievance Procedure

An established grievance procedure is one way an employer can effectively communicate with employees. Employees should be given an opportunity to discuss their problems with their supervisor and the administrator of the facility. A grievance procedure is the outline or procedural guideline on how the employee should communicate with the supervisor. Usually, several steps are involved:

1. The employee who has a complaint or grievance speaks with his or her supervisor within a certain time period. This time period may be 1 to 5 days after an incident occurs. The immediate supervisor should make a written record of the meeting, including the date, time and place of the meeting.
2. If the employee is not satisfied, he or she will reduce the complaint to writing and submit it to the next highest level in the organizational structure (most likely the department head).
3. If the employee still is dissatisfied, he or she may submit the appeal to the administrator. The administrator will make a decision after listening to both sides of the complaint. Generally speaking, the administrator's decision is final. In some facilities, the employee may appeal the administrator's decision directly to the board of directors or to a committee of the board. However, the final decision making should be rested in the administrator from the viewpoint of effective management.

## RECRUITMENT AND INTERVIEWING OF STAFF

Staffing essentially is finding the right person to fill each job in the facility. Job duties and qualifications are determined and job descriptions written to assist with obtaining the levels of staffing required to provide quality services to the residents. Many government regulations (Health Care Financing Administration [HCFA], EEOC, OSHA, state, etc.) apply especially to the numbers required and qualifications of professionals and para-professionals in health care facilities. The administrator must determine the basic types of staff needed (nursing, physicians, social workers, therapists, dietary and others) and the numbers of personnel needed in each category relative to his or her facility's resident needs and size. Present and future needs due to such factors as expansion of the facility and services, employee turnover, and changes in regulations are included in such forecasts.

### Staffing Plans

The administrator must utilize a master staffing plan to assist in drawing up an accurate operating budget and to plan and control effectively. Each department establishes a department staffing plan indicating the number and titles of jobs to be filled. The master staffing plan gives the number and titles of all jobs in the facility and the current annual salaries. It also indicates which positions are filled and which need to be filled during the coming year.

### Manpower Inventory

Used in conjunction with the staffing plan, the manpower inventory will help identify employment needs. The more the census varies in a facility, the greater the need to review manpower requirements. Monthly, weekly or daily manpower inventories are referred to variable periodic staffing plan reviews.

### Recruitment

#### Recruitment and Interviewing Techniques

These techniques include media advertising, applications and interviewing. Health care facilities participating in Medicare and Medicaid must adhere to the ethics mandated by federal guidelines and law. Both the Fair Labor Standards Act of 1968 and Title VI of the Civil Rights Act of 1964 prohibiting discrimination on the basis of race, color or national origin are very important in these areas.

#### Sources of Recruitment

A facility may use a variety of sources in obtaining personnel including:

- **Present Employees**—Present employees may be a good source of personnel. If there is good morale among employees, some may be pleased to recommend applicants when they are aware of openings. Some facilities offer a small bonus to employees who bring in an acceptable applicant, usually paid after the new employee has completed a probationary period of several months. However, social cliques may develop, and discipline may be undermined because of family ties or friendship.

- **Door Applicants**—These constitute the greatest number of applicants and rejections. This is probably the poorest source of recruitment of new personnel because, although there is face-to-face contact, very little screening has been accomplished prior to the interview. This may be a good source of entry level areas (such as housekeeping or kitchen staff).

- **Public Employment Agencies**—In the smaller towns, this may be a valuable source of recruitment for nonprofessional positions where applicants are of higher quality and better known. In urban areas, sometimes those who register with public agencies are not of the highest caliber and are not looking for long-term employment, properly trained or screened by the agency.

- **Private Employment Agencies**—These may be excellent sources of recruitment, especially for professionals where an agency has a large field specific pool to draw on to match openings and qualifications. The private employment agency realizes that to remain in business, a good job of selection must be done. Usually the employment counselors are specialists who are able to judge both the needs of the person seeking the job and those of the employer. An important service of the private employment agency is the screening of applicants and the checking of their references. Ordinarily the applicant is obligated to pay the fee directly to the employment agency. In those job areas where the supply is limited and the demand is great, it is customary that the employer pay the employment fee.

- **Newspaper Advertising**—Placing ads in the classified ad section is a customary way of recruitment. Creativeness and innovation are the keys to good classified ad recruitment. The writing of classified ads should comply with various federal regulations and Title VI. Generally, ads may not specify age, sex, race, religious preference or national origin. Placement should consider what type of personnel is needed. Advertising for nurses may be placed in urban areas where there are nursing training schools. Nonprofessional personnel advertising can be placed in large and/or small community newspapers. Wording can help somewhat to reduce the number of unqualified persons who may apply for an opening.

- **School and College Placement Bureaus**—Professionally trained personnel may be obtained from this source although they may be lacking in work experience. Once experience is gained, this employee may seek upward mobility or move on.

- **Professional Trade Journals**—Ad advertisement in journals such as the *Nursing Journal* or *American Dietetics Association Journal* may reach the professional or technical person required to work in a health care facility. Although these ads reach a wide area, they are usually costly and require placement allowing for a planned open position and time to recruit and fill the position.

Other techniques of good recruitment or "tricks of the trade" include:

- **Recruitment Outside Traditional Working Hours**—In some areas, success in recruitment has been achieved during evening hours when workers are normally free to call for information.

- **Stressing Desirable Working Conditions and Job Titles**—Point out the environmental factors, liberal fringe benefits, good salary.

- **Use of Bulletin Boards**—A list of vacancies posted on the bulletin board may be helpful to those looking for advancement in the same organization, but may pose a problem when it is necessary to say no to a present employee.

- **Recruitment from Special Groups**—Consider recruitment among older workers, handicapped workers or part-time workers (housewives or students).

### Interviewing, References and Employee Documents

The use of a well-constructed application form and good techniques of interviewing are very important in determining the suitability of prospective employees for the facility. Pre-employment tests, interviews and employer references are tools that can be used to measure the applicant's "can-do" or verbal skills. The interview is one of the most effective methods of obtaining desired detailed information about an applicant. The "will-do" or nonverbal skills (motivation, quality of work, commitment to the facility's goals and objectives) are more difficult to measure.

## Application Blank

Proper composition of the application blank will provide a great deal of information to the staff regarding the applicant. This form should be printed on quality paper, inclusive without being too long, and conform with federal and state laws regarding the questions that may or may not be asked. Questions that may be asked include: name, address, telephone number, education, special job training, licenses, experience, references, citizenship, felony convictions and health as it relates to the job. Questions that may not be asked include: age (except under 17 or over 70), birthplace, race, color, religion, marital status, arrest record, sex, height, length of residence and welfare benefits.

## Interviews

Two types of interviews are used: a **preliminary** interview intended to screen out those who are clearly not suitable for the position when the applicant completes a short questionnaire and is interviewed briefly, and an **in-depth** interview when the applicant completes a formal application and is afforded a significant amount of time to determine suitability.

Whether the interview is preliminary or in-depth, it must be conducted so that civil rights and other federal laws are not violated. Federal guidelines suggest that the interviewer may cover the following questions: legal name, present address, age requirement suitability, citizenship, convictions for specific crimes, education, organizational memberships, personal references, work scheduling, health as related to the job and current licenses if required.

The interviewer may not ask questions concerning: titles that refer to sex, color, religion, handicaps or national origin; foreign addresses; birth or baptismal records; race; birthplace; religious background or preference, references from clergy indicating religion, working religious holidays; sex; arrests; pregnancy; marital status; child care plans; or height and weight unless related to the job.

Note that applicants may volunteer information of any type. Once an applicant is hired, much of the excluded information may be included in the personnel records, and a photograph may be obtained if necessary.

## Interviewing Techniques

Either a nondirective or structured interview may be conducted by a person who has a working knowledge of the job requirements. The interviewer should describe the job duties to the applicant. In a nondirective or open-ended interview, the interviewer seeks to avoid influencing the applicant's answers, allowing maximum freedom to ask questions and give information. This allows the applicant to answer questions subjectively and gives the interviewer insight as to the applicant's values, feelings and attitudes concerning the job opening. In a structured interview, specific questions are asked usually in an exact order. Such questions allow little freedom, and the applicant's answers are precise, objective and will give specific information pertinent to the job opening.

## Matching Job Qualifications with Job Requirements

The clinical approach and the statistical approach are two basic methods for matching job qualifications with job requirements. In the clinical approach, the interviewer reviews all information about the applicant and decides whether or not to hire him or her. In the statistical approach, applicants are screened using the predictors of success and then compared using appropriate formulas.

## Verification of Employment History

References are important in assuring the work potential of the applicant and in protecting the facility from corporate negligence. Prior work performance is an excellent indicator of success. Approval must be obtained from the applicant to check his or her references. The best source of reference is from previous employers and, in particular, from the immediate supervisor if the applicant has a work history. At least two references should be checked, preferably by telephone contact.

**Employee Documents**

Every facility participating in Medicare and Medicaid must keep in current form certain records of their employees. Some of the important documents include:

1. Completed application form.
2. Preemployment test results, reference checks, letters, calls.
3. Federal and state withholding forms.
4. Copies of incident and accident reports.
5. Illness and attendance records.
6. Training records.
7. Grievances.
8. Signature by employee relating to: receipt of personnel policies, warnings, job evaluation, and in-service and orientation training.
9. General health records including employee's physical history, copy of a recent physical exam by system and record of any chronic or infectious disease. Such records must be maintained *after* the employee has been hired.
10. General correspondence file.

## EVALUATION PROCEDURES

The administrator plays an important role in establishing and maintaining the employee performance evaluation program in his or her facility. Copies of the codes of ethics for nurses, physical therapists, dietitians and other professionals should be reviewed with these staff members and available for reference. Basic purposes of employee evaluations are to assist:

1. In creating and maintaining a performance level that is satisfactory to the employer.
2. Employees to grow and understand their strengths and weaknesses.
3. Supervisors and line managers to observe the behavior of subordinates.
4. Supervisors in using guidelines for promotion, transfer, layoffs and discharges.
5. In the administration of the wage and salary program.

The immediate supervisor completes the employee's evaluation form, which is then signed by both the supervisor and employee involved. The supervisor signs and makes a note of any employee's refusal to sign, if this is the case.

### *Analysis of Absenteeism and Turnover Rates*

One of the tools management has to measure the effectiveness of administrative procedures in the facility is the analysis of employee absenteeism and turnover rates. These are related to employee morale: high percentages of absenteeism and turnovers are indicators of low morale. Excessive absenteeism must be controlled and the reasons promptly determined. More than 35% turnover in a department is considered too high. Reasons for high turnover rates can occur when employees feel overworked and understaffed or where pay is low (turnover rates are lowest among higher paid employees).

### *Exit Interviews*

Establishing a mechanism for exit interviews will assist management in obtaining insight into employee attitudes. An exit interview gives an employee the opportunity to express himself or herself to the immediate supervisor or other member of administration in private concerning the reasons for voluntarily or involuntarily leaving the facility. This is particularly important to the administrator in the event of voluntary termination. Usually, employees will be honest and open about the reasons for leaving at exit interviews.

### Employee Performance Rating Scales

The principle kinds of rating scales for employee performance are personal traits and behavior, job dimension and behaviorally anchored rating. Rating scales are on a continuum where the rater places a mark along a numerical line or along steps ranging from excellent to poor. Some advantages of rating scales are: a required evaluation of employee performance, ease of use and understanding, and objective statistical information. The disadvantages are that the rating process is subject to the:

1. Halo effect, which is the tendency to let the rating assigned to one characteristic excessively influence the ratings on all subsequent traits.

2. Leniency error where the supervisor has a tendency to be liberal in rating and assigns high ratings constantly.
3. Strictness error where the supervisor consistently rates employees low.
4. Central tendency where the rater seeks to avoid conflict and will rate either high or low so that the ratings will meet in the middle of a continuum.
5. Interpersonal bias where personal feelings, likes or dislikes of the rater are expressed in the ratings.

### Personal Traits and Behavior Scale

Also referred to as the conventional rating scale technique, this scale is one of the oldest and most widely used of all appraisal methods. The rater (usually the employee's immediate supervisor) uses a printed form that contains a number of qualities and characteristics to be rated. For nonsupervisory personnel, typical qualities rated include quantity and quality of work, job knowledge, cooperativeness, dependability, initiative and attitude. For managers, some rating factors are analytical ability, judgment, leadership, creative ability and initiative.

### Job Dimension Scale

This technique requires that a different set of scales be constructed for each job or job family. The factors to be rated are taken from the job description and each task rated from excellent to poor in a straight-line continuum. For example, a job dimension for a nurse might include such tasks as renders first aid treatment, treats job injuries, keeps records of treatment and maintains inventory of supplies. Each item would be rated excellent, good, satisfactory, fair or poor.

### Behaviorally Anchored Rating Scales (BARS)

A separate rating form is used for each job family or dimension. Each job dimension contains 7 or 9 anchors that are specific statements illustrating actual job performance. In developing a BARS program, the following steps are suggested:

1. Identify the key job dimensions or areas of responsibility.
2. Ask the job holders and supervisors to describe desirable examples of job behavior.

3. Classify these examples under the various job dimensions.
4. Ask knowledgeable supervisors and department heads to rate each item of job behavior by assigning a number on a scale of 1 to 9; 1 indicating the lowest level of job performance and 9 the highest level.

### Job Evaluation

Four of the most important basic systems for evaluating jobs are:

- **Ranking or Job Comparison**—This system involves gathering descriptions for all jobs and ranking each job from low to high job requirements. It is used primarily in smaller companies.
- **Grade Description**—This also is known as the classification system and involves dividing the job hierarchy into a number of pay groups or grades. Written descriptions for each grade are developed and every job is then assigned to a particular grade.
- **Point System**—Under the system, job descriptions are prepared for each job in the organization. Each job is divided into factors (such as education, experience, training or judgment), and each factor assigned to a degree. Points are assigned to each degree: the more points, the more specialized the job. This system is most commonly used.
- **Factor Comparison**—This system is the next most popular method after the point system and is used for evaluating white collar, professional and managerial positions. A combination of the ranking and point system, it rates jobs by comparison. The jobs are divided into comparable factors and rated in terms of numbers.

### Wage or Pay Scale Evaluation

Several methods used to determine wage or pay scales are:

- **Increment Plan**—Under this plan, the employee receives a base pay at the time of hiring and receives raises periodically with or without merit reviews.

- **Seniority System**—Here the wage is dependent on how long the employee has worked in the facility.
- **Merit System**—Also referred to as the wage evaluation system, this method is based on the employee's performance.
- **Mixed System**—This combines the seniority and merit systems.
- **Job-Based System**—Everyone performing the same job receives the same pay.
- **Shift Differential**—The rate of pay under this plan is based upon the shift the employee works.

## STAFF DEVELOPMENT AND TRAINING

The health care facility administrator plays a vital role in assuring that adequate training is available for employees and that such programs are implemented and adequately assessed.

To properly implement this mandate of training, the administrator should designate a training director who will be responsible for the orientation and training of employees. One of the training director's first tasks is to conduct organizational, task and personnel analysis. The organizational analysis reviews the goals and policies of the facility; the task analysis examines each job performed; and the personnel analysis assesses employee skills. Such analysis will help identify and define employee weaknesses. Study of accident and incident reports, deficiencies identified by state and federal inspections, and operational problems encountered by department heads may assist in pointing out areas where training is needed. Good communication among the training director, department heads and administrator is very important in determining these training needs.

### Orientation Programs

The purpose of an orientation program is to enable new employees to carry out their work properly and provide information and guided adjustment to the facility and work environment.

Initial orientation should include:

1. A copy of the facility's mission statement, policies and practices.

2. An explanation of the organizational structure.
3. A copy of the personnel policies and explanation of the responsibilities of the employee to the facility and the facility to the employee and the rules of conduct.
4. A tour of the facility with introductions to key department heads and an explanation of the departments' relations to each other.
5. Review of fire and disaster procedures.
6. Review of confidentiality of information.
7. Information on the enforcement of residents' rights.

Job orientation is most effectively accomplished with the new employee's supervisor. This would include a detailed explanation of the job duties, the location of work materials and the importance of proper resident care and treatment.

### In-service and On-the-Job Training

On-the-job training is the most commonly used training technique and consists of assigning an employee to a staff member who assists him or her in learning the basic elements to adequate job performance. This method is appropriate for teaching knowledge and skills that follow a routine and can be learned in a relatively short time when only one or very few employees need such training. Supervisors teach acceptable employee conduct to non-professionals regarding facility policy, procedures and rules in such areas as resident dignity and rights, confidentiality and proper response to resident actions.

In-service training is usually group education carried out in a seminar type of setting within the facility. In-service training required in those facilities participating in Medicare includes the areas of infection control, confidentiality and fire safety. Such training is used to teach concepts, attitudes, theories, problems and depth of knowledge relating to various jobs. Relevant materials are available from educational catalogs for long-term care facilities. Liberal use is made of films, video cassettes and programmed instruction. Such teaching techniques include:

1. **Lecture**—A formal organized talk by an instructor to a group of students.
2. **Conferences**—Small group meetings that are conducted according to an organized plan in which

the instructor, as leader, seeks to develop knowledge and understanding by oral participation of the attendees.

3. **Case Study**—The presentation of actual case problems in which attitudes may be analyzed and their solutions discussed.

4. **Role Playing**—Used in conjunction with lecture or conferences. After being presented with written or oral instruction as to the situation, two or more trainees are assigned the roles to be played before the class. The problems and possible solutions are discussed.

5. **Programmed Instruction**—Used to teach factual information, such as mathematics, foreign language and job routines. The material is broken down into small units where the student gains immediate knowledge of each answer result. The instructor does not have a key role, and each student will learn at his or her own pace.

6. **Computer-Assisted Instruction**—Used to provide drill and practice to help the student learn material that is well structured (such as grammar, mathematics or reading). This is similar to programmed instruction.

7. **Simulation and Games**—Use of equipment and techniques that duplicate the actual conditions encountered on the job.

The effectiveness of training programs can be evaluated in several areas by several methods. A questionnaire passed out to trainees at the end of the program will indicate their opinion as to its worth. The knowledge or skill of each employee can be measured before and after the training. Indexes of work performance before and after such training will measure the program's effectiveness. One of the best methods is to measure performance before and after training for both a central group and an experimental group.

## LABOR RELATIONS AND LABOR LAW

Labor relations and labor law are important in the operation of a long-term health care facility. Two basic areas of labor law to consider are federal and state. Federal labor law is applied only when a federal court has jurisdiction under the United States Constitution. Interstate Commerce Commission (ICC) activity expands the role of the federal government in labor relations. State labor laws applied to those business activities that are intrastate (within the state). Labor laws relating to workers' compensation, child and female labor, and right to work are customarily handled by the state. If a state statute recognizes employees' rights to organize, bargain collectively and strike, broad language usually will extend these rights to state and municipal employees.

### Basic Labor Laws

In the early 1930s during the country's most severe depression, political pressure in Congress increased, and general dissatisfaction arose over judicial restrictions in labor relations. Federal labor laws were passed to protect civil rights and discrimination in three basic areas: protection of the employee's rights to organize, encouragement of collective bargaining and elimination of unfair labor practices.

#### Norris-La Guardia Act

In 1932, Congress passed the Norris-La Guardia Act (also called the Federal Anti-Injunction Act). The act allowed employees full freedom of association, self-organization, designation of representatives of their own choosing, negotiation of terms and conditions of employment, and freedom from employer interference, restraint or coercion. Further, it recognized employees' right to freedom from employer interference (i.e., wrongful use of injunctions) and their efforts toward self-organization and collective bargaining.

#### National Labor Relations Act (Wagner Act)

In 1935, Senator Robert Wagner, then chairman of the National Labor Board, led the fight for this act. It guaranteed the right of employees to join any labor organization and bargain collectively through representatives of their own choosing. The act also detailed specific employer unfair labor practices and created the National Labor Relations Board (NLRB) to enforce its provisions by determining appropriate bargaining units, supervising elections at the request of workers, certifying duly chosen unions, taking testimony about unfair employer practices, and issuing cease and desist orders. In 1937, the U.S. Supreme Court, following the case of *NLRB v. Jones & Laughlin Steel Co.* (301 U.S. 1), declared the Wagner Act constitutional.

## Taft-Hartley Act

Because of the tremendous growth and power of unions for the next 10 years, Congress in 1947 amended the National Labor Relations Act by enacting the Taft-Hartley or Labor Management Relations Act. The act reorganized the NLRB and included union unfair labor practices covering such topics as: closed shop, damages resulting from broken union contracts and/or strikes, 60-day cooling-off periods before strikes, the right to publish financial statements and political contributions, bargaining requirements, boycotts by unions not involved in a dispute, and strikes over work assignments.

## Landrum-Griffin Act of 1959

The Landrum-Griffin Act of 1959 was the result of a congressional investigation of the unions. This law provided for:

- **Union Member Rights**
  1. Equal rights with all members in voting and participating in union activities.
  2. Freedom of union members to express their opinions.
  3. A voice in proposed increases in dues.
  4. Protection against being fired or expelled from the union without a written list of charges.
  5. Freedom to sue, testify and communicate with any legislator without being limited by the union.
- **Elections**
  1. Elections must be by secret ballot.
  2. Members must have reasonable opportunity to nominate candidates.
  3. Members must have sufficient notice of elections.
  4. Voting for each candidate must be reported local by local.
  5. Elections must be carried out according to constitution and bylaws of the unions.
- **Union Reporting**
  1. Required by law to file copies of its constitution and bylaws with the labor secretary and to file annual reports on conduct of its internal affairs.
  2. Must also report in annual fiscal statement compensation to officers and employees of the union making in excess of $10,000.

- **Trusteeships**
  1. Control of a subordinate union by a parent organization can be established and administered only to correct corruption, ensure unions' duties as bargaining representatives are fulfilled, and ensure that union contracts are fulfilled.
  2. A parent union is prevented from usurping power and funds from a subordinate union.

## Protection Regarding Hours, Wages and Child Labor

## Walsh-Healy Act of 1936

This act applies to workers employed by firms that have government contracts in excess of $10,000. Penalties for infractions of the act can be fined up to $10,000 and/or six months in jail. Its two basic provisions are:

1. All work in excess of eight hours each day must be paid at time and a half.
2. Minimum wages based upon the prevailing rates in the community must be paid.

## Fair Labor Standards Act of 1938

The act has been amended many times. These amendments are highly technical and complicated. The 1968 amendment prescribes minimum wages and maximum hours (40-hour workweek) of employment, requires payment of time and a half for overtime, sets minimum age of 16 years for general employment, and requires employers to maintain records of hours worked and wages paid. Penalties for infraction of the provisions can be fines up to $10,000 and/or six months in jail. This act covers all firms or persons engaged in interstate or foreign commerce. It exempts executives, administrative personnel and professionals, farm laborers and domestic servants.

A section specifically addresses employment in hospitals and in establishments caring for the sick, aged or mentally ill. It generally provides that a work period of 14 consecutive days is accepted for purposes of computing overtime, if the employee and employer have agreed to this, and the employee receives overtime for more than 80 hours in any 14-day workweek.

An amendment to the act added a training wage (85% of the minimum wage) for new workers in non-agricultural jobs with less than 60 days of cumulative work experience.

### Equal Pay Act of 1963

This act is an amendment to the Fair Labor Standards Act. It prohibits employers from discriminating on the basis of sex in the payment of wages for equal work. Pay differentials may exist, but they must be justified on the basis of skill, efforts, responsibility, working conditions, seniority, merits or some other factor other than sex.

## Employment Discrimination

### Equal Employment Opportunity Act of 1973

This act amended Title VII of the Civil Rights Act of 1964 and prohibits any form of employment discrimination by companies, labor unions and employment agencies on the basis of race, color, religion, sex or national origin. The EEOC was created to provide enforcement procedures including investigations, attempts at conciliation and suits filed on behalf of the complainant.

### Vocational Rehabilitation Act of 1973 (Section 503)

This act requires holders of federal government contracts in excess of $2,500 to take affirmative action to employ and advance in employment qualified physically and mentally handicapped individuals.

### Age Discrimination in Employment Act of 1967 (as amended in 1978)

This act prohibits employment discrimination against those who are between the ages of 40 and 70, forbids forced retirement based on age before 70, permits compulsory retirement for executives who are entitled to pensions of $27,000 per year or more, and authorizes jury trials in certain cases.

### Social Security Act of 1935 (as amended)

This act establishes two national systems of Social Security for protection against loss of income due to unemployment, old age, disability and death:

1. Retirement services, disability insurance and health insurance for persons over age 65.
2. Unemployment insurance for persons over age 65 and unemployment insurance that operates under a state-administered, federal-state plan in which operating costs are paid by the federal government.

## National Labor Relations Board

The NLRB carries out the policies of the National Labor Relations Act. The board includes a five-member board and its staff; the general counsel and its staff; and 50 regional and field offices located in major cities. The board has two major functions:

1. Supervising and conducting representation elections.
2. Adjudicating employer and union unfair labor practices.

The NLRB activities are set in motion only when requested in writing and filed with the proper NLRB office. Such requests are called petitions in the case of elections and charges in the case of unfair labor practices.

### Procedure of NLRB Regarding Unfair Labor Practice

A charge is filed with the NLRB regional director by an employee, employer, labor union or individual alleging an unfair labor practice. The party charged is called the respondent and is notified that an investigation of the alleged violation will be conducted. If no settlement is reached, an unfair labor practice hearing is conducted before an administrative law judge, who makes findings and recommendations to the NLRB based on the record of the hearing.

All parties are authorized to appeal the administrative law judge's decision directly to the board. The board considers the information provided and the data collected. If it believes an unfair labor practice has occurred, an order to cease and desist such practices and to take appropriate affirmative action is issued. A cease and desist order directs the violators to stop whatever activities were deemed unfair labor practices.

The board exercises some discretion in determining appropriate affirmative action by issuing such orders to employers and may direct them to:

1. Disestablish an employer-dominated company union.
2. Offer employees immediate and full reinstatement to their former positions and pay them back their wages with interest.
3. Upon request, bargain collectively with the exclusive bargaining representative of the employees.

Unions may be directed to:

1. Refund excessive or illegally collected dues plus interest.
2. Upon request, bargain collectively in good faith with the prescribed employer.

### Federal Courts and NLRB Proceedings

The U.S. District Courts under the enforcement provisions of the act serve two major purposes: to provide injunctive relief by issuing a temporary restraining order (TRO) where appropriate and to review appealed decisions and orders of the NLRB. A U.S. Court of Appeals may enforce an order upon reviewing the orders of a U.S. District Court, return it for reconsideration, alter it or set it aside. The final appeal is to the U.S. Supreme Court.

### Health Care and NLRB

The NLRB's jurisdictional standards relating to the health care industry (as of July 1, 1976) apply to privately operated health care institutions such as hospitals (with at least $250,000 total annual volume of business); nursing facilities, visiting nurses associations and related facilities (at least $100,000 total annual volume of business); and all other types of private health care institutions (at least $250,000 total annual volume of business). The statutory definition includes "any hospital, convalescent hospital, HMO, health clinic, nursing facility, skilled nursing facility, or other institution devoted to the care of the sick."

## UNION ORGANIZATION

One of the prime considerations of the nursing facility administrator regarding labor relations in the nurs-

ing facility is the reasons why employees in a facility would want to organize. Generally speaking, employees unionize due to poor supervision, job dissatisfaction, or a lack of good employee benefits and personnel policies that are clearly written and distributed to all employees. Poor policies in this area that are improperly communicated can lead to problems of inconsistent treatment of personnel, misunderstandings, unrest, rumors, jealousy and high turnover. Personnel policies should include an explanation of the facility's standard wage program, vacations, paid holidays, sick leave hospitalization benefits, funeral leave, grievance procedures, promotion policies and discipline procedures as a minimum. These should be reviewed and updated periodically to remain competitive in the area. Administrators need to be familiar with personnel policies and benefits being paid in their own areas and throughout the state.

Internal communication is of prime importance as well. If a lack of communication exists, employees may not feel part of the team, be insecure in their jobs or feel that no outlet is available for grievances. Suggestions for improving communications include:

1. Regular monthly department head meetings with the administrator.
2. Regular department head meetings with employees.
3. Publication of an internal "house organ" or newspaper.
4. Use of suggested programs for input by the employees.
5. Recognition programs where outstanding employees are identified and given public recognition.

## Representation Election Procedure

### Campaign Initiations

Union organizing campaigns usually start at the "grassroots level" of employees. Either the workers themselves ask the union to help, or union organizers identify a facility with problems and get in touch with the workers by handbill or personal contact. The vital first step is to establish a two-way communication between the facility employees and the union. Next comes the educational process in which the union points out employees' problems, compares wages at their facility to wages at unionized facilities, and explains the role of the union in helping to satisfy their job-related needs (see Exhibit 4–1).

The union will make every attempt to convince the workers to complete union authorization cards and to support the forthcoming organizing campaign by wearing union buttons, attending meetings and signing up others. Some of the most effective ways to do this are one-to-one contact, peer contact, persuasion and high-quality professionally designed written communications.

### Filing a Petition for Election

The procedure for unionization is started when the potential bargaining representative for the employees files a petition with the NLRB for an election where the employees in a bargaining unit will vote on whether a union will represent them. The NLRB is authorized to conduct an election only when such a petition has been filed by an employee, group of employees, any individual or labor organization or an employer. If filed by an employee or on behalf of employees, the petition must be supported by evidence (usually by authorization cards) that a substantial interest in union representation exists (30% of the bargaining unit). Further, it must show that the employer has denied a request by the union to recognize it as an employee representative.

After receiving a petition, the NLRB will promptly notify the facility and request a list of employees; a facility is not required to submit a list of employees but usually will comply as an act of good faith. Next, the NLRB will arrange a conference with the facility and union to discuss the possibility of a "consent election." Here, if both sides agree to the appropriate bargaining unit, voter eligibility, ballot, and time and place for the election, a consent election will be held. If either party refuses to agree on any of these items, a formal hearing to settle these matters will be requested and conducted.

### Election Investigation and Hearing

If the union and management officials do not agree to a consent election, the NLRB must investigate the petition, hold a hearing if necessary and then direct an election if it finds there is a question of employee representation. Some of the questions to be answered by the investigation include:

1. Does the board have jurisdiction?
2. What is an appropriate bargaining unit?
3. Does substantial interest in representation (30%) exist among employees in the unit?
4. Are there any barriers to an election in the form of existing unions, prior elections or present labor agreements?

---

**Exhibit 4–1** Union Solutions to Employee Problems

| | |
|---|---|
| Desire for improvement of present fringe benefits | Negotiate better benefits for bargaining unit employees |
| Earns less than deserved compared to others doing similar work | Emphasize comparable wages (local, regional, national), provide data from other unions, Department of Labor and wage surveys |
| Desire for additional fringe benefits | Negotiate new benefits, such as dental insurance or legal aid |
| Difficult to get work days and hours changed | Negotiate work schedule procedures with rules and policies that are administered fairly and in accordance with the contract |
| Inadequate time for leisure activities | Attempt to obtain shorter hours and workweek, more holidays and longer vacations for time worked |
| Skills underutilized in present job | Negotiate promotion policies and procedures |
| Unpleasant work environment | Negotiate working conditions and transfer opportunities, institute safety and health committees |

### Appropriate Bargaining Unit

The bargaining unit is a grouping of jobs or positions in which two or more employees share common employment interests and conditions, and which is eligible for union representation and to bargain collectively. Determination of the appropriate bargaining unit is left to the discretion of the NLRB. The NLRB's determination of a bargaining unit strongly influences whether the union will win the election. Therefore, the composition of a bargaining unit is of vital importance to nursing facility administrators. A bargaining unit may include registered nurses (RNs), professional employees, technical employees such as licensed practical nurses (LPNs), service and maintenance employees (such as housekeeping or dietary) or office and clerical staff.

The NLRB's discretion has been somewhat limited by the fact that professional employees cannot be included in a unit composed of both professional and nonprofessional employees unless a majority of the professional employees vote to be included in a mixed unit. Agricultural laborers, public employees, independent contractors, supervisors and managers are excluded from bargaining units.

Under the National Labor Relations Act (NLRA), the term supervisor means any individual having authority in the interest of the employer: to hire, transfer, suspend, layoff, recall, promote, discharge, assign, reward or discipline other employees. Supervisor also means having responsibility to direct such employees to adjust their grievances, or to recommend effectively such action if, in connection with their jobs, the exercise of such authority is not of routine or clerical nature, but requires the use of independent judgment. The importance of supervisory status is that supervisors are not "employees," within the meaning of the act, and have no right to vote in elections for determination of bargaining representatives. As expected, times arise when the question of whether an employee is a professional, a supervisor or perhaps not either is very close.

In the case of *University Nursing Home, et al.* (168 NLRB 53), the employer sought to exclude an LPN from a bargaining unit composed of housekeeping, kitchen and maintenance employees on the basis that she was a professional employee. The NLRB never specifically determined the LPN's status as a professional person, but instead found that the nurse was a supervisor and as such was to be excluded from the housekeeping bargaining unit. The board noted that the practical nurse was in charge of one of three wings that comprised the facility, supervised the work of three nurses aides and one orderly, carried out orders and treatments prescribed by residents' doctors, reviewed residents' charts to make certain that proper medications and diet had been given, and observed and reported symptoms to the head registered nurse.

### Eligibility of Voters

Usually those employees on the payroll just before the date of the elections are eligible. There are exceptions made to allow employees who are on sick leave, vacation, temporarily laid off or on temporary leave to vote in the election.

### Administration's Dos and Don'ts During a Union Organizational Drive

Administrators often learn of union organizing attempts from department heads or from rank and file employees and through actual observation before they receive the official notification (by letter or telegram) from the union demanding recognition. Some facilities react violently; others do little to acknowledge any union attempt to organize the employees. Some administrators may tell their employees about their opposition and urge them not to sign union authorization cards.

Generally, the employer should not intimidate or retaliate against employees who are interested in working with a union. It is recommended not to:

1. Ask employees for an expression of their thoughts about a union or its officers.
2. Prevent employees from soliciting union members on their free time on company premises, as long as the literature does not interfere with the work being performed by others.
3. Threaten loss of jobs, reduction of income or discontinuance of any privileges or benefits presently enjoyed by the employees.
4. Use intimidating language that may be designed to influence an employee in the exercise of his or her right to belong or refrain from belonging to a union.
5. Threaten or actually discharge, discipline or layoff an employee because of his or her activities on behalf of the union.

6. Ask employees whether they intend to sign a card.

7. Discriminate against employees actively supporting the union by intentionally assigning undesirable work to the union employee.

8. Exhibit conduct that would indicate to employees they are being watched to see if they are participating in union activities.

9. Promise employees an increase in pay, a promotion or any special favors or benefits if they stay out of the union or vote against it.

10. Suggest to employees that they will be discharged if they work for the union.

11. Urge employees to try to persuade others to oppose the union or to stay out of it.

Generally, the employer has the right to deal honestly with staff, give correct information, and express opinions as to why the facility does not want to deal with a union. It is recommended that the employer may:

1. Inform the employees of the disadvantages of belonging to a union, outlining such things as the loss of income because of strikes, the requirements for them to serve on a picket line, the expense of having to pay dues, and the expense of fines and assessment.

2. Tell employees that the nursing facility prefers to deal directly with them rather than through an intermediary or the union organization.

3. Point out to the employees the pay and fringe benefits they now enjoy.

4. Let employees know they are free to join or not join the union, and, that if they do join, the facility will not be prejudiced against them.

5. Express opinions regarding unions and union leaders, even though those opinions may be uncomplimentary. However, it should be very clear that these are just the employer's personal opinions.

6. Inform employees about any misleading statements or any statements considered to be untrue or a misrepresentation that have been issued to employees by a union organizer.

7. Tell employees that if the union belongs to an international union, the probability will be that the international union will try to dominate the local union.

8. Layoff, discipline or discharge any employees for cause as long as such action is the customary practice and there is no discrimination between union and nonunion members.

9. Tell employees that no union can make a company agree to anything it does not wish to or pay any more than it is willing or able to pay; that all clauses in a collective bargaining agreement must, in fact, be agreed upon by both parties to the agreement.

10. Let employees know how their wages, benefits and working conditions compare with other nursing facilities in the area.

11. Relate to employees any experiences the employer may have had with unions.

### The Representation Election

The election to determine whether the majority of the employees in an appropriate bargaining unit want to be represented for collective bargaining purposes is conducted by NLRB officials within 45 days of the petition filing. Usually the voting draws up to 90% of the eligible voters. Using a ballot with the appropriate company and union designations, a secret ballot election usually is conducted under NLRB supervision during working hours at the employer's location. The majority rules. The act defines majority as a simple majority rule—50% plus one vote of those voting. If the majority votes "no union," no representation election can be held for 12 months. If the union receives the majority of the votes, the NLRB will certify it as the exclusive bargaining agent of the employees in the bargaining unit. After the votes have been counted, either party has five days to file objections alleging misconduct or to challenge the ballots of voters that one party believes should not have voted in the election.

### Duties of the Exclusive Bargaining Agent and Employer

The bargaining representative chosen by the majority of the employees in the appropriate unit has the duty to represent equally and fairly all employees in that unit. The employer has a comparable obligation to bargain in good faith with the exclusive bargaining agent and to refuse to bargain with another union seeking to represent the employees.

### Decertification Procedures

Whenever employees believe that the union is not representing the interest of the majority, a decertification procedure is available. Any employee, group of employees or an employee representative may file a petition for a decertification election 12 months after the union has been certified or upon expiration of the labor agreement, not to exceed 3 years. The facility cannot petition for a decertification election; however, they can question the union's majority status and petition the NLRB for a representation election.

## Labor Agreements and Collective Bargaining

If a union is successful in obtaining representation, the next step in the labor negotiations process is the collective bargaining agreement. The National Labor Relations Act imposes mutual obligations on the facility and the union to bargain collectively.

### Collective Bargaining Agreement

A bargaining team consisting of nursing facility and union representatives is established, and an initial meeting is scheduled with the union to establish procedures and proposals to be included in the labor agreement. Available collective bargaining agreements relating to similar health care facilities in its area are reviewed. All activities that take place are recorded. The facility usually first negotiates nonmonetary items (such as recognition, management rights, grievance procedures, union rights, seniority rights, arbitration agencies and subject matter). It then considers monetary items (such as wages, vacations, paid holidays and sick leave). Other subjects negotiated include compensation of employees on union committees during negotiation periods (not a facility responsibility), composition of the bargaining team (including members of the employee committee representing the union not on facility bargaining team), time and frequency of future meetings, and settlement of disputes. State statutes usually provide that the preferred method of resolving labor disputes between nursing facilities and their employees is through voluntary negotiation.

### Administering the Agreement

Once the labor agreement has been negotiated, great care must be given to its execution; facility rights established at the bargaining table may be lost if the contract is haphazardly administered.

Unions generally administer labor agreements within the facility through "shop stewards." Stewards are employees who are either appointed by the union or elected by fellow employees to supervise the labor agreement on behalf of the union. Employees turn to their departmental steward or to the facility's "chief steward" for advice about whether or not to file a grievance to protest an alleged contract violation. If a worker is called by a department head for an interview, which the employee believes may result in disciplinary action, the employee has the right to insist upon the presence of the union stewards.

Top administration must assure that its own representatives understand the significant aspects of the agreement. Department heads who are unaware of the central aspects of the agreement may unintentionally violate unions' rights, and the contract may thus be eroded. One of the best ways to communicate the terms of a newly negotiated labor agreement to the key personnel in the facility is through an extensive in-service training program. The problem of discipline is of singular concern. Quite often department heads believe that workers may not be discharged under a collective bargaining agreement. To deal with this misconception and to assure that discipline is administered for appropriate reasons, department heads need to be trained in the use of progressive discipline.

### Notice Requirements

The NLRA includes notice requirements that must be satisfied before a contract can be modified or terminated:

1. The act requires that the party seeking the change must give written notice at least 60 days prior to the time that the agreement expires, or if there is no expiration date, 60 days prior to the time it desires to make such termination or modification.
2. If no agreement is reached within 30 days, the party wishing to terminate or modify the agreement must notify the Federal Mediation and Conciliation Service (FMCS) that a labor dispute exists. The service will help mediate the dispute if called by one of the parties to do so.

## Subject Matter of Negotiations

The NLRA requires parties to bargain over the subjects within the three broad categories of:

1. **Wages**—Shift differentials, severance pay and rents for facility owned housing.
2. **Hours**—Number, length and hours of a shift, and length of workday.
3. **Other Terms and Conditions**—Price of food in facility cafeteria, work loads, union access to the premises, management rights, promotions and compulsory retirement.

Subjects falling within these categories are called the "mandatory" or "statutory" subjects of bargaining; it is illegal for either party to refuse to negotiate about them.

Subjects that fall outside mandatory categories are known as "permissive or discretionary." Although they are not legally bound, the parties may bargain over these subjects. It is illegal to precondition agreement negotiations upon a permissive subject or to bring negotiation to an impasse because of insistence upon a permissive subject. Furthermore, it is illegal for a union to strike or for management to lock-out employees because of a disagreement over a permissive subject.

## What is Bargaining in Good Faith?

The most subtle and complicated requirement of the NLRB is that parties negotiate in good faith. The NLRB defines the obligation to bargain in good faith as: "The performance of the mutual obligation of the employer and the representative of the employees to meet at reasonable times and confer in good faith with respect to wages, hours, and other terms and conditions of employment." Both the NLRB and the courts have said that a good faith attitude is one that has an open mind and a sincere desire to reach agreement. Although one ingredient of good faith bargaining is willingness by each party to discuss the other's proposals, mere discussion is not enough. "Surface" or "shadow" bargaining is where one party engages in extensive discussion, but never reaches agreement on anything. Tactics designed solely to delay negotiations may violate the act.

The failure to reach agreement or to make a concession is not bad faith bargaining. However, unwillingness to reach common ground on any significant issue may be viewed "in totality of the circumstances" or in combination with other factors (i.e., evidence that party lacks good faith).

The facility is not helpless in collective bargaining when the parties reach an impasse. It is entitled to "lock-out" employees in order to compel a union to accede to management's position where mandatory subjects are involved in the negotiations. From a practical viewpoint, a facility rarely will lock-out its employees.

## Duty To Furnish Information to a Union

The duty to furnish necessary information to a collective bargaining representative is made clear by case law and the NLRB. The fundamental general principle is that a facility must furnish a union, upon request, sufficient information to enable it to bargain intelligently and police the administration of an existing agreement. However, the duty to supply information is not absolute. A facility is not required to supply information on wages, hours or other conditions of employment merely because of union request; the union must show that the requested information is relevant to the bargaining process or to the administration of the agreement.

Compliance with a request for relevant information by a union must be made promptly. Whether a delay in the furnishing of the requested information is so unreasonable as to constitute unlawful refusal depends upon the individual facts of the situation. In one case, the NLRB held that a two-month unexplained delay in providing relevant information was unlawful.

## Unilateral Changes

The duty to bargain is a continous obligation. If the facility seeks to make a substantive change in the agreement, such change must be negotiated with the union before it is implemented. An impasse is the inability of the parties to agree upon one or more issues. When an impasse has been reached, the duty to bargain is suspended. The facility is then free to make unilateral changes consistent with its offers to the union. The union may waive its rights to bargain about certain issues.

## Strikes, Picketing and Secondary Activity

Some state statutes are clear in allowing strikes to occur. Before the passage of the NLRA in 1935, strikes and other job-related acts were governed solely by state laws (with the exception of the Federal Anti-Injunction Laws). Although most state laws did not expressly prohibit strikes by employees, neither did they expressly permit strikes, and frequently a facility could persuade the state courts to enjoin a strike. The NLRA now protects the right of employees to engage in "concerted activities," including the right to "a concerted stoppage of work by employees" or strike.

Employees may engage in three types of strikes: primary economic, unfair labor practice and recognitional. The NLRA requires labor organizations to give written notice to health care institutions and the FMCS at least 10 days before engaging in any strike, picketing or other concerted refusal to work. The union is guilty of an unfair labor practice if it fails to give this notice.

### Economic and Unfair Labor Practice Strikes

Two major kinds of lawful strikes are economic and unfair labor practice. Under the NLRA, strikers retain their "employee" status while on strike. However, a striker's rights to reinstatement to a job may depend on whether the strike is economic or unfair labor practice.

An **economic strike** usually concerns wages, hours or working conditions. When employees engage in a lawful primary economic strike against the facility, they may not be disciplined or discharged because they have engaged in such activity. The facility may replace them either temporarily or permanently, because it must continue to operate. Economic strikers are generally disenfranchised for 12 months after a strike begins. Economic strikers who have been temporarily replaced are generally entitled to reinstatement at such time as they make an unconditional offer to return to work. Economic strikers who have been permanently replaced are not entitled to automatic reinstatement when the strike is over. They do not lose status as "employees." They must be placed on a preferential hiring list and offered reinstatement when future vacancies arise, unless they refuse an unconditional offer of reinstatement after a strike is over, abandon the job or have been discharged for serious strike misconduct.

An **unfair labor strike** is one that protects a facility's labor practices. Unlike economic strikers, unfair labor practice strikers have a legal right to reinstatement and may not be permanently replaced. The facility must reinstate them upon their unconditional application for reinstatement, even if their jobs have been filled. An unfair labor practice striker is entitled to vote in any election held at any time.

### Illegal Strikes

Certain strikes are unlawful because their purpose is illegal or because the means used during the strike are illegal and are not protected under the NLRA. Employees who participate in an illegal strike are not protected by the NLRA; they will lose their employee status. They may be discharged with no right to reinstatement and are ineligible to vote in any representation election. Examples of strikes that are illegal or unprotected under the NLRA are:

1. Sit-down strikes where strikers remain on the facility premises and refuse to leave after being instructed to do so.
2. Strikes not complying with notice periods outlined in the NLRA.
3. Partial or intermittent strikes or slow downs.
4. Strikes with illegal aims.
5. Work assignment strikes.
6. Strikes in violation of a "no strike" clause in a collective bargaining agreement.

### Picketing

Picketing is the act of patrolling by one or more persons of a place related to a labor dispute. Picketing may be conducted by employees or nonemployees. Like strikes, some picketing may be subject to regulations.

The 1974 amendments to the NLRA added requirements with respect to strikes and picketing in an attempt to reduce the interruption of health care services. The Board of Inquiry was created and is called in if a dispute threatens to interrupt health care in a particular community. This board is appointed by the FMCS director within 30 days after notification of either party's intention to terminate a contract. The board investigates and reports its findings of fact and recommendation for settlement within 15 days. Once the report is filed with FMCS, both parties are expected to maintain the status quo for an additional 15 days.

A 90-day notice must be given to the facility by the union prior to the expiration of a collective bargaining agreement, and a 60-day prior notice to the FMCS.

## *Remedies for Illegal Strikes and Picketing*

Peaceful strikes and picketing are subject to regulation exclusively by the NLRB and the NLRA. Violent strikes and picketing are subject to regulation both by the NLRA and by the state courts. Violent strikes are primarily police matters that are left to the states. Only peaceful strike and picketing activity is federally preempted. The facility that is confronted with a violent labor dispute has a number of options. It may:

1. Seek an injunction and damages from a state court.
2. File an unfair labor practice charge under the NLRA.
3. Request the NLRB to seek an injunction from a federal court.
4. File a criminal complaint if criminal statutes are violated.

Although a facility may find it difficult to secure injunctive relief in the federal courts, such relief is available if a union violates a "no strike" clause of a collective bargaining agreement, which contains mandatory grievance and arbitration procedures. An injunction is an order issued by a court directing that a certain act be done or not done. Persons failing to comply with court orders are in contempt of court and may be subjected to fines or imprisonment.

## BIBLIOGRAPHY

Allen, J.E. 1992. *Nursing home administration*, 2nd ed. New York, NY: Springer Publishing.

Beach, D.S. 1985. *Personnel—Management of people at work*. New York, NY: Macmillan.

Code of Federal Regulations, Title 42, Parts 430 to end, 1998.

Davis, W. 1994. *Introduction to health care administration*, 4th ed. Bossier City, LA: Publicare Press.

Department of Health and Human Services, Health Care Financing Administration. 1992. *Interpretive guidelines: State operations manual #250*. Baltimore, MD.

Department of Labor. 1984. *Fair Labor Standards Act of 1938, as amended*, WH Publication 1318. Washington, DC.

Department of Labor. 1983. *Handy reference guide to the Fair Labor Standards Act*, WH Publication 1282. Washington, DC.

Department of Labor. 1985. *Fair Labor Standards Act of 1938, as amended*, WH Publication 1318-A. Washington, DC.

Holley, W., and K. Jennings. 1980. *The labor relations process*. Hinsdale, IL: Dryden Press.

Leslie, D.L. 1991. *Labor law in a nutshell*. St. Paul, MN: West Publishing.

Macdonald, M. and Essig. 1994. *Health care law: A practical guide*. New York, NY: Matthew Bender Co.

National Association of Boards of Examiners—NHA. 1997. *NAB study guide*, 3rd ed. Washington, DC.

Vaccaro, P., and M. Bryant. 1995. Are you covered by FMLA? *Provider*. April, 1995.

# Appendix 4-A

## Glossary

**Adverse Impact ("Four-Fifths Rule")**—Under the Civil Rights Act of 1964 and its amendments, adverse impact occurs whenever the selection rate for any protected group (racial, ethnic or sexual) is less than 80% of the rate of selection for the non-protected group.

**Affirmative Action**—Review of hiring practices by the federal government for facility conformity to the 1964 Civil Rights Act and its amendments.

**Arbitration**—The submission for determination of a disputed matter to private unofficial persons selected in a manner pursuant to law.

**Bargaining Unit**—A grouping of jobs or positions in which two or more employees share common employment interests and conditions.

**Benefits**—Compensation to employees other than cash, such as vacations or sick leave.

**"Can-Do" Factors**—Job applicant factors involving tests, interviews and background checks to measure knowledge, aptitude or skills.

**Career Ladder**—Paths or promotion routes established by the organization along which employees can seek progress.

**Career Paths**—Defined avenues of upward mobility available to employees within an organization (similar to career ladder).

**Check List**—In employee orientation, a step-by-step specification of activities to be completed before employee orientation is considered completed.

**Clinical Approach to Hiring Decisions**—A hiring technique in which the employer makes the decision after reviewing all the information in hand about the match of the applicant and the job.

**Code of Ethics**—Set of principles or rules that do not usually apply to the general public.

**Collective Bargaining**—The making of collective agreements between employers acting through their management representative and organized labor.

**Compensation Management**—Determining and administering wage and benefit programs for a facility.

**Compensation Theory**—Ideas or approaches to the functions of wages and benefits in motivating employees to meet requirements of the employer. (See **equity theory**.)

**Conciliation**—When a neutral party calls the parties together, encourages communication and serves as a procedural facilitator.

**Content Validity**—Degree to which a test or interview procedure measures the skills or performance requirements needed in the position for which a person is applying.

**Construct Validity**—Extent to which a selection tool measures a trait or behavior important to the job performance.

**Cost of Living Increases**—Increasing wages during inflationary times to assist worker's purchasing power.

**Credit Reports**—Under the federal Fair Credit Reporting Act, credit reports will be requested. If the applicant is rejected because of a poor credit report, the applicant must be so informed and given the name and address of the reporting credit agency.

**Discrimination**—The use of any selection procedure that has an adverse impact on hiring, promotion or other employment or membership opportunities for members of any race, sex or ethnic group.

**Employee Handbook**—A compilation of the facility policies that directly relate to work conditions. Often treated as a binding contract by the courts.

**Equal Employment Act of 1972**—An amendment to Title VII of the Civil Rights Act of 1964 intended to cover all employers of 15 or more persons and numerous other groups and educational institutions.

**Equal Employment Opportunity Commission (EEOC)**—The organization created by the Civil Rights Act of 1964 to carry out the provisions of that act.

**Equity Theory**—Concept that employees seek an exchange in which their wages and benefits are equal to the work effort, especially when compared to wages and benefits being paid to similarly situated co-workers.

**Error of Central Tendency**—Error made by supervisor in using rating scales when he or she gives only moderate scores to employees on performance appraisals regardless if the employee is a poor or superior performer.

**Expectancy Theory**—The belief that the level of motivation to perform is a mathematical function of the expectations individuals have about future outcomes multiplied by the value employees place on the outcome.

**Fair Labor Standards Act**—Sets minimum wage, overtime, equal pay, child labor and record keeping requirements for over 50 million employees, including those in nursing facilities.

**Federal Mediation and Conciliation Service (FMCS)**—A federal agency making government facilities available for conciliation, mediation and voluntary arbitration of labor disputes.

**Flex Time**—A program allowing employees to choose the hours they work so long as they put in the expected number of hours per time period.

**Global Rating**—A summary score based on the components of a performance appraisal.

**Goal Setting**—Setting of objectives to be achieved by an employee before the next performance appraisal.

**Grievance Procedure**—Established method by which an employee can have any decision of a supervisor reviewed by higher level management in an organization.

**Halo Effect**—Error made by supervisors using the rating scales who value one particular type of job behavior and permit the presence or absence of that one trait to color several or more other trait ratings.

**Health Insurance**—A benefit given to most employees. Typically the employee is covered free and can obtain family coverage for an additional periodic payment.

**In-Depth Interview**—An interview in which substantial structure is provided on a form of specific questions to be covered.

**Individual Bargaining**—Individuals with skills especially needed by a facility may be able to negotiate a higher wage than other employees in similar positions.

**In-Migration/Out-Migration**—Movement of labor into or out of a geographic area within which a facility is recruiting for specific positions.

**In-Service Training**—Education offered during work career of the employee.

**Intrinsic Needs**—Needs arising out of the essential nature of an individual's personality (i.e., the need for authority over people).

**Job**—A position in which one is employed. A collection of tasks performed by an employee undertaken in order within the scheduled work time to accomplish the work goal.

**Job Analysis**—The process of defining a position in terms of tasks or behaviors required and specifying the qualifications (behavior, knowledge and skill required) of the employee to be assigned that responsibility. Done before a job description is written.

**Job Bidding**—The practice of posting available jobs on bulletin boards and encouraging employees to apply (bid) for openings.

**Job Classification**—The systematic arrangement of particular duties for each individual job or position such as nurse, housekeeper or dietitian.

**Job Descriptions**—A statement of duties and responsibilities in order of importance of the position, authority and qualifications based on the job analysis, usually including the education, training and experience required.

**Job Evaluation**—The process of assessing and rating all jobs in an organization by considering, for instance, skills and education as a basis for the wage and salary system. There are four evaluation methods: ranking, classification, factor comparison and point system.

**Job Factors**—Include such items as skill, education and training, effort, responsibility and working conditions.

**Job Family**—A group of two or more jobs that have similar duties.

**Job Posting**—Same as job bidding in which the job is posted on the bulletin boards inviting employees to bid.

**Job Specification**—Includes the personal characteristics a worker must possess for a job.

**Job Title**—Naming of the job to distinguish that job from all other jobs, often indicating level (for example, supervisor II).

**Job Worth**—Establishing the value of a job by comparison to other jobs in the facility.

**Key Job Comparison**—A method of establishing wage rates for jobs based on comparing all jobs in the organization to a touchstone job (such as nursing) in the facility.

**Labor Market**—The geographic area from which applicants for positions are to be recruited.

**Layoffs**—Temporary dismissals of workers from their jobs.

**Leniency Error**—An error made by managers using rating scales to avoid conflict by giving consistently high ratings to employees.

**Mediation**—The act of a governmental third person who interposes between parties in disputes for the purpose of reconciling them.

**Nepotism**—Favoring one's family members in hiring practices.

**Nondirective Interview**—Interviewer refrains from influencing applicant remarks, allowing maximum freedom for applicants to ask questions and give information.

**On-the-Job Training**—Assignment of employee to one staff member who assists the employee to acquire the capabilities required in a position in the facility.

**Patterned Interview**—Approach in which all questions are sequential and highly structured, allowing no or little variation.

**Performance-Centered Objectives**—Stated training goals in terms of behaviors that can be learned and observed by instructors or others; for example, ability to demonstrate proper procedures for turning a patient suffering from decubitus ulcers.

**Performance Evaluation**—Occurs daily as supervisors observe workers, monitoring the degree to which goals are being achieved, and is formalized into written appraisals given periodically to employees, evaluating current performance and setting work goals for the next period.

**Personnel Manager**—A staff function. Assists line managers in record keeping, recruitment, selection, training and retaining employees, as well as compensation management and performance evaluation.

**Position**—The responsibilities and duties performed by one individual. There are as many positions as employees.

**Preliminary Interview**—A short questionnaire and interview used by some facilities to help screen out unsuitable applicants for a position.

**Prevailing Wage Rate**—The wages paid by the predominant number of facilities in a community. Most businesses indicate they pay the prevailing wage rate.

**Progressive Discipline**—Use of a specified number of verbal and then more stern written warnings for each offense of the same rule before suspending or firing an employee.

**Rating Scale**—Listing a number of characteristics, traits and/or requirements of an employee's position on a line or scale. This list is checked off by the rater as the degree to which the employee does or does not possess a specific characteristic or trait or fulfill a stated requirement.

**Ratio Hiring**—Requirement by a government agency that an employer increase the proportion of women or minority persons in the employer's workforce.

**Referrals**—Recommendations by others of a person for a position at a facility.

**Search Firm**—A type of employment agency focusing on middle- or upper-level positions by conducting national searches for any prospective employee.

**Staffing**—Finding the right person for each defined job which involves recruitment, interviewing and offering the job.

**Statistical Approach to Hiring**—Identifying the most valid predictors of job success, and then using weights in a complicated formula to choose among applicants for position.

**Task**—A coordinated and aggregated series of work elements used to produce an output such as making beds.

**Task Analysis**—Review of job descriptions and activities essential for performing each job. (Step 2 of establishing training needs.)

**Transfer**—Placement of an employee in another position that is approximately equivalent to the employee's present position.

**Uniform Guidelines on Employee Selection Procedures**—A publication of four federal agencies in 1978 setting standards by which federal agencies determine the acceptability of validation procedures used for written test and other selection devices.

**Validity**—A test or selection procedure is valid when it actually measures what it is intended to measure and does it well.

**Wage and Salary Surveys**—A continual process followed by many health organizations to identify pay scales of specific job categories.

**Wage Class**—Establishment of pay grades and rates by employers to both achieve equity and offer some flexibility to supervisors in setting employee's wages.

**Wage Mix**—Determination of wage rates by considering the labor market, prevailing wage rates, cost of living, ability to pay, collective bargaining agreements, individual bargaining agreements and value of the job.

**Wage Policy**—Decisions by management on the rate of pay for the facility staff, the amount of discretion supervisors may use in setting individual salaries, the spread between pay rates for long-time and new employees, and the period between pay raises together with the weight given seniority and merit.

**"Will-Do" Factors**—The more difficult to predict job applicant factors such as level of motivation, interest in the facility and other personality characteristics that will affect employee performance on the job.

# CHAPTER 5

# Financial Management

## ACCOUNTING

This chapter relates the functions of accounting and an accounting system to management. One purpose of the planning function of management is to make very basic decisions concerning the types of service to be provided by the nursing facility. Administrators must be concerned with fiscal objectives in order to have adequate funds to carry out the established mission and goals and to see that the facility resources are used effectively and economically. Fiscal objectives take into consideration income and expenditures within the various organizational units or departments and are expressed in monetary or statistical terms to allow coordination of operations throughout the organization.

Planning and controlling that are meaningful to the facility require a sound organizational structure for fiscal operations. Some sort of information and statistical data relating to each department must be available to assist the administrator and other key personnel in making intelligent management decisions. Such an accounting system accurately reflects detailed aspects of the business. Elaborate methods of accounting are not necessary, but the system should be sophisticated enough to carry on and permit basic cost analysis so that the administrator will be aware of expenditures and income relating to the vital departments. The accounting system also should document procedures that are taking place, such as the number of admissions, discharges and transfers.

Accounting is the set of rules and methods by which financial and economic data is collected, processed and summarized into reports that can be used in making decisions. Accounting involves accumulation of data of a quantitative nature relating to the activities taking place in the facility, interpretation of the results of the data, and communication. Accumulation is the mechanical process of actually recording financial transactions. Interpretation is analysis of the data to assist in making sound financial decisions. Communication is the reporting of information to administration and department heads.

The National Corporations Act was passed in England in 1845 to regulate business. One of the effects of the act was to develop accounting principles. Since that time American accountants have formed societies and encouraged legislation leading to the formation of authoritative accounting bodies, including:

- The **American Institute of Certified Public Accountants (AICPA)** was created in 1936 and played a very active role in the development of guidelines for accounting from 1937 to 1973.
- The **Financial Accounting Standards Board (FASB)**, an independent private body, assumed responsibility for the issuance of financial accounting standards in mid-1973. The FASB began to issue standards at that time and is now the independent non-governmental body that develops and issues standards to financial accounting. By mid-1986, the FASB had issued 88 standards and six concepts

statements so that today accountants look to a mixture of Accounting Research Bulletin (ARB), the Accounting Principles Board (APB) and FASB statements for authoritative guidelines.

- The **Securities and Exchange Commission (SEC)** has the legal authority to prescribe accounting methods for firms whose shares of stock are sold to the investing public.

By following the standards and precepts of the above-mentioned voluntary and governmental regulatory agencies, the financial accounting information will conform to those standards called Generally Accepted Accounting Principles (GAAP).

## Basic Concepts of Accounting

Accounting is a discipline based upon well-founded concepts that should be understood by the administrator. Some of the basic concepts are as follows:

1. The nursing facility is considered a legal entity capable of buying, selling and carrying on other business activities.
2. The facility is capable of a continuity of activity. It has a business life of its own and that business life is divided into segments or time measurements that determine the amount of money earned and the expenses paid in each one.
3. The facts ascertained by the accounting process must be capable of being objectively documented. For example, whenever the nursing facility disburses money, it is fundamental that these disbursements be documented by various evidence of the disbursement. For example, the payment for an item purchased by the facility should be supported by a receipt slip of the item, a purchase order, invoice and voucher, and check issued in payment of the invoice. The reliability and the accuracy of the accounting system is based upon such necessary documentary evidence for the various transactions which have taken place.
4. The accounting system should be consistent; standardization and uniformity of methods are used in the accounting process from one period to another. Many states require uniform accounts and reporting in a nursing facility. These may include a standardized chart of accounts, a mandatory

statistical collection method, and annual reports to state regulatory agencies.
5. Full disclosure relating to accounting procedures is also important. This concept requires that the facility report all significant data used in establishing its accounting reports.
6. Historical cost is the accounting term for the evaluation of assets and the recording of most expenses. It involves the cost of acquiring a depreciable asset, including the purchase price, taxes, shipping, storage, assembly, installation and calibration, and initial training.
7. Nursing facilities and other health care providers sometimes acquire properties by way of donation. In a technical sense, the acquisition of property in this way does not involve cost. However, such property should be recorded at the fair market value when it is received. Failure to do this may result in understatement of assets, revenues and expenses in the facility.
8. Basic internal controls should be in place and include separation of certain record keeping functions from the operating functions of a department, periodical reports comparing current activities and historical patterns with a method to note deviations for closer inspection, a system of authorization for all department and major transactions.

## The Accounting Cycle

The accounting cycle is as follows:

1. First the transactions is recorded in the general journal on a daily or chronological basis.
2. From the general journal, there is a posting to the general ledger.
3. From the ledger, a worksheet is made.
4. From the worksheet, various reports (i.e., profit and loss statement, equity statement, balance sheet) are produced.

### General Journal

The journal is a chronological record of decreases and increases affecting transactions. Adjusted entries and closing entries are made at the end of each month to reflect the facility's financial standing and equity. It does not reflect the account balances that are needed in order to prepare various financial statements for the facility at the end of the month. The information in the journal must be transferred to a book called the ledger.

### Ledger

A ledger account is kept for each account in the chart of accounts. At the end of the month, the information recorded in the general journal is transferred to each of the accounts in the ledger. This procedure is called posting.

### Worksheet

After all transactions for the month have been journalized and posted, and after the balances have been determined for each ledger account, a worksheet is prepared. The worksheet is the statement from which the accountant compiles important financial statements, such as the profit and loss statement and the balance sheet.

### Chart of Accounts

Before a financial transaction can be recorded, a classification of the information to be recorded must be established. The manner in which the information is recorded and classified is known as a chart of accounts (see Exhibit 5–1 for a sample chart of accounts). In addition to helping to systematize and categorize information of a financial nature, the chart of accounts will assist in meeting the requirements of the Internal Revenue Service (IRS), legal criteria and other regulatory agencies.

## THE ACCOUNTING SYSTEM

There are two basic systems of accounting. One of these is the **cash basis of accounting** system where revenues are recognized when the cash is actually received. All expense and asset items are not recorded until cash is actually dispersed. The operating statement, or profit and loss statement, established as a result of this system amounts to little more than a summary of cash receipts and disbursements or a recording of cash flow. Accrued income, accrued expenses, revenue and revenue deductions, expense ac-

**Exhibit 5–1** Sample Chart of Accounts

**Assets**—Assets are items of value owned by the nursing facility:
101 Cash (money in banks)
102 Accounts Receivable (due from residents or services rendered)
103 Inventory (the cost of unused supplies)
104 Prepaid Insurance (insurance premiums paid in advance)
105 Land (cost of land)

**Liabilities**—Liabilities are the debts of the nursing facility:
201 Accounts Payable (the amount of money owed to creditors for supplies and services)
202 Salaries and Wages Payable (the salaries and wages earned by employees but not yet paid)
203 Mortgage Payable (the amount owed to an insurance company or bank on the mortgage)

**Capital**—Capital is the equity of the owner in the enterprise, or the amount of the owner's investment. In the event of a corporation, this would be the corporate ownership rather than a proprietary ownership:
301 Owner's Capital
302 Owner's Withdrawals
303 Revenue and Expense Summaries

**Revenues**
401 Daily Service Revenue (room, board, nursing service)
402 Special Service Revenue (physical therapy department, pharmacy, rehabilitation department, etc.)

**Expenses**
501 Salaries and Wages
502 Supplies
503 Utilities and Telephone
504 Advertising
505 Depreciation
506 Insurance

counting and depreciation are not taken into consideration.

The **accrual basis of accounting** system is the one recognized for use in nursing facilities and required for those participating in Medicare because the information provided can be developed into more meaningful data that gives the administrator a more complete picture of the overall obligations and prospects of the business. The accrual system of accounting gives recognition to all revenues in the time period when they are actually earned and to all expenses when they are actually incurred. The cash flow has very little to do with this type of recording transactions, because they are reflected when they take place irrespective of the flow of cash between the nursing facility, its residents and its suppliers. For example:

> Resident X is admitted to the nursing facility and receives services at a per diem charge of $80. This resident brings an advance deposit of $80. Under the cash system of accounting, the $80 income would be recorded in full the date it is received; the fact that the resident has not received any services is irrelevant. Under the accrual system, however, the $80 income would be recorded when that amount of service is given and earned (i.e., first day at $80).

> There is a three-year liability insurance policy costing $3,000. Under the cash system, the payment of the insurance policy would be recorded in the books when it is paid, whether in the first year or in the third year. Under the accrual system, the payment would be recorded on the basis of when that expense is incurred, most likely at the end of each of the three years.

This system takes into consideration accrued income (income earned but yet received in cash), accrued expenses (expenses incurred but not yet paid in cash), revenue, deductions from revenue, expense accounting and depreciation.

## Revenue

Revenue is income received at the facility's established rates or charges for all services rendered to the resident whether or not these amounts have actually been paid to the facility by the resident or by a third-party payer. The purpose of revenue accounting is to keep accurate records of gross revenue earned. The revenue is allocated to the various departments that earn it, and a meaningful comparison as to the earning ability of the various departments in the nursing facility

can be made. Those departments with earning ability also may be compared in terms of expense to determine which departments are making net income for the nursing facility.

### Reimbursement Mechanisms

Most nursing facility bills are paid using personal funds, purchased long-term care insurance and Medicaid; Medicare pays a small fraction of these bills. Within the mission and goals of the facility, the administrator must pursue the best mix of private pay and third-party payers of revenue for routine and special (i.e., pharmacy or physical therapy) services. Other sources of operating revenue, such as employee meals, beauty and gift shops and other concessions, also are considered. Nonoperating revenues, such as the sale of property and campaigns for grants or donations, also are taken into account.

Nursing facilities increasingly are targeting the private pay market by offering special care units for residents with Alzheimer's and other dementias, added services where premium rates are charged for elegant decor or hotel-like services, assisted living, adult day care and/or meals on wheels.

In the private pay section, the rates set should be enough to recover costs and some level of profit. Decisions must be made as to whether to charge an inclusive rate that is the same for all residents or a rate that varies with individual care costs. Decisions also must be considered on how to handle extra charges for separate services and/or items. In making these determinations, considerations should be weighed such as resident satisfaction, record keeping and billing costs, marketing position in relation to other facilities, and incentives for caregivers in ordering services and supplies.

If the nursing facility participates in Title XVIII (Medicare), Title XIX (Medicaid) and/or other third-party reimbursement systems, the administrator has to deal with fixed rates and rate maximums set by formula and needs to be familiar with the methods of reimbursements under such regulations.

Fiscal intermediaries pay the facility for direct and indirect costs and some auxiliary charges related to resident care (i.e., nursing, administrative and maintenance costs, interest expense, depreciation, dietary, drugs and laboratory test). The fiscal intermediary for Medicare is usually an insurance company (such as Blue Cross and Blue Shield) selected by the federal government; the fiscal intermediary for Medicaid is selected by the state. Different billing procedures are used for Medicare and Medicaid. Some Medicaid programs pay nursing facilities a higher rate for certain residents requiring a higher degree of care (i.e., ventilator-dependent residents, trauma victims and those afflicted with AIDS).

To maximize the facility's reimbursement under the governmental programs, the administrator should screen residents for eligibility in the various programs, keep good records of financial and statistical data, compute all cost reports accurately, and make sure that the billing practices are followed. A system of appropriate appeal procedures should be put in place in the event of a denial of claims.

### Reimbursement by Medicare

With its goal of reducing Medicare funding and skilled nursing care, home health and outpatient service costs, the Balanced Budget Act of 1997 established:

1. A price-based system which eliminates the reasonable cost-based system previously used for Medicare reimbursement.
2. Consolidated billing which ships the responsibility for the billing of ancillary services to the skilled nursing facility (SNF). Medicare Part B services provided to a resident in a Medicare certified facility will be paid only to the facility. The price will be the same for each resident in a particular rehabilitative classification, regardless of the amount of therapy provided or if the service is provided in-house or under contract.

Starting in July 1998, implementation of payments to SNFs phases in over a four-year period from facility and federal per diem blends to a 100% national rate in the year 2001. Generally, a prospective payment system (PPS) considers all inclusive per diem rates, routine and ancillary services and capital expenses. The federal per diem rate includes cost (from the 1995 Medicare cost report), estimated cost for certain Part B services, adjustments for case mix and geographical area wage indexes, and an inflation factor. Routine and ancillary services (pharmacy, contract rehabilitation services) are bundled into the case-mix-adjusted federal per diem and provide over 40 levels of care, using the MDS assessment tool. The federal per diem also

includes a per-beneficiary annual cap for services under Part B. Services excluded from coverage by federal statute included physician services to SNF residents, physician assistants working under physician supervision, and nurse practitioner and clinical nurse specialist.

Antifraud and abuse measures in this area include penalties that suspend provider participation in federal care programs for 10 years or life (repeated violations), criminal and civil penalties, or denial of participation (conviction of felony). Surety bonds (requiring ownership disclosure) must be posted by companies providing home health care, medical equipment, ambulance service and rehabilitation services.

Under PPS, Medicare eligibility and coverage guidelines will not change. Facility transition will involve an identification of cost versus payment rates, evaluation of the utilization of group categories (such as special rehabilitation, extensive and special care), an accurate and timely MDS process, and education of personnel. The facility needs both to manage cost within the reimbursement price and to control and monitor vendor and contract services.

### Deductions from Revenue

On many occasions, the facility will receive less than its full charges for services rendered to the residents. It is important that the comparisons between potential revenue and revenue losses due to fees paid at less than full charges be recorded in the accounting system. These revenue losses or deductions from revenue are of three basic types:

- **Contractual Adjustments**—A contractual adjustment is the uncollectable difference between the full-established charges and what is actually paid by a third-party payer. For example, the per diem charges are $80, and the welfare department offers $60 per day. The $20 per day difference is considered a contractual adjustment and thus a deduction from revenue. The same kind of situation exists with Blue Cross, Medicare and Medicaid.
- **Services of a Charitable Nature**—All charity is a deduction from revenue that is recognized at full-established rates. However, an item cannot be categorized as charity service if any attempt is made to collect a bill from a third-party payer or from the resident.

- **Provision for Bad Debts**—Basically, this is an estimate of an amount of the accounts receivable that cannot be collected and become credit losses. If any attempt is made to collect a bill from a resident or third-party payer and the attempt is unsuccessful, revenue is reduced by applying the provision for bad debts.

## Expense Accounting and Cost Finding

The purpose of cost finding is the determination of the costs of doing business by gathering on an accrual basis a meaningful record of the expenses in a manner that relates them to the operation of a particular unit or department. It plays an important role in the operation of a nursing facility and provides a reliable source of information in managing costs. An administrator should be aware of the requirements of cost finding, including an order of allocation and a unit of revenue for each department's volume.

Costs are classified as direct costs, which are traceable to a specific department, and indirect costs, which are incurred for the joint benefit of several departments and relate to overhead expenses such as laundry, housekeeping, dietary or general administration departments, which provide some services to the revenue producing departments.

Total cost is the sum of fixed costs and the variable costs for a certain volume of business. A break-even analysis is necessary to determine when the cost of the operation equal the income and computes how many resident days or other units a facility must produce to break even. The person doing this analysis must know the revenue per unit, the month-cost per unit and the fixed costs.

Under Medicare, a nursing facility must file annual cost reports. The levels and ceilings of these rates may be directly related to data from a previous year's cost report. Settlements often are determined by comparing the allowable costs separated by the facility to the amount it already has received. An adjustment is then made either upward or downward in the per diem rate the facility may receive.

## Depreciation

All assets the nursing facility owns, whether purchased or donated, must be included in the balance sheet. All assets (except land) depreciate or lose value through use, wear and tear, and obsolescence. The asset eventually to be replaced and is considered as an operating expense reflecting the cost of replacement; depreciation is recorded as an operating expense. If the asset was recognized and the depreciation expense ignored, the real cost of operating the facility would be significantly understated.

Several methods of depreciation that are recognized by the IRS are:

- **Straight-Line Depreciation**—The straight-line method provides for equal periodic charges to expenses over the estimated life of the asset. For example, assume that the cost of a depreciable asset is $16,000 and its life is 4 years. The depreciated amount is $4,000 per year ($16,000 divided by 4 equals $4,000).
- **Units of Production Method**—This method yields a depreciation charge that varies with the amount of asset usage. The life of the asset is expressed in terms of hours, miles or number of operations. Assume that a machine with a cost of $15,000 is expected to have an estimated life of 10,000 hours; the $15,000 cost divided by the 10,000 hours life is $1.50 hourly depreciation.
- **Declining (Double Declining) Balance Method**—This method yields a declining periodic depreciation charge over the estimated life of the asset. The most common method is to double the straight-line depreciation rate and apply the resulting rate to the cost of the asset. Assume an asset cost of $8,000, double the 10% straight-line depreciation rate, thereby depreciating 20% of the $8,000 which equals $1,600 first year depreciation expense. At the end of the second year, the depreciation formula would be $8,000 - $1,600 = $6,400 x 20% = $1,200, which is the amount depreciated. The original cost minus previous depreciation times 20% is applied each year thereafter.
- **Sum-of-the-Years Digit Method**—The periodic charge for depreciation declines steadily over the estimated life of the asset, because a successively smaller fraction is applied each year to the original cost of the asset. For an asset with an estimated life of five years, the denominator is 5 + 4 + 3 + 2 + 1 or 15. For the first year the numerator is 5, for the second year 4, and so on. For example:

| Year | Cost | Rate | Depreciation for Year |
|------|------|------|------|
| 1 | $15,000 | 5/15 | $5,000 |
| 2 | $15,000 | 4/15 | 4,000 |
| 3 | $15,000 | 3/15 | 3,000 |

- **Accelerated Depreciation**—Accelerated depreciation, such as the declining balance and the sum-of-the-years digit, provides for a higher depreciation charge in the first year of use of the asset and a gradually declining charge thereafter. This is a preferred method of depreciation because increased depreciation in the early years may reduce taxable earnings.

## FINANCIAL REPORTS

### Profit and Loss Statement

The purpose of the profit and loss statement (see Exhibit 5–2) is to reflect the results of the financial operations in the terms of the amount of revenues the facility has earned (current assets or cash and property usually consumed in one year such as cash, accounts receivable or inventory) and the amount of expenses the facility has incurred (current liabilities or obligations to be paid in one year such as accounts payable, wages and salaries or taxes payable) for a given period of time. It is sometimes called an operating statement or a statement of income and expenses, and is usually prepared monthly. The statement of expenses should be departmentalized thus enabling the administrator to determine the income and expense of each department for better analysis of worth, efficiency and so on. The percentage of occupancy figure is important because the administrator can better determine how many residents are required in the facility to operate in the black.

### The Balance Sheet

The balance sheet is used to portray the entire financial operation of the facility in terms of its assets, liabilities and capital at a given moment in time (i.e., January 1, 1999, June 30, 1999 or December 15, 1999). It usually is prepared once a month. Assets include current assets, long-term investments (i.e., stocks or bonds) and fixed assets that have a value to the facility over a long period of time (i.e., buildings or equipment). Liabilities include current liabilities, long-term liabilities (debts becoming due in a period over one year such as mortgages or long-term notes). Capital or owner's equity is the amount of funds supplied by the owner(s) of the facility. This can come from the sale of stocks, retained funds (earned by the facility for the owner[s] but left in the business) or equity funds (considered as a long-term and/or permanent investment by the owner[s]). Total assets less the total liabilities represent the owner's equity or net worth. Thus the total liabilities plus the owner's equity must equal the assets. See Exhibit 5–3 for an example.

## ACCOUNT PROCEDURES

### Cash

The importance of cash in any kind of business is important because it is obvious that this is a way of financing the business operation. Cash transactions occur more than any other kind of transaction in a health care facility. Cash is the asset that is the most susceptible to fraud and misappropriation. Cash is easily concealed, and its ownership is determined mainly on the basis of possession. As part of the financial management of the facility, therefore, some type of internal control is necessary for cash receipts. The American Health Care Association recommends that the following items and procedures be practiced as an internal control relative to cash receipts:

1. Incoming mail should be opened by someone who does not have access to accounting records and who is not responsible for making bank deposits.
2. Whoever is charged with opening the mail should prepare a remittance list of all cash items received by mail. One copy of this remittance slip should be given to the person making the bank deposits.
3. All persons who are handling cash should be bonded.
4. Bank reconciliations should be prepared by persons who do not handle cash or who do not record cash transactions.
5. Cash received by the facility should be handled as follows:
   a. Cash receipts are prepared for all cash received by the facility.
   b. The original of the receipt slip goes to the person paying the cash, and the copy is sent to accounting.

**Exhibit 5–2** Profit and Loss Statement, Statement of Expenses

|  | Month 3/99 | Month 3/98 | Year To Date 3/99 | Year To Date 3/98 |
|---|---|---|---|---|
| **Salaries—General Nursing** |  |  |  |  |
| **Nursing Wing A** |  |  |  |  |
| Salaries & Wages—RNs | $ 8,000 | $ 6,000 | $24,000 | $18,000 |
| Salaries & Wages—LPNs | 4,000 | 3,000 | 12,000 | 9,000 |
| Salaries & Wages—Others | 2,000 | 2,000 | 6,000 | 6,000 |
| **Total Salaries Wing A** | 14,000 | 11,000 | 42,000 | 33,000 |
|  |  |  |  |  |
| **Nursing Wing B** |  |  |  |  |
| Salaries & Wages—RNs | 8,000 | 6,000 | 24,000 | 18,000 |
| Salaries & Wages—LPNs | 4,000 | 3,000 | 12,000 | 9,000 |
| Salaries & Wages—Other | 2,000 | 2,000 | 6,000 | 6,000 |
| **Total Salaries Wing B** | 14,000 | 11,000 | 42,000 | 33,000 |
|  |  |  |  |  |
| **Salaries—Special Services** |  |  |  |  |
| Pharmacy | 8,000 | 7,000 | 24,000 | 21,000 |
| Recreation | 5,000 | 4,000 | 15,000 | 12,000 |
| Rehabilitation | 7,000 | 4,000 | 21,000 | 12,000 |
| Physical Therapy | 7,000 | 4,000 | 21,000 | 12,000 |
| **Total Salaries Special Services** | 27,000 | 19,000 | 81,000 | 57,000 |
|  |  |  |  |  |
| **Salaries—Administrative** |  |  |  |  |
| Administrator | 2,500 | 2,400 | 7,500 | 7,200 |
| Secretarial | 1,500 | 1,400 | 4,500 | 4,200 |
| **Total Salaries—Administrative** | 4,000 | 3,800 | 12,000 | 11,400 |
|  |  |  |  |  |
| **Total Salaries** | 59,000 | 44,800 | 177,000 | 134,400 |
|  |  |  |  |  |
| **Statement of Supplies and Expenses** |  |  |  |  |
| Administrative | 5,000 | 4,000 | 15,000 | 12,000 |
| Nursing Service | 5,000 | 4,000 | 15,000 | 12,000 |
| Dietary | 8,000 | 7,000 | 24,000 | 21,000 |
| Housekeeping | 5,000 | 4,000 | 15,000 | 12,000 |
| Operation of Plant | 5,000 | 4,000 | 15,000 | 12,000 |
| **Total Supplies and Expenses** | 28,000 | 23,000 | 84,000 | 69,000 |
|  |  |  |  |  |
| **Plus Total Salaries** | 59,000 | 44,800 | 177,000 | 134,400 |
|  |  |  |  |  |
| **TOTAL NET EXPENSES** | $87,000 | $67,800 | $261,000 | $203,400 |
|  |  |  |  |  |
| **Gross Earnings from Nursing Home Services** |  |  |  |  |
|  |  |  |  |  |
| **Routine Daily Services** | $85,000 | $65,000 | $255,000 | $195,000 |
|  |  |  |  |  |
| **Special Services** |  |  |  |  |
| Physician Care | 1,200 | 1,000 | 3,600 | 3,000 |

*continues*

**Exhibit 5–2** continued

| | Month 3/99 | Month 3/98 | Year To Date 3/99 | Year To Date 3/98 |
|---|---|---|---|---|
| Recreation | 500 | 400 | 1,500 | 1,200 |
| Rehabilitation | 500 | 400 | 1,500 | 1,200 |
| Day Care/Beauty Parlor | 500 | 400 | 1,500 | 1,200 |
| **Total Special Services** | 2,700 | 2,200 | 8,100 | 6,600 |
| | | | | |
| **Total Gross—Services** | 87,700 | 67,200 | 263,100 | 201,600 |
| | | | | |
| **Deductions from Gross Earnings** | | | | |
| Medicare | 300 | 300 | 900 | 900 |
| Blue Cross | 100 | 100 | 300 | 300 |
| Charity | 100 | 100 | 300 | 300 |
| Provisions for Losses | 200 | 100 | 600 | 300 |
| **Total Deductions** | 700 | 600 | 2,100 | 1,800 |
| | | | | |
| **Net Income from Residents** | 87,000 | 66,600 | 261,000 | 199,800 |
| | | | | |
| **Other Operating Income** | | | | |
| General Contributions | 500 | 500 | 1,500 | 1,500 |
| Grants | 1,000 | 800 | 3,000 | 2,400 |
| Donated Services | 400 | 300 | 1,200 | 900 |
| Purchase Discounts | 500 | 400 | 1,500 | 1,200 |
| Income from Investments | 1,500 | 1,000 | 4,500 | 3,000 |
| **Total Other Income** | 3,900 | 3,000 | 11,700 | 9,000 |
| | | | | |
| **TOTAL REVENUES (total income before depreciation)** | 90,900 | 69,600 | 272,700 | 208,800 |
| | | | | |
| **Deduct Prov for Depreciation** | 500 | 300 | 1,500 | 900 |
| **Net Income from Operations** | 90,400 | 69,300 | 271,200 | 207,900 |
| | | | | |
| **Net Expenses from Operations (from statement of expenses)** | 87,000 | 67,800 | 261,000 | 203,400 |
| | | | | |
| **Excess-Income Over Expense (Nonprofit) or Profit** | $ 3,400 | $ 1,500 | $ 10,200 | $ 4,500 |
| | | | | |
| **Percentage of Occupancy** | 95% | | | |

c. All cash receipts are recorded in the appropriate accounting records at the earliest time practical.

d. Cash received is deposited daily.

6. Immediately upon receipt of checks, endorsement is made by indicating on the back of the check "For deposit to the account of Prairieweed Nursing Facility."

7. The accountant records all cash received in a cash receipts journal on a daily basis. These receipts are then posted to the residents' ledger.

**Exhibit 5–3** Balance Sheet, Prairieweed Nursing Facility, December 31, 1998

*Assets*

**Current Assets**

| | | |
|---|---|---|
| Cash | $10,000 | |
| Accounts | 4,000 | |
| Inventory | 9,000 | |
| Prepaid Insurance | 2,000 | |
| Total Current Assets | | $25,000 |

**Fixed Assets**

| | | |
|---|---|---|
| Land | | 15,000 |
| Building | 71,000 | |
| Less Accumulated Depreciation | 1,000 | 70,000 |
| Equipment | 16,000 | |
| Less Depreciation | 1,500 | 14,500 |
| Total Fixed Assets | | 99,500 |
| | | |
| Total Assets | | $124,500 |

*Liabilities and Capital*

**Current Liabilities**

| | | |
|---|---|---|
| Accounts Payable | $13,500 | |
| Salaries and Wages Payable | 35,000 | |
| Total Current Liabilities | | $48,500 |

**Long-Term Liabilities**

| | | |
|---|---|---|
| Mortgage Payable, etc. | 50,000 | |
| Total Long-Term Liabilities | | 98,500 |
| | | |
| Total Liabilities | | 98,500 |
| | | |
| Owner Capital (net worth) | | 26,000 |
| | | |
| Total Liabilities | | $124,500 |

In addition to the profit and loss statement and the balance sheet, a well-managed facility will use additional financial reports concerning supplies and expenses. Such reports to use as guides in the fiscal operation are a report of cash receipts and disbursements, an accounts receivable report and an accounts payable report.

**Cash Report**

This report gives the administrator a working knowledge of the amount of cash on hand. It is usually prepared monthly.

| | |
|---|---|
| Cash on Hand, 8/31/98 | $30,000.00 |
| Add Cash Receipts | 50,000.00 |
| Total | 80,000.00 |
| Deduct Cash Disbursements | 40,000.00 |
| | |
| Cash on Hand, 9/30/98 | $40,000.00 |

**Accounts Receivable Report**

This report is a controlling device checking fiscal operations from the income point of view. It includes only income from residents and third-party payers and points out the effectiveness of collection procedures, billings and whether good cash flow is maintained. It also is prepared monthly.

| | |
|---|---|
| Accounts Receivable, 8/31/98 | $100,000.00 |
| Add Resident Charges | 40,000.00 |
| Total | 140,000.00 |
| Deduct Resident Payments | 70,000.00 |
| | |
| Accounts Receivable, 9/30/98 | $70,000.00 |

**Accounts Payable Report**

This monthly report is also a controlling device assisting the administrator in keeping operating expenses (such as outstanding debts by vendors) in line with the monthly cash flow. The operating expenses included on this report are only those payable within one year. Such items as mortgages, loan interest payments, wages and salaries are not included.

| | |
|---|---|
| Accounts Payable, 8/31/98 | $75,000.00 |
| Add Purchases | 30,000.00 |
| Total | 105,000.00 |
| Deduct Payments | 60,000.00 |
| | |
| Accounts Payable, 9/30/98 | $45,000.00 |

## Purchasing and Accounts Payable

Because supplies and equipment are a major source of expenditure in a nursing facility, the administrator is responsible for implementing sound purchasing procedures. Materials management is an important consideration in the operation of a facility.

Some of the steps involved in effective purchasing procedures are considering:

1. Quality standards for supplies and equipment being purchased. The purchasing agent or other authorized person in the facility should consider the size, performance, ease of use and the ways the goods increase or decrease the hours of staff time.
2. Vendor selection systems. Some of the items that should be considered in selecting vendors are payment terms, delivery times and charges, packaging, record for delivering orders on time, record on current billing, instructions, maintenance agreements, and willingness to provide staff of the facility with operating assistance.
3. Requisitioning systems. This would include standardized procedures for placing and processing orders, receiving goods, approving invoices, and authorizing and recording payments. The procedures for placing orders may include preparation of specifications, getting bids and comparing prices. A prohibition should be placed on the staff accepting kickbacks or gifts from vendors.
4. Discounts related to purchase volume and early payment. Group purchasing with other nursing facilities may be considered to maximize discounts for purchase volume.
5. Leasing agreements. The administrator may want to consider whether leasing would be more advantageous than purchasing major equipment if monthly payments on a lease are lower than those required on a bank loan. Some items to consider in a leasing agreement are monthly payments, insurance coverage and equipment upkeep and repair.

An accounts payable account is a creditor of the nursing facility. A procedure for handling these accounts is as follows:

1. Start a file folder for each company that the nursing facility does business with regarding the purchase of supplies and services.
2. Issue a purchase order number or write a purchase order for all purchases.
3. Have a central storeroom where all goods are received.
4. When supplies or goods are received, a receiving slip should accompany the items. Make certain the number of cartons received corresponds to the items on the receiving slip. Make a notation of any items that are backordered.
5. The receiving slip, after being checked by the storekeeper or other person handling this function, should then be sent to the bookkeeper.
6. When the facility receives the invoice from the vendor, either the accountant or the accounts payable clerk should check the invoice for the following items.
   - Find the purchase order signed by the person in authority to order the item.
   - Check the invoice against the purchase order to determine if the unit price and extensions are correct.
   - Check the invoice against the receiving slip to determine if all ordered goods were received.
   - Submit the above information to the individual responsible for authorizing payment.
   - Place all approved invoices in an accounts payable file in alphabetical order by the name of the vendor.
   - Prepare checks.

## Accounts Receivable

Because the survival of the nursing facility depends upon adequate revenue, the procedure for establishing rates and recording revenue plays a vital role in the operation of the facility. The majority of all revenue received will be from residents' revenue for room and board and revenue from special service departments. A procedure for handling these accounts is as follows:

1. Review and establish the rate structure for room, board and special services at least on an annual basis.
2. At the time of admission, set up a ledger card in the name of the resident, noting such essential information as name, room, number, source of payment (i.e., private pay, Medicare, Medicaid or welfare) and daily service charge.

3. At the end of the week or month, prepare an accounts receivable journal for resident income. This will act as a check and balance on the ledger.

4. Gather all charge slips from the various departments involved in special services (i.e., pharmacy, physical therapy or special charges) that are not included in the daily rate. Keep a special service revenue journal to act as a check and balance. Charge tickets should be summarized and reviewed on a daily basis.

5. At the end of the month, the totals in these journals should be posted to the general ledger and the resident's ledger card. Bills for room, board and special services are then prepared and submitted to the responsible parties.

6. Record payments as received and check that these are timely.

## Credits and Collections

The accumulation of accounts receivable that are uncollected can cause concern and financial crisis in a nursing facility. For this reason, an effective credit and collection procedure must be instituted. A suggested procedure is as follows:

1. Financial data on the source of payment should be obtained from the resident or family upon admission to the facility. If third-party payers (Medicare or other insurance companies) are to pay for the resident's stay, verify this coverage as soon as practicable.

2. Determine if the resident is eligible for welfare or other governmental assistance.

3. Determine if there is someone other than the resident who has legal access to his or her financial resources.

4. Explain to the resident the types of services and the charges for them at the time of his or her admission.

5. Explain the nursing facility's billing procedures and collection policies.

6. Prepare an accounts receivable aging schedule for each resident. If an account is a month old, write a letter informing the resident of the past due account.

A great deal of tact and diplomacy must be used in collecting accounts. Reportedly, 66% of all negligence cases against health care facilities start when a resident is dunned for a bill. The facility should determine policy concerning the use of any collection agency or an attorney to collect unpaid bills.

## Resident Account Management

One of the earliest procedures in accounting for resident property is the establishment of means for safeguarding resident valuables. With the advent of Title XVIII (Medicare) and Title XIX (Medicaid), the quantity of resident funds and accountability of these funds by the facility has increased.

A procedure should be established in the facility whereby a legal document creates a trustee relationship between the facility and the resident. A pooled or individual resident trust fund separate from the facility accounts must be established to record cash transactions, receipts and disbursements for each resident account in accordance with generally accepted accounting principles.

At least quarterly, a statement of resident receipts and disbursements must be available to each resident or designated legal representative. (More detail on related federal law under Medicare and Medicaid is included under resident rights in Chapter 6.) The resident fund transactions should be filed annually with the appropriate state agency.

## Payroll

Because salaries and wages are likely to represent 60% to 70% of a long-term care institution's operating expenses, adequate records and procedures must be maintained.

### Time Keeping

A method of time keeping should be used for hourly employees and salaried employees. Manual time and earnings records may be used. Some facilities pay biweekly, whereas others pay weekly. Assuming a biweekly pay period is utilized, the following procedure might be considered:

1. At the first day of the pay period, the employee's name and the date of the pay period is recorded on the record.

2. The record is then given to the employee's supervisor. (If time cards are used, the supervisor places them in the appropriate slots.)
3. At the end of each day, the employee or supervisor enters the number of hours the employee worked in each department.
4. At the end of the pay period, the record is returned to the accountant who calculates the hours worked, gross pay and deductions.

### Payroll Journal

The employee time and earnings record serves as a basis for entries into the payroll journal. Two separate accounts may be maintained: one named "Cash in Bank—General Checking"; the other named "Cash in Bank—Payroll Checking." Accounts payable and wages and salaries should not be paid out of the same account.

Once the total net payroll for the period is determined from the payroll journal, a single check for the total net payroll is written out of the general account and put into the payroll checking account. When the payroll clears the bank, the payroll checking account should have a minimal balance. Different colored checks should be used for the payroll checking and the general checking accounts.

### Payroll Procedure

Payroll procedure should have as its goal the following considerations:

1. Identification and calculation of the various payroll deductions and payroll taxes that apply to the long-term care industry.
2. Recognition of the major portions of the Social Security program.
3. Computation of net pay due.
4. Recording of periodic payroll and employer payroll taxes.
5. Effective control of payroll.

### Payroll Deductions

Payroll deductions from the gross pay of the employee are grouped into two basic categories—payroll taxes and voluntary deductions.

Payroll taxes are of prime importance. They are:

- **Social Security Taxes Under the Federal Insurance Contributions Act (FICA)**—Under this act, both employees and employers contribute equal amounts based upon a stated percentage of taxable wages paid. The employee portion must be withheld by the employer from each payment of taxable wage until the current taxable wage base has been reached.
- **Federal Income Tax Withholding**—Each employee's taxable earnings are subject to federal income tax withholding as required by law and by IRS regulations. The amount of taxes withheld depends upon the employee's earnings, the frequency of the payroll period and the number of income tax deductions claimed by the employee. At the start of employment and when the deductions change, each employee fills out an employee withholding allowance certificate (Form W-4).

  At the end of the calendar year, each employee must be provided with a wage and tax statement (Form W-2). This form shows the amount of taxable wages paid to the employee during the year, the federal taxes withheld, FICA taxes withheld and the state income taxes withheld (if applicable).
- **Other Tax Deductions**—A number of states and some cities levy income taxes on the gross earnings of the employee subject to withholding.

### Voluntary Deductions

Voluntary deductions include amounts withheld for such purposes as pension and retirement benefits, group health insurance, life insurance or union dues. The employee usually makes arrangements with the employer to deduct these amounts from the gross pay received.

### Employer Taxes

Employer taxes include:

- **Federal Unemployment Tax Act (FUTA)**—This established a joint federal and state program for payments to persons who became unemployed. The program is administered locally by each state. Under it, a full tax is levied on employers only. No employee withholding occurs for this program.
- **State Unemployment Compensation Tax**—All states require employers to pay state unemploy-

ment compensation taxes. Each state is allocated part of the FUTA taxes by the federal government for use in administering the program locally. Unemployed persons who qualify for unemployment benefits are paid by a state agency. The amount of unemployment benefits and the number of weeks payable depend on wages earned and the amount of time worked by an employee.

State unemployment tax laws vary in their application. The basic unemployment tax rate paid by the employer may be reduced according to a merit program. If the employer's annual contributions are sufficiently greater than unemployment benefits paid to a discharged employee, the basic rate of the employer is reduced.

### Personnel File

An individual folder should be maintained for each employee. It should contain all the personnel information such as references, physical exam results, pay increases, advancements, awards, reprimands and payroll information (earnings records or W-2 form). Some facilities post from the cards to employee's individual earnings records. Others prepare payroll checks and duplicate and file the duplicate copy in the employee's folder.

## Inventory Control

The primary objective of maintaining inventory control is to make sure that supplies are kept at an optimum level for use by the various departments and to discourage theft and embezzlement. To establish any kind of an inventory system, it is necessary to have a centralized storeroom set up with one person assigned for its operation and the storing and issuing of supplies. A purchase requisition system also should be established whereby the department heads requesting supplies complete a purchase requisition form and submit it to the central storeroom supervisor or other person responsible for this function.

### Perpetual Inventory System

A perpetual inventory system should be considered along with the inventory control system. This system involves keeping on a set of cards or other records a daily record of supplies received, supplies issued and supplies in inventory. The system requires that all issues from the storeroom be substantiated by a requisition slip. The requisition forms are then used by the accountant to make appropriate charges to the various departments in the nursing facility.

The perpetual inventory system provides a day-by-day record of the amount of supplies on hand and is usually required in the pharmacy department. It helps the administration in planning by establishing maximum and minimum inventory levels, thereby avoiding shortages of supplies that are desperately needed. This system also provides a ledger card balance at the year's end to serve as a check against the fiscal inventory that should be taken on an annual basis.

## Ratio Analysis

Solvency is the ability of a business to meet its formal obligations as they become due. Solvency analysis focuses primarily on balance sheet relationships that point out the ability to liquidate current and noncurrent liabilities. To be useful, ratios relating to a firm's solvency must show the firm's ability to liquidate its liabilities. The use of these ratios pointing out the ability to liquidate current liabilities is called current position analysis and is of particular interest to short-term creditors. Types of ratios are:

- **Current Ratio**—This ratio also is called working capital ratio or banker's ratio and is a more dependable indicator of solvency than is working capital. It indicates the strength of the working capital position.

  | | |
  |---|---|
  | Current assets ÷ Current liabilities | |
  | Current assets | $550,000 |
  | Current liabilities − | $210,000 |
  | Current capital | 340,000 |
  | Current ratio | 2:62 |

- **Acid Test Ratio**—This is a ratio that measures the "instant" debt paying ability of a company. It is the ratio of the sum of cash, receivables and marketable securities (also referred to as quick assets) to current liabilities.

  | | |
  |---|---|
  | Quick current assets ÷ Current liabilities | |
  | Quick current assets | $1,300,000 |
  | Current liabilities − | $ 650,000 |
  | Working capital | 650,000 |
  | Current ratio | 2:1 |

- **Price Earnings Ratio**—The price earnings ratio indicates the relationship of the price to the earnings of a share of common stock.

  Price earnings ratio—divide the market price per share by annual earnings.

  | | |
  |---|---:|
  | Market price | $20.50 |
  | Earnings per share | $ 1.64 |
  | Price earning ratio | 12:5 |

## BUDGET PREPARATION AND EXECUTION

The lifeblood of the nursing facility is financial solvency. One of the most important aids for administration in sound financial planning and controlling is the budget. The budget is defined as a projection of fiscal data for a specific period of time (usually one year). It provides a set of standards by which to measure and control fiscal performance. A budget should not be completely restrictive. After periodic administrative review of the budget, it may be necessary to make an adjustment of revenues and expenses, either upward or downward.

Three kinds of budgets are basically used: an operating budget, a capital (plant and equipment) budget and a cash budget. Those nursing facilities maintaining all three kinds are said to have a comprehensive budget.

### The Operating Budget

This is a projection for the 12 months of revenues, deductions from revenues and expenses.

To establish the revenue budget, the monetary and statistical data concerning income by each department in the facility is carefully reviewed. Trends should be noted, established, evaluated and then projected for the coming year. The anticipated volume changes in the internal operation should be reviewed for such items as:

1. Changes in the bed complement.
2. New services.
3. New or amended bylaws to be placed into effect.
4. Projection of resident days on a realistic basis.
5. Projection of the volume of services in each department for the budget period.

After all of the above items have been reviewed, a rate structure may be established for the coming year and a revenue budget for each department projected for 12 months.

To view revenues realistically, deductions from revenue also should be budgeted and include the following steps:

1. Relate the past experiences to the total budgeted resident service revenue.
2. Take into consideration changes in law relative to Medicare, Medicaid, welfare, admissions relating to fiscal matters and so on.
3. Develop a percentage of deductions to gross revenue classified by each type of deduction.

In establishing a budget regarding expenses, the administrator and each department head discuss the projected budget figures for expenses in the particular department. Department head participation in this fiscal planning encourages acceptance of responsibility and provides sufficient information and knowledge as to what is expected in the department. Steps in budgeting expenses include:

1. Make salary projections for a 12-month period in each department, using a master staffing plan with authorized titles of all positions in the nursing facility.
2. Determine supplies for each department based on last year's expenditures with an inflation ratio.

### The Capital (Plant and Equipment) Budget

This budget provides for major (not operating budget) items to upgrade and expand buildings, to provide equipment to upgrade services and to meet state, federal and local regulations. Capital expenditures are generally a minimum of $500 with a minimum useful life of over 1 year. To establish a plant and equipment budget, each department head submits proposals to the administrator for anticipated purchases of equipment in his or her particular department. The proposal should indicate what equipment is needed, why it is needed and what it will cost.

A requested capital expenditure needs to be carefully reviewed by administration in terms of cost, benefit to the residents, technological obsolescence of the physical plant and/or equipment, and relation to the long-term mission and goals of the facility. The administrator may apply one of the several methods that have been developed for capital investment decision making if two or more competing requests are made for a long-term capitalization expenditure. These methods consider such issues as the estimated level and probability of cash inflows and outflows associated with the capital item; the useful life of the item; opportunity costs (difference between the return on one investment and the return on an alternative); and interest-bearing instruments and the distribution of cost over the estimated life of the item by depreciation. Expenditures for compliance with regulatory standards of a state agency would appear justified. If review and approval by state agencies are required, a clear need for the capital expenditure must be outlined with the facility's statement of financial feasibility.

The administrator also must review the source of long-term capital financing. Debt financing is raising funds through interest-bearing instruments that include conventional mortgages, issuance of taxable and tax-exempt revenue bonds, and participation in state and federal housing administration loan programs. Some factors considered to evaluate debt financing alternatives are:

1. Amount of periodic debt service payments.
2. Effective cost of financing.
3. Repayment schedule.
4. Prepayment procedures.
5. Various tax laws.
6. Medicare and Medicaid reimbursement policies.

Proprietary and for-profit facilities may consider equity financing (sale of stock), government grants, drawing upon income or investment cash or conducting philanthropic fund-raising drives. Nonprofit facilities also may participate in the latter fund-raising drives. The facility should review the advantages of borrowing on an unsecured versus a secured basis. Monitoring of interest rate trends is also important to determine when it is advisable to refinance debt at a lower rate.

### The Cash Budget

For a facility to continue to operate, it must have adequate working capital so that necessary purchases can be made during the period of rendering a service and receiving income for that service. Working capital is the excess of current assets over current liabilities.

The cash budget reflects projections of cash for each month, cash disbursements and cash receipts from all services. Prediction of cash receipts is based in part on historical trends in such areas as slowdown of collections during the holiday season, time lapse between the billing for resident services and the receipt of payments, and year-end settlements with third-party payers. A schedule of disbursements should be made monthly to predict cash disbursements in such areas as wages and salaries, and quarterly, annual or other payments such as real estate taxes, insurance premiums and dividends.

The cash budget forces the administration and governing body to direct their attention to the flow of cash in a given month. For instance, it may point out that a shortage of cash will occur in the seventh and eighth months of the upcoming year. The facility then can plan to either borrow money to supplement this shortage or to make other adjustments (i.e., raising rates, cutting expenses or postponing capital equipment purchases). Most cash receipts will come from the following sources:

- **Cash Receipts from Residents**—A review of residents' accounts will provide the administration with a guide to budgeting cash receipts from residents or third-party payers. For example, if past experience shows that 75% of current billings are collected in the month billed, 10% the following month, and 15% the subsequent month, an idea of the cash flow will be apparent.
- **Cash Receipts in the Form of Interest and Dividends on Investments**—Estimated income from these can be based on such information as the rate of interest, the probable yield in the investments and a determination of what month the dividends and investments are paid.
- **Bank Loans**—Bank loans sometimes are budgeted for periods when cash flow is low. If the facility needs to borrow money from a bank, a cash budget will help; very often banks require that the prospective borrower submit a cash flow report as part of the application for the loan.

If any cash flow is left over after payment of current debts, it should be invested in such items as certificates of deposit, commercial paper or treasury securities.

The generation of profit for a nursing facility is a reality of operations, whether the entity is a proprietary or nonprofit facility. A surplus of profit is required to make major renovations, to provide replacements or expansions of plant and equipment, to repay debts, for working capital, and to cover the cost of charity not reimbursable by third-party payers.

If income does not meet the demands of obligations owed, the administrator needs to consider obtaining short-term loans, step up collections or postpone payments of accounts payable.

## RISK MANAGEMENT

Some of the potential hazards in a health care facility relate to employees. Injuries and illness can possibly result from the lifting and moving of residents, slipping and falling, and encountering communicable diseases among residents. The federal government mandates that the facility carry workers' compensation liability coverage and adhere to the applicable rules and regulations of the Occupational Safety and Health Act. Another area of possible liability is with the residents, their guests and others who come to the facility to legally conduct business.

In addition to necessary insurances, the facility should have an operational safety plan, a safety committee and periodic evacuation drills. Any accident and incident reports should be reviewed by the administrator with the safety committee on a regular basis to determine causes and apply any required remedial steps. Orientation and in-service training programs also should emphasize safety precautions regarding residents and other individuals using the facility.

### Insurance

Risks for which a health care facility should be insured fall generally into two classes:

- Liability risks where the insured may be liable to others because of his or her own actions or those of his or her employees and agents.
- Property loss risks where the insured may suffer loss or injury to property due to his or her own actions or the actions of others.

### Liability

Most liability coverages are divided into two separate sections: bodily injury and property damage. The health care facility is exposed to lawsuits for its own negligence and the negligence of others. The most common liability coverage policy provides coverage only for sums that the insured becomes legally obligated to pay resulting from accidents. It does not provide coverage for occurrences that are not considered accidents (such as illness caused by repeated exposure to unsanitary conditions). Other occurrences for which the insured is legally obligated to pay that are not covered in a basic policy include liabilities for which the insured is not obligated under negligence law until fault is proven and liabilities where the insured voluntarily admits fault. Broader coverage may be obtained on basic policies for additional premiums and by substituting such words as "occurrence" for "caused by accident." Comprehensive general liability and other policies will offer broader coverage.

Various types of basic liability coverages for health care facilities are:

- **Owners and Directors Liability Coverage**—The basic policy insures against claims resulting from the ownership and operation of the facility. This is usually a scheduled policy inasmuch as it names the particular properties and risks insured against. The comprehensive general liability policy offers similar coverage on a nonscheduled basis.
- **Workers' Compensation**—This is designed to cover employees who have been injured while working in the scope of their employment.
- **Professional Liability**—Originally called malpractice insurance, this insurance covers the area of malpractice, error, and negligence in rendering or failing to render medical, nursing or other professional treatment. It does not cover the liability of individuals working in the home unless provided in a schedule.

In addition to satisfying money claims, liability insurance can provide a number of valuable services and other benefits. They include:

- **Defense of Law Actions**—The insurance company will defend in the insured's name all suits or actions brought against him or her—even if false or groundless. The policy will pay all costs including investigating the claim, procuring witnesses and legal defense. It also pays for bonds required in the appeal of any suit and bonds to release attachments.

- **Medical Payments Coverage**—This can be added to liability policy for an additional premium. It covers all reasonable medical, surgical and funeral expenses incurred within one year of an accident to each person who sustains bodily injury, sickness or disease caused by an accident—regardless of whether the insured is legally liable or not. Normally, the insured or employees of the insured are not covered for these medical payments without this addition.

In summary, some risks to be protected against in regard to liability insurance are shown in Table 5–1.

### Property

Direct loss to tangible property has various coverages:

**Table 5–1** Liability Insurance Risk Protection

| Risk | Liability to Others | Loss to Insured | Policy |
|---|---|---|---|
| Tort (False Arrest, Libel, Slander) | X | | Personal Injury Liability Coverage |
| Employee Accident or Disease | X | | Workers' Compensation |
| Accident on Premises | X | | Comprehensive General Liability |
| Accident on Elevators | X | | Comprehensive General Liability |
| Malpractice, Negligence | X | | Professional Liability |
| Auto Accidents (Insured's Auto) | X | Property Damage, Bodily Injury | Auto Comprehensive Liability |
| Injury to Persons or Property on the Premises | X | | General Liability |

*Fire Insurance.* This covers direct loss by fire and lightning. It also covers certain types of damage by smoke, such as that caused by a hostile or intentionally set fire either involving insured or uninsured property. Smoke damage caused by defective heating apparatus is not usually covered by a basic fire policy

*Extended Coverage.* Coverage for other perils can be added by endorsement to the fire policy. The extended coverage endorsement insures against:

1. **Windstorm and Hail**—Damage to the interior of a building and/or its contents resulting from water, rain, sand, snow or dust is covered but the building must be damaged by the force of wind and hail as well.
2. **Explosion**—Excludes steam boiler usually.
3. **Riot or Civil Commotion**—Includes direct loss due to theft or pillage.
4. **Aircraft**—Includes objects falling from aircraft or being hit by a plane.

*Additional Extended Coverage Endorsement.* The extended coverage must be written for the same amount as the fire policy, thus not increasing the face amount of the policy. They merely extend the coverage to include the added perils. Some of the following coverages also may be written separately:

- Collapse.
- Explosion of steam or hot water boiler.
- Falling trees.
- Glass breakage.
- Vandalism.
- Vehicles owned or operated by the insured.
- Water damage.
- Ice, snow and freezing.

*Other Coverage.* Additional coverages to be considered as endorsements to the fire policy or as separate coverages are:

- Earthquake insurance.
- Sprinkler leakage.
- Automobile damage (includes all risks of damage and collision of vehicles owned by the facility).
- Steam boiler and machinery (narrow form limited to damage caused by explosion, cracking, bulging, etc., to the boiler alone; broad form covers all

damage caused by explosion to the boiler and surrounding property).

### Consequential Loss Insurance

This is an indirect loss following destruction preventing the use of all or certain facilities:

*Business Interruption Insurance.* This provides a source of recovery for loss of income because of a reduction of business due to destruction or breakdown of the facility or part thereof.

*Extra Expense Insurance.* This covers costs of emergency operations.

*Accounts Receivable Insurance.* This protects against physical destruction of the accounts receivable records. A pattern of previous accounts receivable must be established to determine the amount of coverage.

### Theft Insurance

Two broad categories of theft insurance are burglary and theft, and fidelity bonds.

*Burglary and Theft.* The following are various forms of burglary and theft insurance:

1. **Open Stock Burglary Policy**—Insures against loss by burglary of merchandise, furniture, fixtures, equipment and damage to the premises because of the burglar by all but the nursing facility employees or agents. It does not cover the loss of money, securities, records and accounts.
2. **Mercantile Safe Burglary Policy**—Covers loss of money, securities, other property and damage resulting from the burglary of a safe.
3. **Money and Securities Broad Form Policy**—A comprehensive coverage for most mercantile risks providing coverage for all risk of money and securities.
4. **3D Policy**—Protects against comprehensive dishonest, disappearance and destruction.
5. **Blanket Crime Policy**—Like 3D but provides a single amount for all coverages.

*Fidelity Bonds.* This insurance covers an employer against the loss of any kind of property (money, securities, raw materials, merchandise or equipment) resulting from dishonest acts of employees. Some bonds insure only the named individuals; others cover all employees of a firm. If the insured is a partnership, the fidelity bonds will not cover the accounts of the partners because they are not employees. In a corporation, all officers are covered because they are employees, but the directors are excluded unless they are also officers or employees.

### Multiple Peril Coverage

These are sometimes called package policies and combine into one policy many different coverages. Advantages of multiple peril coverage are broader coverage, elimination of overlapping coverage and claims, and lower cost. Some policies cover all risks, whereas others insure specified perils.

## MEDICARE

Run by the Health Care Financing Administration (HCFA) of the Department of Health and Human Services, Medicare (Title XVIII) is a federal health insurance program for people age 65 or older and some disabled persons. State Social Security Administration offices provide information and registration for the program. This plan provides basic protection against the cost of health care but does not pay all medical nor most long-term care expenses; supplements to the program are sold by private insurance companies.

The Medicare program has two parts: **hospital insurance (Part A)**, which helps pay for inpatient care in hospitals and skilled nursing facilities, home health care and hospice care, and **medical insurance (Part B)**, which helps pay for doctors' services, outpatient hospital services, home health care and other medical services and supplies not covered under Part A. Before Medicare begins to pay for covered services and supplies, the insured must pay certain out-of-pocket expenses which include deductibles per benefit. (Part A) and per year (Part B), and coinsurance payments set each year by Congress.

Private insurance companies make the Medicare payments to the insured by contract with the federal government. Fiscal intermediaries are the insurance companies making coverage and payment decisions for the services under Part A; carriers are those insurance companies handling claims for services by doctors and other suppliers under Part B.

For services to be covered under Medicare, the providers of care from a hospital, skilled nursing facility (SNF), home health agency, hospice or outpatient rehabilitation service must be certified by Medicare. Other services that must be certified include ambulatory surgical centers, independent physical/occupational therapists, clinical laboratories, portable X-ray suppliers, dialysis facilities, rural health clinics and durable medical equipment suppliers. Medicare may pay for emergency care in a qualified nonparticipating (not certified by Medicare) hospital.

Doctors' services must be medically necessary and delivered in the most appropriate setting for the insured to be covered under Medicare. **Peer review organizations (PROs)** consist of doctors and other health care professionals paid by the federal government to review the hospital care of Medicare patients and are located in each state. They also review notices of noncoverage, individual complaints and hospital request for reconsideration of former PRO decisions.

Medicare benefits, protection and appeal rights are retained whether the beneficiary chooses fee-for-service or managed care. Under the fee-for-service program, the beneficiary receives services from Medicare certified providers of choice, and Medicare pays its share of the bill and the beneficiary the balance. Under the managed care plan, the beneficiary receives all services (except emergency) from the providers participating in the plan and may have to pay a monthly premium and co-payment at each visit.

## FEE-FOR-SERVICE SYSTEM

Following is an explanation of how Medicare benefits are received under the fee-for-service system.

### Hospital Insurance—Part A

Medicare Part A helps pay for most (but not all) services received from a hospital (inpatient), SNF following a hospital stay (inpatient), home health agency and hospice. Providers must inform those receiving services of the purposes of and their rights under advanced directives. The use of services under Part A in hospitals and skilled nursing facilities is measured by benefit periods; a benefit period starts upon first entry to a hospital and ends 60 days from the day of discharge. A new benefit period starts with each admit-

tance and the beneficiary must pay a new inpatient hospital deductible. There are no limits to the number of benefit periods.

### Hospital Inpatient Care

Medicare hospital insurance can help pay for up to 90 days of medically necessary inpatient hospital care if all of the following four conditions are met:

1. A doctor prescribes inpatient hospital care for treatment of the illness or injury.
2. The kind of care required can only be provided in a hospital.
3. The hospital is participating in Medicare.
4. The utilization review committee of the hospital or peer review organization approves the stay.

During each benefit period, Part A will pay for the 1st through the 60th day less the deductible and the 61st through the 90th day less the coinsurance. An additional 60 hospital inpatient reserve days are available to those needing a hospital stay of more than 90 days for which Part A will pay after a coinsurance payment. These days are for a lifetime and may be used at the patient's discretion.

Most inpatient hospital care is paid by Medicare under the prospective payment system (PPS), where, generally, fixed amounts based on the principle diagnosis are paid for each hospital stay. Participating hospitals must accept Medicare payments as payments in full and cannot bill Medicare patients for anything except the unpaid deductible amounts and noncovered items or services (e.g., telephone, private duty nursing, cosmetic surgery).

Medicare hospital insurance can pay for these inpatient services:

1. A semiprivate room (2 to 4 beds in a room).
2. All meals, including special diets.
3. Regular nursing services.
4. Costs of special care units (intensive or coronary care).
5. Drugs furnished by the hospital during the stay.
6. Blood transfusions furnished by the hospital during the stay except for any non-replacement fees.
7. Lab tests included in the hospital bill.
8. X-rays and other radiology services (including radiation therapy) billed by the hospital.

9. Medical supplies (casts, surgical dressings, splints).
10. Use of appliances (wheelchair).
11. Operating and recovery room costs including hospital costs for anesthesia services.
12. Rehabilitation services (physical/occupational therapy, speech pathology).

Medicare hospital insurance will not pay for these inpatient services:

1. Requested personal convenience items (e.g., television, radio, telephone).
2. Private duty nurses.
3. Any extra charges for a private room, unless it is determined to be medically necessary.

### Care in a Psychiatric Hospital

Hospital insurance can help pay for no more than 190 days of care in a participating psychiatric hospital in a lifetime. However, a special rule applies if the patient is in a participating psychiatric hospital. Any Social Security office can give the information about this special rule.

### Inpatient Care in a Skilled Nursing Facility

Medicare hospital insurance can help pay for inpatient care in a Medicare-certified SNF if all of the following conditions are met:

1. Daily skilled nursing or skilled rehabilitation services are required, which can only be provided in an SNF as a practical matter.
2. There is a three-day (not counting the date of discharge) stay in a hospital before admittance.
3. Admittance is within 30 days after leaving the hospital.
4. The required care is for a condition treated in or related to the condition treated in the hospital.
5. A medical professional certifies that skilled nursing or skilled rehabilitation services are needed and received on a daily basis.

Medicare hospital insurance will not pay for skilled nursing or rehabilitation services needed only occasionally and which are available outside the SNF, no longer improving the condition or may be carried out by someone other than a physical therapist or physical

therapist assistant. Custodial care (primarily for meeting personal needs and provided by non-professionals) is not covered even if received from participating providers.

Medicare hospital insurance can help pay for 100 days of needed daily skilled nursing care or rehabilitation services in a participating SNF, even if the insured is discharged and readmitted more than once during the benefit period. Part A pays for all covered services for the first 20 days; a daily coinsurance payment applies for the 21st day through the 100th day.

Medicare hospital insurance can pay for these major skilled nursing facility services:

1. A semiprivate room (2 to 4 beds in a room).
2. All meals, including special diets.
3. Regular nursing services.
4. Blood transfusions furnished during the stay (except any nonreplacement fees).

### Home Health Care

If part-time skilled health care is needed in the home for the treatment of an illness or injury, Medicare can pay for covered home health visits furnished by a participating home health agency—a public or private agency that specializes in giving skilled nursing services and other therapeutic services (such as physical therapy) in the home. A facility that mainly provides skilled nursing or rehabilitation services cannot be considered a home.

Medicare can pay for home health visits only if all of the following four conditions are met:

1. The care needed includes part-time or intermittent skilled nursing care, physical or speech therapy.
2. Confinement to the home.
3. A doctor determines the patient's need for home health care and sets up a home health plan.
4. The home health agency providing services is participating in Medicare.

Once these conditions are met, either hospital insurance or medical insurance can pay for medically necessary home health visits. Medicare pays the unlimited approved cost of all covered home health visits. There is no deductible. Any services or costs that Medicare does not cover may be charged to the recipient.

Part-time or intermittent home health services covered by Medicare include:

1. Nursing care.
2. Home health aides.
3. Medical social workers.
4. Various therapist (physical, occupational, speech).
5. Medical supplies.
6. 80% of the approved cost of durable medical equipment (such as oxygen equipment or wheelchairs).

### Hospice Care

A hospice is a public or private agency primarily providing pain relief, symptom management and supportive services to the terminally ill and their families. It includes both home and inpatient care (when needed) and a variety of services not otherwise covered under Medicare (i.e., everyday services, appropriate custodial care, homemaker's services or counseling).

Medicare can help pay for hospice services as long as a physician certifies the need if the following three conditions are met:

1. A doctor certifies that the patient is terminally ill.
2. A patient chooses hospice care over standard Medicare benefits for the terminally ill.
3. Care is provided by a Medicare-certified hospice program.

Hospital insurance can pay for up to 210 days of hospice care or longer in some cases. While the insured is receiving hospice care, Medicare will help pay for covered services under the standard benefit program for necessary treatment of a condition not related to the terminal illness; in this instance, deductibles and coinsurance must be paid. Under the hospice benefit, no deductibles are used, and Medicare pays the full cost of services except for the coinsurance on drugs and inpatient respite care where limited amounts apply. Inpatient respite care gives temporary relief to the provider of regular home care.

### Medical Insurance—Part B

Part B medical insurance picks up where Part A hospital insurance leaves off—to pay for doctors' services and a wide range of medical services and supplies.

A one-time yearly medical insurance deductible is paid by the insured. This can be met with any combination of the covered expenses related to doctors, health care providers and suppliers. Generally, Medicare medical insurance will pay 80% of the approved charges for any additional services received during the year. The Medicare carrier in each area determines the approved or reasonable charge for each service in accordance with Medicare law. The insured is usually responsible for the remaining 20% of the charges and all charges and services not covered by Medicare.

### How Medical Insurance Payments are Made

Payments are made two ways under Medicare medical insurance. After meeting the yearly medical insurance deductible, the medical insurance payment can be made to the doctor, supplier (by assignment), or to the patient:

- **Assignment**—The assignment method can be used only if both the patient and physician or supplier agree to it. When the assignment method is used, the doctor or supplier agrees that the total charge for the covered service will be the charge approved by the Medicare carrier. Medicare pays the doctor or supplier 80% of the approved charge, after subtracting any part of the yearly deductible not met. The patient is charged only for the part of any deductible not met, the co-insurance (the remaining 20% of the approved charge) and any services that Medicare does not cover.
- **Payment to the Patient**—Under this payment method, Medicare pays the patient 80% of the approved charge, after subtracting any part of the yearly deductible not met. The doctor or supplier can bill the patient for the actual charge, even if it is more than the charge approved by the carrier. The amount a physician may charge is limited; if he or she charges over this amount, the sanctions are severe. Doctors providing elective surgery and/ or services he or she believes Medicare will determine medically unnecessary—and therefore not cover—must inform the patient of this and the estimated charge in writing.

Doctors and suppliers can sign agreements to become Medicare-participating doctors or suppliers— thus agreeing to accept assignment on all Medicare claims. Hospitals, SNFs, home health agencies, comprehensive outpatient rehabilitation facilities, and providers of outpatient physical/occupational therapy and speech pathology services are all participating providers and must submit their claims directly to the Medicare carrier; the patient is billed for the 20% coinsurance and any unpaid part of the yearly deductible.

### Part B Coverage

*Physicians' Services.* Medicare medical insurance can help pay for medically necessary services provided by a doctor of medicine or a doctor of osteopathy in the office, hospital, SNF or other location in the United States. (Coverage is limited for services provided in Canadian or Mexican hospitals.) Second opinions involving surgery are recommended; Medicare will help pay for these.

*Other Medical Services and Supplies.* Benefits in these areas have special requirements. Some are more limited than others. Included are:

- Outpatient hospital services—helps pay for diagnosis or treatment of illness or injury received from participating hospitals or SNFs, or from Medicare-approved home health, rehabilitation or public health agencies or clinics.
- X-rays and laboratory tests.
- Ambulance transportation—can help pay for medically necessary ambulance transportation if the ambulance, equipment and personnel meet Medicare requirements and if transportation in any other vehicle would endanger the patient's health. This covers ambulance transportation between a patient's home and a hospital or SNF.
- Breast prostheses following mastectomy.
- Services of certain specially qualified practitioners (not doctors)—includes certified registered nurse, certified nurse midwife, clinical psychologist, clinical social worker, nurse practitioner and clinical nurse specialist. Medicare will help pay for services of chiropractors, podiatrists, dentists and optometrists under very limited circumstances.
- Physical and occupational therapy.
- Speech language pathology services.
- Home health services—if patient does not have Part A of Medicare.

- Blood—helps pay for the costs of blood received during an inpatient hospital or SNF stay. The annual blood deductible is the first three pints that must be paid for or replaced.
- Flu, pneumonia and hepatitis B shots.
- Pap smears for detection of the cervical cancer—once every three years.
- Mammograms to screen for breast cancer—every 24 months.
- Outpatient mental health services.
- Artificial limbs and eyes.
- Eyeglasses for corrective lenses after cataract surgery.
- Arm, leg and neck braces.
- Durable medical equipment—can help pay for durable medical equipment (oxygen equipment, wheelchairs, home dialysis systems and other medically necessary equipment) prescribed by a physician for use in the home and provided by an approved supplier.
- Kidney dialysis and kidney transplants.
- Heart and liver transplants—under limited circumstances in approved facilities.
- Medical supplies—includes ostomy bags, surgical dressings, splints, casts, and so on.

*Services in Special Health Care Facilities.* Medicare Part B covers a variety of services from providers other than hospitals and skilled nursing facilities. These include:

- Ambulatory surgical centers—for certain types of surgery performed at approved ambulatory surgical centers.
- Rural health clinics—services provided by doctors, nurse practitioners, doctor assistants, nurse midwives, clinical psychologists and social workers who are part of the clinic.
- Comprehensive outpatient rehabilitation facilities (CORFs)—if prescribed by a physician and the facility participates in Medicare.
- Community mental health centers—for specially qualified programs providing partial hospitalization for mental health care.
- Federally qualified health centers—a full range of services provided by community health centers, Indian health clinics, migrant worker health cen-

ters and centers for the homeless located in inner-city and rural areas.

- Certified medical laboratories—all charges (except in Maryland) for clinical diagnostic tests provided by a certified laboratory participating in Medicare.

Medicare medical insurance does not pay for many services and items, including:

1. Routine physical examinations and tests.
2. Routine foot care.
3. Most dental care and dentures.
4. Eyeglasses or hearing aids.
5. Most prescription drugs.

## MANAGED CARE PLANS

Each managed care plan has its own network of hospitals, skilled nursing facilities, home health agencies, doctors (of whom the beneficiary may choose a primary care physician) and other professionals who provide services at one or more centrally located health facilities and in private offices. With Medicare managed care plans, Medicare generally pays for all care received directly through the plan or from health care professionals referred by the plan. According to the plan selected, the beneficiary may have to pay a fixed monthly fee and a copayment each time a service is received. The managed care plans have varying contracts with Medicare as to where covered services can be received and percentages charged for services received outside the plan's provider network. The Part B premium to Medicare must be paid, but no deductibles or coinsurance are paid to Medicare for care received under a managed care plan.

### Medicare+Choice—Part C

Under the Balanced Budget Act of 1997, widespread changes in the federal program of health care for the elderly were made from financing the unmanaged care provided by traditional Medicare plans toward a variety of managed care plans. Managed care is directed toward reducing overuse and excesses in the fee-for-service system by offering appropriate individualized medical interventions (including some coverage of outpatient prescription drugs, hearing and visual care) at competitive costs. These plans are required to implement quality assurance programs, using outcome and patient satisfaction measures that will apply to the contracting health care providers. Provision of current fee-for-service benefits and a percentage of profits and requirements for additional services are mandated.

Beginning in 1999, an open enrollment period will be held each year for beneficiaries to choose how their Medicare benefits will be provided. Options are:

1. **Original Medicare**—Beneficiaries can use any hospital or doctor who accepts Medicare patients. The government regulates the doctors' fees and most other aspects of the program.
2. **HMO (health maintenance organization)**—Patients must use doctors, hospitals and suppliers approved by the HMO. The plan may pay for prescription drugs and other items not covered by Medicare. (See above the general explanation of managed care plans.)
3. **PPO (preferred provider organization)**—This plan pays a percentage of costs for health care while the beneficiary is responsible for the rest. A larger percentage is paid for using health care providers on the PPO's preferred list than for selecting providers outside this network.
4. **POS (plans with point of service options)**—When combined with a basic HMO package, this plan will pay some for care from health care providers outside of the HMO's network selected by the beneficiary. There will be higher out-of-pocket expenses to the beneficiary.
5. **PSO (provider-sponsored organization)**—The beneficiary receives care from hospitals and doctors who are the owners of the PSO and agrees to have his or her care managed by this plan. This form of managed care works much like an HMO.
6. **PFFS (private fee-for-service plan)**—The Medicare beneficiary chooses an insurance plan other than Medicare, which determines how much to reimburse for the provided services. Medicare pays this private plan a premium to cover the traditional benefits; the beneficiary pays whatever the plan does not cover and for any additional premiums.

## BIBLIOGRAPHY

Davis, W. 1994. *Introduction to health care administration*, 4th ed. Bossier City, LA: Publicare Press.

Department of Health and Human Services Health Care Financing Administration. 1997. *The Medicare handbook* (publication 10050). Baltimore, MD.

Elsey, D. 1998. *An introduction to the Medicare prospective payment system*. Minneapolis, MN: Larson, Allen, Weishair & Co.

Fisher, C. 1998. Crossing over to PPS. *Provider*.

Hawryluk, M. 1997. Reforms create a la carte Medicare. *Provider*.

National Board of Examiners of Nursing Home Administrators. 1997. *NAB study guide*, 3rd ed. Washington, DC.

Reynolds, I., N. Hillman, A. Douglas, and R. Kochanek. 1987. *Principles of accounting*, 4th ed. Hinsdale, IL: Dryden Press.

Wolver, R. 1998. All roads lead to skilled nursing facilities. *Provider*.

# Appendix 5-A

## Glossary of Accounting and Medicare-Related Terms

### GENERAL ACCOUNTING TERMS

**Acid Test Ratio**—Also called quick rate or quick current ratio, it measures the immediate solvency or debt-paying ability of a company.

**Accelerated Depreciation**—A method of computing depreciation, such as sum-of-year's digits or double-declining-balance, at a more rapid rate than would occur by the straight-line method.

**Accounting**—Record-keeping system and preparation analysis and interpretation of financial reports of a business.

**Accounting Equation**—An equation that is both the basic formula for the balance sheet and the foundation of double entry accounting. Assets = Liabilities + Fund Balances (stockholder's equity or capital).

**Accounting Period**—A period of time covered by an income statement. This period generally is not less than one month or longer than one year.

**Accounting Principles**—A body of rules, standards and conventions that determines the manner in which transactions are recorded and in which data are presented in financial statements.

**Accounting Reports**—Must have both fidelity and significance.

**Accounts Payable**—Amount owed to suppliers for goods or services purchased on credit.

**Accounts Receivable Aging Schedule**—An analysis of accounts receivable by length of time the accounts have been outstanding.

**Accounts Receivable Turnover**—Charges to residents' accounts during a given period divided by the amount of accounts receivable.

**Accumulated Depreciation**—The accumulation to date of depreciation expense, or the total portion of the original cost of depreciable assets that already has been allocated to expense in prior and current periods.

**Accrual Basis of Accounting**—Revenues and expenses are recognized in the period they are actually earned and consumed; assets and liabilities are reported in the time period purchased and incurred.

**Activity Ratio**—These divide various types of assets into net operating revenue.

**Adjusting Entry**—An entry that is necessary to adjust book account balances to conform with the actual balances and accrual basis at the end of the accounting period.

**Aging Schedule**—Separates and categorizes accounts according to the length of time they are outstanding.

**Allowable Charge**—The maximum fee a third-party payer will use in reimbursing a provider.

**Allowable Costs**—Costs that are reimbursable by a third-party payer.

**Amortization**—The systematic allocation of an item to revenue or expense over a determined number of accounting periods.

**Amortization of Debts**—The repayment of a loan over a period of time by making regular payments of principal and interest.

**Annuity**—Rents (receipts or payments) to be received or paid periodically in the future.

**Assets**—Property that an organization owns.

**Audit**—Checking and reviewing the accuracy of account records by an independent agency or person.

**Auditors**—Accountants who cross-check the bookkeepers to make certain records are accurate.

**Balance Sheet**—Financial statement summarizing assets, liabilities and net worth.

**Bank Statement**—Statement made by a bank to checking account customers, showing deposits, expenses, balances, interest earned and any service charges.

**Bidding**—Requesting a response to written specifications for goods or services (a price list) from vendors.

**Bill of Lading**—A document issued by a carrier to a shipper upon acceptance of goods for shipment, representing a receipt for the goods and the contract stating the terms for carriage.

**Bill of Sale**—A receipt signed by a seller, stating that a particular property has been transported to a specific buyer.

**Board-Designated Funds**—Unrestricted funds set aside by action of the nursing facility's governing board for specific purposes.

**Bond**—A written promise under seal to pay a sum of money at some definite future time.

**Bond Discount or Premium**—The difference between the par or face value of a bond and the amount received (by the issuer) or paid (by the investor) when a bond is issued or purchased.

**Bond Indenture**—The contract between the bondholders and the nursing facility issuing the bonds.

**Bond Sinking Fund**—A fund in which assets are accumulated in order to liquidate bonds at their maturity date or earlier.

**Book Value**—The amount at which a specific asset or liability is carried in the accounting records of the nursing facility.

**Break-Even Point**—The volume of revenue where revenues and expenses are exactly equal (i.e., the level of activity at which there is neither a gain nor a loss from operations).

**Capital**—Funds acquired for use in the business.

**Capital Expenditure**—An expenditure chargeable to an asset account where the asset acquired has an estimated life in excess of one year and is not intended for sale in the ordinary course of operations.

**Capital Expenditure Budgeting**—The process of planning and controlling expenditures for property, plant and equipment items.

**Capital Structure Ratios**—These show the relationship of long-term debt to total assets or to capital.

**Cash Basis of Accounting**—Revenue and expenses are not recognized until cash is received or paid out.

**Cash Disbursement Journal**—Records expenditures of cash.

**Cash Flow Statement**—Financial report showing cash receipts and disbursements leading to a change in cash position.

**Certificate of Deposit**—A certificate issued by a bank for a form of time deposit under which the depositor agrees to leave funds or deposit for a specified period of time in return for a rate of interest usually higher than a savings account.

**Charity Care**—Care provided to a resident knowing that the full cost will not be reimbursed either by the resident or any third-party payer.

**Chart of Accounts**—Complete listing of names of the accounts in the general ledger.

**Chattel Mortgage**—A mortgage on personal property, excluding real estate.

**Coinsurance Clause**—An insurance policy clause that limits the liability of the insurance company to a determinable percentage of the loss suffered by the insured.

**Collateral**—Assets that are pledged to secure a loan.

**Commercial Banking System**—Important source of funds for financing a business.

**Common Stock**—A form of ownership of a company.

**Compensating Balances**—Cash deposits required by a bank as personal compensation for lending or other services it provides to a nursing facility.

**Composition Ratio**—Shows the relationships between various types of assets and current or total assets.

**Compound Interest**—Interest that is computed on the principal amount invested or borrowed and on any interest earned (on such principal) that has not been paid.

**Computer Core**—This is the part of the memory unit that stores the computer's instructions and data.

**Consignee**—A person or party to whom merchandise is consigned or shipped.

**Contingent Liabilities**—Possible future liabilities that may arise due to some future event that is considered possible but not probable.

**Contra Account**—An auxiliary account that is an offset to a related account (i.e., allowance for uncollectable accounts offsets accounts receivable).

**Contractual Discount**—The uncollectable difference between the amount the facility charges for its services and the lower amount the facility has agreed to accept as reimbursement for Medicare or Medicaid.

**Contributed Capital**—Amount paid into the nursing facility by donors.

**Contribution Clause**—An insurance policy clause that limits the liability of the insurance company to a pro rata portion of a loss of property insured by more than one company.

**Control Account**—A general ledger account, the detail of which is contained in a subsidiary ledger (e.g., accounts receivable).

**Controllable Cost**—A cost in which the amount is controllable by someone in the organization (usually a variable cost).

**Controller**—The title usually given to the executive responsible for the accounting function in the organization.

**Corporation**—An artificial person or legal entity, created by law, with the capacity of perpetual succession.

**Cost**—The present value surrendered in cash or cash equivalent (or promised to be surrendered in the future) determined at the time of sale, in exchange for goods and services received. Expired costs are expenses; unexpired costs are assets.

**Cost Basis**—The use of historical, objectively determined cost as the basis of accounting for most assets.

**Cost Center**—An organizational unit whose costs are separately accumulated in the accounts.

**Cost Control**—The attempt to maintain actual costs at or below budgeted levels.

**Cost Finding**—The process of allocating indirect costs to cost centers to determine the true costs of services.

**Cost or Market, Lower Of**—A valuation basis for inventories and temporary investments.

**CPA's Purpose**—To provide impartial documentation as to the financial condition of the organization.

**Current Assets**—Assets that can be converted into cash within one year.

**Current Liability**—Obligations in which payment is expected to require use of current assets, usually paid within a one-year period.

**Current Ratio**—The ratio of current assets to current liabilities to measure the borrower's ability to meet current obligations.

**Day's Revenue in Receivables**—The average number of days of billings in accounts receivable and uncollected at a given point in time.

**Debenture Bond**—A bond not secured by specific assets but by the general credit standing of the issuer.

**Debit**—Amount shown in the left side of a T account, increasing assets and expense accounts and decreasing owner's equity and liability.

**Debt-to-Equity Ratio**—Long-term liabilities divided by total assets. Debt-to-equity ratio of 0.5 or more is considered good.

**Debt Financing**—Raising funds through interest bearing instruments.

**Department of the Treasury**—Internal Revenue Service operates under this department.

**Depreciation**—Decrease in value of an asset due to obsolescence.

**Depreciation Types**—Declining balance and straight line, and sum of the digits.

**Desirable Feature of Debt Financing**—Interest payments are deductible.

**3/10 N 30**—A discount of 3% if paid in 10 days; bill is net if paid in 30 days.

**Discounting of Receivables**—A method of short-term financing in which patient receivables are used to secure a loan from a financial institution.

**Discounted Note**—A note issued at a discount in which the interest is deducted in advance.

**Discretionary Costs**—Advertisement, sales promotion, donations, etc.

**Dishonored Note**—A note that is not paid at maturity.

**Dividends**—Earnings distributed to stockholders.

**Double Entry Accounting**—A system of recording both the debit and credit aspect of each transaction.

**Earnings**—Revenues not recognized until all activities to create them have been completed.

**Economic Order Quantity (EOQ)**—The optimum (least cost) quantity of goods that should be purchased in a single order.

**Endowment Fund**—Funds donated to a tax-exempt organization.

**Equity Financing**—Raising funds by issuing capital stock or ownership shares in a corporation.

**Expenses**—Cost of operating a business, including capital, administrative and other operating expenditures.

**Extraordinary Gains and Losses**—Gains or losses unusual in amount and nonrecurring in nature.

**Factoring**—The process of selling or assigning receivables to a factor as a means of obtaining short-term financing.

**FICA**—Federal Insurance Contributions Act commonly known as Social Security.

**FICA Taxes**—Current liability.

**FIFO**—First-in, first-out; a method of inventory costing.

**Financial Ratio Analysis**—The analysis of quantitative indicators of the financial health of the organization. These are ratios showing liquidity or the ability to satisfy short-term obligations.

**Fixed Assets**—Real estate, fixtures and equipment.

**Fixed Cost**—An operating or capital expense that does not vary with business volume. Examples: rent, real estate tax and depreciation.

**Flexible Budget**—A budget prepared in such a manner that it can be adjusted by interpolation to reflect what expenses should be at any level of activity within a relevant range.

**FOB (Free on Board) Destination**—A shipping arrangement under which the seller of goods bears the cost of transportation to buyer's location. It is at this point that the title of the goods passes from the seller to the buyer.

**FOB (Free on Board) Shipping Point**—A shipping arrangement under which the buyer of goods bears the cost of transportation from the seller's location to the buyer's location. The goods while in transit are the property of the buyer.

**Freight**—Property carried by a transporter.

**Functional Classification**—The groupings of expenses according to the operating purposes (such as administrative, property and related) for which costs are incurred. Revenues also are classified functionally.

**Fund**—A self-contained accounting entity set up to account for a specific activity.

**Fund Balance**—The excess of assets over liabilities (net equity). An excess of liabilities over assets is known as a deficit in fund balance. Term is used for tax-exempt entities.

**Funded Debt**—Long-term debt.

**Funded Depreciation**—The setting aside of a portion of retained earnings in a special account to be used for the purpose of new or replacement capital assets.

**FUTA**—Federal Unemployment Tax Act that established the federal unemployment insurance program.

**Garnishment**—A legal proceeding directing employers or others to withhold a designated amount of pay or other assets for the plaintiff.

**General Ledger**—A book that summarizes all journal entries for an accounting period in order to arrive at a trial balance.

**Goodwill**—Intangible asset. A fixed and favorable consideration of residents arising from a well conducted facility.

**Gross Income**—Gross receipts of a business before deduction or expenditures.

**Gross Margin Method**—A method of estimating the amount of inventory at a given point in time.

**Historical Cost**—Cost of acquiring a depreciable asset.

**Imprest Cash Fund**—(See Petty Cash Fund.)

**Increase an Asset**—Debit the account.

**Insolvency**—The inability to meet matured obligations.

**Installment Note**—A method of financing the acquisition of new equipment by installment payments over a period of months. The seller retains title until all payments have been completed.

**Intangible Asset**—An asset not having apparent physical existence (e.g., patents, copyrights and goodwill).

**Interest**—A charge for the use of money.

**Interim Financial Statements**—Financial statements prepared at a date other than the end of the fiscal year (e.g., monthly balance sheets and income statements).

**Inventory**—Amount of goods and materials on hand that are currently used in producing services.

**Inventory Turnover**—Cost of supplies used divided by the average inventory for the period.

**Inventory Valuation**—Accurate measurement of the cost of ending inventory to calculate net earnings. Inventories should be valued at a lower of cost or market. Inventory valuation methods are:

- *Average Cost*—This method determines a new unit cost for each item in stock every time new stock is received. The value of the old stock on hand is added to the cost of the new stock. The total stock value is divided by the total quantity on hand.
- *FIFO (First In, First Out)*—This method assumes that the older supplies are used first. In the event of inflation, this makes the value of the goods remaining in inventory higher than that of the goods used to provide service.
- *LIFO (Last In, First Out)*—This method assures that inventory added last to stock is used first. This makes the value of goods remaining in the inventory lower than that of the goods used to provide services.

**Invested Capital**—Equity capital that is supplied by the owner of a nursing facility.

**Invoice**—A document showing the details of a sale.

**Journal**—Book of original entry.

**Lease**—A contract in which the lessee (user) pays the lessor (owner) for use of an asset.

**Ledger**—A collection of all accounts payable and receivable used in the business.

**Lien**—A claim on particular property for payment of a debt or obligation.

**LIFO**—Last in, first out. An inventory costing method.

**Line of Credit**—An arrangement whereby a financial institution commits itself to lend a specified maximum amount during a specified period.

**Liquidity**—A nursing facility's financial position and its ability to meet currently maturing obligations. This denotes how quickly an asset can be converted to cash.

**Long-Term Investments**—Investments, generally in securities, which the nursing facility intends to hold for longer than one year from the balance sheet date.

**Long-Term (fixed) Liability**—An obligation not due for more than one year.

**Low Acid Test Ratio**—Can be explained by a seasonal fluctuation of service.

**Marginal Customers**—Customers who are poor credit risks.

**Marginal Return**—The point at which income equals expenses: the break-even point.

**Marketable Security**—Short-term financial instruments that can be readily purchased or sold without loss in principal.

**Matching**—An accounting principle that requires the recognition of related revenues and expenses in the same period.

**Material Management**—The integration of the processes of planning, acquiring, moving and controlling materials.

**Maturity Date**—Day on which a note becomes due and payable.

**Mortgage**—A pledge of designated property as security for a loan (e.g., mortgage bonds).

**Natural Expenditure Classification**—A method of classifying expenditures according to their natural classification such as salaries, utilities and supplies.

**Net Income**—Excess of revenue over related expenses during an account period.

**Net Worth**—Equals assets minus liabilities.

**Note**—An unconditional written promise to pay a definite sum of money at a certain date.

**Notes Receivable Discounted**—Notes receivable that have been discounted with recourse at a financial institution.

**Occupancy Rate**—The ratio of actual number of patient days to the total possible patient days.

**Operating Budget**—Includes anticipated income by source and anticipated expense by category.

**Operating Cycle**—The amount of time necessary for a facility first to convert cash into resident services, then resident services into receivables and then receivables into cash.

**Operating Ratio**—Total operating expenses divided by total operating revenues.

**Opportunity Cost**—The measurable advantage forgone in the past or that may be sacrificed as a result of a decision involving alternatives. Profits lost when capital is invested elsewhere.

**Owner's Equity**—Owner's investment which is the assets minus the liabilities.

**Par Value**—Face amount of a share of stock.

**Partnership**—An association of two or more people to operate a business for profit.

**Payback Period**—Time (in years) for a capital investment to pay for itself.

**Payroll Journal**—Record of payment of salaries and wages to employees.

**Periodic Inventory System**—A system of accounting for purchased goods and supplies by which items purchased are charged to expense accounts rather than to inventory.

**Perpetual Inventory**—System of inventory control based on keeping continuous records of supplies on hand.

**Petty Cash Fund**—A small fund of cash maintained for the purpose of making minor disbursements for which the issuance of a check would be impractical.

**Physical Inventory**—The actual inventory as determined by physical count, usually at the end of a reporting period.

**Pledging of Receivables**—Use of account receivables as security or collateral for a loan.

**Position Control Plan**—A management tool for controlling the number of employees on the nursing facility payroll and for assuring the utilization of each employee to the point of maximum effectiveness. Also termed a **staffing plan**.

**Posting**—Transfer from general journal to the ledger.

**Preemptive Right**—The right of existing stockholders to purchase a new issue of capital stock before it is offered to the general public.

**Preferred Stock**—Utilizes a fixed interest rate of corporate earnings.

**Prepaid Expenses**—Expenses paid in advance for a future period of time.

**Profitability or Performance Ratios**—Used in the study of income and revenues.

**Promissory Note**—This involves at least two parties and represents a promise to pay.

**Proprietary**—Ownership of property or business usually by one person.

**Purchase Order**—Document issued by a purchaser authorizing a seller to deliver goods with payment to be made later.

**Qualified Audit Report**—An audit report including one or more qualifications or exceptions.

**Quantity Discount**—A reduction in unit purchase cost received by those who purchase supplies in a quantity in excess of a certain amount.

**Ratio**—Expression of the relation of a numerical item to another.

**Real Estate**—Property in the form of land, buildings and hereditaments (things capable of being inherited).

**Reconciliation**—The procedure of checking bank accounts, deposits and withdrawals against the bank statement.

**Reserve for Bad Debts**—Reserve for uncollectable accounts.

**Responsibility Accounting**—A system of accounting that compiles financial and statistical data according to the organizational units producing the revenues and incurring the expense. The purpose is to attain optimum management control.

**Restricted Funds**—Funds restricted by donors for specific purposes. The term refers to specific purpose and endowment funds. This term applies specifically to tax-exempt organizations.

**Retained Earnings**—That portion of stockholders' equity attributable to profitable operation.

**Revenue**—Income or the inflow of assets from sale of services or products.

**Revenue Expenditure**—An expenditure charged against operations, as opposed to capital expenditure.

**Revolving Loan**—Bank loan expected to be renewed at maturity.

**ROP (Reorder point)**—In inventory management, the point in time at which a new order should be placed for supplies.

**Safe Harbor Regulations**—Federal regulations describing investment interest and other business transactions that are not violations of the Medicare and Medicaid anti-fraud and abuse regulations.

**Salvage Value**—The estimated amount for which a plant asset can be sold at the end of its useful life. Also called scrap value.

**Self-Pay Resident**—A resident who pays either all or part of the bill from his or her own resources as opposed to third-party payment.

**Semi-variable Costs**—Costs that are partly variable and partly fixed in behavior in response to changes in volume.

**Serial Bond**—This is a bond assigned a particular date after which it may be redeemed.

**Sinking Fund**—Funds required by external sources to be issued to meet debt service charges and the retirement of indebtedness on plant assets.

**Specific Purpose Fund**—Funds restricted by donors to tax-exempt organizations for a specific purpose. Board-designated funds do not constitute specific purpose funds.

**Stale Check**—An outstanding check of over 180 days usually.

**State of Changes in Financial Position**—A financial statement summarizing the movement of funds (working capital) within a nursing facility for a given period of time.

**Stock Authorization**—Maximum number of shares allowed for issuance by corporate charter.

**Stock Dividend**—A dividend paid in the form of additional shares of stock.

**Stockholders' Equity**—The excess of assets over liabilities, consisting mainly of invested capital and retained earnings.

**Stock Right**—A transferable subscription warrant issued by a corporation in connection with sale of a new issue of stock.

**Stock Split**—An action taken by a corporation to increase the number of shares outstanding, other than by sale, in order to reduce the market price of the stock to a level more attractive to investors.

**Straight-Line Method of Depreciation**—Also a method of amortizing bond premium and discount.

**Subordinate Debentures**—Bonds having a claim on assets only after the senior debts have been paid off in the event of liquidation.

**Subchapter S Corporation**—A corporation that is taxed as a private individual.

**Subsidiary Ledger**—A group of accounts that is contained in a separate ledger and supports a single account (a control account) in the general ledger.

**SYD (sum of years' digits)**—A method of accelerated depreciation.

**T Account**—A form of account resembling the letter "T." Credit is on the right-hand side, and debit is the left-hand side. Used in double entry accounting.

Account Name

| Debit an account to: | Credit account to record: |
|---|---|
| Increase an asset | Decrease an asset |
| Decrease a liability | Increase a liability |
| Decrease an owner's equity | Increase an owner's equity |

**Tangible Asset**—One that has physical characteristics such as equipment, land and buildings.

**Temporary Investments**—Investments, generally in marketable securities, that a nursing facility does not intend to hold for more than one year from the balance sheet date.

**Term Loan**—A loan generally obtained from a bank or insurance company with a maturity greater than one year. Term loans are generally amortized.

**Terms of Sale**—Conditions controlling the payment for a sale. For example: the term 4/10 net 30 means that if payment is made within 10 days of the invoice date, the seller will allow a 4% discount, or that the invoice must be paid within 30 days or it becomes overdue. The term 4%/10 E.O.M. means that a 4% discount may be taken if the invoice price is paid by the 10th day of the following month.

**Third-Party Payer**—Someone paying for the bill other than the patient. May be a commercial insurance company, Medicare or Medicaid.

**Trade Credit**—Debt arising from transactions in which supplies and services are purchased on credit from suppliers.

**Trial Balance**—A statement showing name and balance of all ledger accounts that are arranged according to whether they are debits or credits. Debits must equal credits.

**Turnover Ratios**—Emphasize the efficient management of assets by indicating the number of times assets (i.e., inventories, accounts receivables) are replaced during a period.

**Unamortized Bond Discount (Or Premium)**—That portion of bond discount (or premium) that has not yet been amortized.

**Unemployment Taxes**—Taxes levied by federal and state governments to finance payments to the unemployed. Paid by the employer.

**U.S. Treasury Security**—Security backed by the full faith and credit of the federal government.

**Unrestricted Funds**—A term used in tax-exempt organizations for funds that bear no external restrictions as to use or purpose (i.e., funds that can be used for any legitimate purpose designated by the governing board). They are distinguished from funds restricted externally for specific operating purposes, for plant replacement and expansion, and for endowment.

**Useful Life**—An estimate of the number of years an item of plant and equipment will be used by a nursing facility.

**Variable Cost**—An operating cost that varies in direct proportion to changes in volume such as salary costs and supplies.

**Variance Analysis**—Managerial control technique that identifies and investigates deviations from a budget's original projections.

**Voucher System**—A system for the processing and control of cash disbursements.

**Weighted-Average Costing**—A method determining the cost of supplies used and the valuation of inventory.

**Working Capital**—Generally, the excess of current assets over current liabilities.

**Write Off**—Removing a bad debt by reducing its value to zero.

**Yield**—The actual rate of return on an investment as opposed to the nominal rate of return.

## ACCOUNTING AND FINANCE TERMS FOR LONG-TERM CARE FACILITIES

**Accommodation**—The type of room a resident occupies. It can be a one-bed private room, a two-bed semiprivate room, or a three- to six-bed ward. In nursing facilities, the two-bed room is generally the accommodation provided.

**Apportionment (Allocation)**—This is a term coined by the Medicare program. It is the term used for describing a cost accounting procedure that distributes overhead costs to the departments producing revenue.

**Balanced Budget Act of 1997 (BBA)**—Established prospective payment system for nursing facilities.

**Bed Turnover Rate**—The number of times the bed complement of a facility changes residents during a given period of time. This is determined by dividing the average occupied beds by the total discharges for the same period of time.

**Cost Reimbursement**—The procedure used by Medicare to pay providers for the services provided to their beneficiaries. It determines the costs incurred and pays on a basis specified by law.

**Department**—A distinct service unit that is designated as such for the purpose of assigning costs and/or management responsibilities.

**Direct Cost**—The cost of providing the services that can be assigned to a specific department without cost finding. For example, payroll costs are assigned to a specific department based on the actual staff assigned. No assumptions or cost spreading are required.

**Donated Services**—The value attributed to services provided to a facility by employees who receive no compensation or only part compensation. The concept is usually applied to services rendered by members of religious orders to tax-exempt institutions.

**Indirect Cost**—An overhead cost that is not directly assignable to the production of the service; however, it must be allocated to various services based on its assumed contribution to the production of revenue.

**Inpatient**—A resident who is provided with room, board and nursing supervision or nursing care as prescribed by a physician in a long-term care facility.

**Inpatient Admission**—The formal acceptance of an inpatient by a long-term care facility for an overnight stay.

**Inpatient Bed Count**—The number of beds available for admission of inpatients as specified by license.

**Inpatient Bed Days Available**—The unit of measure designating the potential number of patient days that could be serviced in a 24-hour period.

**Inpatient Occupancy Rate**—The number of beds occupied in relation to the number of beds available. Calculated by dividing the inpatient bed days occupied by the inpatient bed days available in the specified period.

**Level of Care**—The degree of nursing supervision or nursing care required by an inpatient.

**Long-Term Care Facility**—Any facility licensed as a nursing facility, residential facility, shelter care home, convalescent home, intermediate care facility, skilled nursing facility or assisted living facility.

**Luxury Items**—Items not related to general resident care. This is a phrase coined by Medicare and Medicaid to designate items that are not reimbursable (for example, telephones and televisions).

**Medicaid**—The state-administered health program for the indigent. Reimbursement is shared by state and federal governments, and was required to be cost-related effective July 1, 1976.

**Medical Services**—The services provided by physicians, dentists, optometrists, nurses and other medical professionals.

**Mentally Disordered Resident**—A resident with chronic psychiatric impairment whose adaptive functioning is impaired. This resident requires continuous supervision and normally will benefit from rehabilitation.

**Nonoperating Revenue**—Revenue received from sources other than from operations.

**Occupancy Expense**—Expenses related to use of property (e.g., rent, utilities, depreciation, maintenance and real estate taxes).

**Operating Cost (or Expense)**—An expense incurred in providing resident care services.

**Outpatient**—A resident who is provided with services without being admitted as a bed patient.

**Overhead**—A cost of doing business that does not contribute directly to the production of revenue such as housekeeping, laundry and maintenance.

**Prospective Payment System (PPS)**—Method of Medicare reimbursement for nursing facilities.

**Resident Care Services**—General nursing care including nursing services, activities, social services, disability services and ancillary services.

**Resident Care Point**—The use of a relative value method of determining level of care. Nursing time is converted to point values for various resident care needs. The criteria for valuing level of care normally relates to activities of daily living and administration of medications.

**Resident Day**—Care of one resident for a 24-hour period starting and ending at midnight. In maintaining statistics, the day of admission is counted as a day of care but the day of discharge is not. A bed that is reserved and held for later occupancy is not included as a regular inpatient day. They are accumulated separately and called **bed-hold days**. If the bed-hold days are paid for by someone they are then included in the inpatient day statistics.

**Residential Facility**—A facility that provides room and board with personal services, protection, supervision, assistance in transportation, guidance and training to sustain the person in the activities of daily living. Medications and nursing are not provided.

**Revenue-Producing Cost Centers**—Departments providing direct service to resident for which they are charged, such as nursing, physical therapy, medications and medical supplies.

**Resource Utilization Group (RUG)**—Categories under PPS for medical reimbursement.

**Skilled Nursing Facility (SNF)**—A nursing facility or distinct part of a hospital that provides continuous nursing care to residents who are primarily immobile and need medications and restorative therapies. The intensity of licensed nursing care and medication is more than that provided in a nursing facility. The specifications for the minimum standards of nursing care are regulated by law.

**Stepdown Method of Cost Finding**—A method of cost finding to ultimately assign overhead costs to the revenue production departments. The departments that support the resident care departments are allocated in a rational and systematic manner to the nursing and ancillary departments.

**Swing Bed**—A hospital bed that has been certified as a long-term care bed. It can be used either way according to need in hospitals of less than 50 beds.

## MEDICARE-RELATED TERMS

**Actual Charge**—The amount a physician or supplier actually bills a patient for a particular medical service or supply. (This may differ from the customary, prevailing and/or reasonable charges under Medicare.)

**Assignment**—A process through which a doctor or supplier agrees to accept the Medicare program's payment in full except for specific coinsurance and deductible amounts required to the patient.

**Benefit Period**—Measures the use of service in hospitals and skilled nursing facilities under Medicare Part A.

**Carrier**—A private insurance organization that contracts with the federal government to handle claims from doctors and suppliers of services covered by Medicare medical insurance.

**Claim**—A request to a carrier or intermediary by a beneficiary or a provider acting on behalf of a beneficiary for payment of benefits under Medicare.

**Coinsurance**—A cost-sharing requirement that provides that a beneficiary will assume a portion or percentage of the costs of covered services.

**Comprehensive Outpatient Facility Services (CORFs)**—Services in areas of physical, occupational and other therapies for prevention, betterment and restoration of functional impairment.

**Customary Charge**—The amount that a doctor or supplier most frequently charges for each separate service and supply furnished.

**Deductible**—The amount of expense a beneficiary must first incur before Medicare begins payment for covered services.

**Durable Medical Equipment (DME)**—Wheelchairs, crutches, etc.

**Excess Charge**—The difference between the Medicare-approved amount and the actual charge for service or supplies, where the actual charge is greater.

**Health Maintenance Organization (HMO)**—A prepayment health care plan. HMOs with Medicare contracts offer Medicare beneficiaries all services covered by fee-for-service Medicare.

**Home Health Agency**—A public or private organization that specializes in giving skilled nursing services and other therapeutic services (such as physical therapy) in a beneficiary's home.

**Hospice**—A program operated by a public agency or private organization that engages primarily in providing pain relief, symptom management and supportive services for terminally ill people and their families.

**Hospital Insurance**—The part of Medicare that helps pay for inpatient hospital care, some inpatient care in a skilled nursing facility, home health care and hospice care.

**Intermediary**—A private insurance organization that contracts with the federal government to handle Medicare payment for services by hospitals, skilled nursing facilities and home health agencies paid through the hospital insurance program.

**Limiting Charge**—The maximum amount a doctor may charge a Medicare beneficiary for a covered service if the doctor does not accept assignment of the Medicare claim.

**Medical Insurance**—The part of Medicare that helps pay for medically necessary doctors' services, outpatient hospital services, a number of other medical services and supplies that are not covered by the hospital insurance part of Medicare, and some home health services.

**Medigap Policy**—Private health insurance designed to supplement Medicare.

**Outpatient Facility**—A facility designed to provide health and medical services to individuals who are not inpatients.

**Participating Physician or Supplier**—A physician or supplier who agrees to accept assignment on all Medicare claims.

**Peer Review Organizations (PROs)**—Groups of participating doctors and other health care professionals under contract to the federal government to review the care provided to Medicare patients.

**Prepayment Health Plans**—Health care providers such as HMOs and competitive medical plans (CMPs).

**Prevailing Charge**—Based upon the customary charges for covered medical insurance services or items, the prevailing charge is the maximum charge Medicare can approve for any item or service.

**Prospective Payment System (PPS)**—A process started in 1983 (using diagnosis-related groups or DRGs) under which hospitals are paid fixed amounts based on the principal diagnosis for each Medicare hospital stay.

**Qualified Medicare Beneficiary (QMB) Program**—Where Medicare pays premiums, deductibles and coinsurance for those with incomes below the national poverty level and very few resources.

**Quality Review Organizations (QROs)**—Groups of practicing doctors and other health care professionals under contract to the federal government to review the care provided to Medicare patients.

**Reasonable Charges**—Amounts approved by the Medicare carrier that will be either the customary, prevailing or actual charge, whichever is lowest.

**Skilled Nursing Facility (SNF)**—A specially qualified facility that has the staff and equipment to provide skilled nursing care or rehabilitation services and other related health services.

**Specified Low-Income Medicare Beneficiary (SLMB) Program**—Medicare pays Medicare Part B for those whose annual incomes are slightly above the national poverty level (up 20%).

**Supplemental Health Insurance**—Also termed "Medigap insurance"; private insurance designed to fill some of the gaps in Medicare.

**Supplier**—Person or organization, other than physicians or health care facilities, furnishing covered equipment or services.

# CHAPTER 6

# Resident Care Management: Facility Organization

## ADMISSIONS AND TRANSFER

Admissions determines the case mix (such as proportions of light/medium/heavy care, private/public pay or age range) of the residents in the facility. This affects resident orientation (for example, degree of physical illness and pain or contact with reality) and the general atmosphere, work load of the various services and facility income. Admissions usually are handled by the social services worker and the director of nurses, or by only the director of nurses.

### Preadmission Screening for Mentally Ill Individuals and Individuals with Mental Retardation
### 42 CFR, Sec. 483.100, Ch. IV (10-1-98)

Medicare/Medicaid law requires that the following conditions are complied with relating to admissions.

A nursing facility must not admit any new resident with:

1. Mental illness unless the state mental health authority has determined, based on an independent physical and mental evaluation performed by a person or entity other than the state mental health authority, prior to admission that:
   a. Because of the physical and mental condition of the individual, the individual requires the level of services provided by a nursing facility, and
   b. The individual requires active treatment for mental illness.
2. Mental retardation unless the state mental retardation or developmental disability authority has determined prior to admission that:
   a. Because of the physical and mental condition of the individual, the individual requires the level of services provided by a nursing facility, and
   b. The individual requires active treatment for mental retardation.

The nursing facility is required to notify the state mental health, mental retardation or developmental disability authority promptly after a significant change in the physical or mental status of a resident who is mentally ill or mentally retarded.

At the time each resident is admitted, the facility must have physician orders for the resident's immediate care. (For additional detail on admission requirements, see "Resident's Rights" in this chapter.)

### Notice of Legal Rights

The nursing facility must provide written information to each resident on his or her legal rights as a resident (see "Resident's Rights" in this chapter) in the following areas:

1. Notification of the name, specialty and method of contact for the **attending physician** responsible for his or her care. The provision of this information must be documented.
2. Formulation of **advance directives**, including the facility's policy regarding the implementation of these directives.
3. Protection and handling of **personal funds**. (See "Resident's Rights" in this chapter.)
4. Oral, written and posted information on how to apply for **Medicare and Medicaid benefits** and receive payment for covered services.
5. Requirements and procedures for establishing **eligibility for Medicaid**, including a request for assessment of nonexempt resources at the time of admission to the facility and any share of resources allowed a spouse living in the residence, which are not available for payment toward the cost of care for husband or wife residing in the facility.
6. Filing **complaints** with the state surveys certification agency, concerning abuse, neglect and/or misappropriation of resident property.
7. Posting names, addresses and telephone numbers of **state advocacy groups**, including state certification, survey and licensing offices, ombudsman program, Medicaid fraud control unit, and protection agencies for developmentally disabled and mentally ill.

## Advance Directives and Informed Consent

The **Patient Self-Determination Act of 1990** mandates that health care facilities accepting Medicare and Medicaid funds from the federal government inform individuals upon admission to the facility that they have the right to participate in and to direct the health care decisions that affect them.

Under the legal theory of the presumption of "sweetness and light," every individual is deemed to be competent unless adjudicated by a court of law to be otherwise. Thus, an individual has the right to be informed about his or her medical care, to accept or refuse medical or surgical treatment, and to communicate wishes concerning present treatment and future treatment by prior selection of a person to make health care decisions in the event of his or her incapacity or incompetence. Legal instruments for such advance directives, which are recognized under state law for implementing PSDA-90, include informed consent, living wills and durable powers of attorney for health care.

### Informed Consent

Informed consent ensures that an individual, guardian or agent receives adequate and full information to make a knowledgeable decision as a competent adult concerning any proposed medical or surgical treatment before agreeing to proceed with that treatment.

To give or withhold informed consent, the following information must be provided by the attending physician or other personnel of the health care facility as a minimum:

- The nature and purpose of the proposed treatment or procedure. The caregiver must explain the steps involved and the diagnostic or therapeutic results that are sought.
- The risks and likelihood of success of the treatment or procedure.
- Any alternative courses of treatment, including the option of no treatment (informed refusal).

PSDA-90 ensures the individual of the right to give or withhold consent for any medical or surgical procedure. Part of an informed consent includes the right to decide personal quality of life and whether to employ artificial life support systems when there is no reasonable hope of getting better.

### Living Will

A living will is concerned with personal health care decisions. This document gives precise instructions to the attending physician and health care provider (such as hospital or nursing facility) directing the life-sustaining medical treatment wanted or not wanted in the event of incapacity and a terminal condition or illness. The form and validity of living wills are covered by statutory law which may vary from state to state.

This written document may control life or death, and becomes effective when signed by a competent adult 18 years or older usually in the presence of two subscribing witnesses. Copies are given to the attending physician and/or health care providers. Copies also often are given to the declarant's attorney, clergy and/or family members. The living will should become part of the declarant's medical record pursuant to state statute. It will become operative when the attending physician makes a determination of a terminal illness or condition (as prescribed by state law) and the declarant is incompetent and/or incapacitated.

The living will remains valid and in effect until revoked by the declarant. It may be amended or revoked at any time by notifying the attending physician and health care providers of the changes or revocation, and a notation is made in the medical record. Periodic (every 2 years) review will ensure that this instrument continues to reflect the principal's wishes.

It is important to note that the living will is not operative when the declarant becomes unable to make health care decisions unless he or she also has been determined by a physician in accordance with state law to have a terminal condition or disease. It also does not deal with the many health care decisions other than life-sustaining treatment that must be made should the principal become incapacitated or incompetent and/or terminally ill.

### Durable Power of Attorney

Durable power of attorney deals with the decisions a person wishes to have carried out should he or she become incapacitated. It is drawn up so that another person (agent or attorney-in-fact) can make health care decisions and/or conduct business matters should the principal become unable to do so. Prior to the development of this special legal device, when an individual became unable to manage his or her property or person, it was necessary for someone to petition the court for appointment of a guardian or conservator to make these decisions. Another possibility was for a competent individual to create a funded revocable trust and transfer title of his or her property to someone to manage during any periods of incapacity or incapacitation; this, however, may or may not take care of decisions about one's person or health care. The Uniform Durable Power of Attorney Act provided an alternative for court-oriented procedures, such as conservatorship, guardianship and funded revocable trusts.

The durable power of attorney is a device authorized by state statute under which the principal, while competent, expresses his or her intent concerning the durability of his or her power through an agent to survive any incapacitation or incompetency. The document itself must contain a statement, such as: "This power of attorney shall not be affected by subsequent disability or incapacity of the principal," or "This power of attorney shall become effective upon the incapacity or incompetency of the principal," to be valid and to show the intent of the principal that the authority given to another can be used if the principal is unable to act for himself or herself.

A power of attorney, which only becomes operative upon the incapacity and/or incompetency of the principal, is termed "springing power." An advantage of a springing power is that it leaves the principal, while competent and able, in complete and sole control of his or her property and person as the agent cannot act. However, while one is competent and capable, there still may be difficulty in going to the bank, writing checks or otherwise conducting business. It is sometimes necessary to appoint someone with the power to perform these functions. Questions also can arise concerning just when the principal becomes incompetent or incapacitated and when this power really comes into being. This determination generally is made by the attending physician.

The execution of a durable power of attorney should be undertaken with care. It seems that the powers provided to an agent might be likened to those of a trustee, guardian or conservator. Although considerable power is put into the hands of the agent, he or she has a duty to obey the will of the principal and must act in accordance with the principal's expressed wishes and/or with what he or she understood the principal's wishes would be under the particular circumstances. The agent may have powers if expressly set forth in the instrument that would permit the making of gifts, creation of a trust, disclaimer of interested property and changing of beneficiaries under insurance, annuity policies and directives as to artificial life support systems and/or artificial hydration or nutrition.

The powers granted to an agent will last indefinitely, for a certain number of years as determined by state law, or may be limited within the document itself. However, the durable power of attorney can be revoked orally or in writing at any time so long as the principal is a competent adult, and this is done in accordance with state statute. At the point of incompetency or incapacity, the principal is unable to undo what he or she has done. Review of the durable power of attorney is usually recommended every few years to check that the decisions made are still appropriate.

If no advance directive for health care is available, the attending physician—with the advice and consent of the family or next of kin—will try to make medical care decisions based on what he or she feels is best for the incapacitated or incompetent person, taking into account any expressed wishes known. Many states have statutes that outline the priority followed in picking someone to act for the incapacitated or incompetent person usually in this order: spouse, adult children, father/mother and brother/sister.

## Advance Directives
### 42 CFR, Sec. 489.102, Ch. IV (10-1-98)

Federal regulations define advance directives as written instruments, such as living wills or durable powers of attorney for health care, relating to the provision of health care when an individual is incapacitated. These are recognized under state law and/or by the state courts.

Skilled nursing facilities (SNFs) and nursing facilities (NFs) are among those health care providers who must maintain written policies and procedures concerning advance directives in regards to all adult residents. Facilities are required to provide written information at the time of admission regarding:

1. The right under state law to make decisions concerning medical care, refuse medical or surgical treatment and formulate an advance directive. If state law changes, the facility must inform the resident within 90 days.
2. The facility's written policies to implement these rights and a clear precise statement concerning any limitation as to implementation on the basis of conscientious objection including the:
   a. Difference between the institution-wide conscientious objections and those of individual physicians.
   b. State legal authority allowing such objections.
   c. Medical conditions or procedures covered.
3. Documentation in a resident's medical record on whether the individual has executed an advance directive.
4. Ensure compliance with state law (statutory or recognition by the courts).

5. Educate staff concerning facility policies and procedures in this area.
6. Provide (or participate with other providers or organizations) for community education, including what advance directives are and the state laws involved. Written materials may be developed. Documentation of community education efforts is required.

This advance directives information is given to the family, surrogate or other concerned persons (under state law) should the individual be incapacitated at the time of admission. Follow-up procedures must ensure that such a resident is directly informed once he or she is no longer incapacitated.

Facilities are not to provide care that conflicts with an advance directive. They are not required to implement an advance directive if there is an institution-wide conscientious objection and the state law allows such an objection.

## Transfer of Residents

The transfer of a resident is done only upon request of a physician or the family. Arrangements for transportation are made by the facility when a resident is transferred to the hospital. Records are sent regarding the resident's medications and other pertinent information ensuring continued care until the physician gives orders to the hospital. Needed clothing is sent with the resident, whereas other personal belongings will be transferred to the resident's relatives or kept in safekeeping until proper arrangements can be made to transfer them elsewhere.

Two kinds of transfer agreements exist: a community-wide agreement that is entered into with a group of hospitals and nursing facilities and an individual agreement that is entered into with one or more hospitals. The transfer agreement is one that provides in writing for the transfer of residents and their medical records between the hospital and the nursing facility whenever such action is medically indicated as determined by the attending physician. The community-wide transfer agreement may include not only general health services or resources, but general hospitals, long-term care facilities, outpatient clinics, home care programs, public and voluntary health, welfare and rehabilitation agencies, and mental health services. A nursing facility must have a transfer agreement with at least one hospital.

The objectives and purposes of a formal transfer agreement between the nursing facility and general hospital are:

1. Develop procedures of a standardized nature for transfer of residents from one facility to another.
2. Get the medical staff of the institutions who are parties to the transfer agreement involved in the care of the resident at an early stage.
3. Help to make prompt decisions about shared services between the facilities.
4. Help in recruitment of personnel in both facilities.
5. Assist in conducting educational programs in the facilities.

The major elements of a transfer agreement are:

1. Identification of each institution and of the officers who are legally authorized to sign the agreement.
2. General statement and a listing of specific purposes of the agreement.
3. Designation of any committee composed of the participating institutions who will implement the agreement, conduct periodic reviews and make revisions of the plan as necessary.
4. Procedure for settling disputes arising under the agreement.
5. Statement that the agreement may be terminated by either party if certain qualifications are not maintained by either of the participating institutions.
6. Procedure for changing or terminating the agreement.
7. Procedure for actual transfer and responsibilities and liabilities of each facility.

In the health care field, effective communications are essential between facilities meeting the medical needs of residents and involve timing, intensity of therapy and choice of action. From the viewpoint of giving continuous medical and nursing care, communication is extremely important if the resident is to maintain or advance any recovery in a rehabilitation center or hospital.

## Transfer Agreements
### 42 CFR, Sec. 483.75, Ch. IV (10-1-98)

Medicare and Medicaid law requires that the facility have in effect a written transfer agreement with one or more hospitals approved for participation under the Medicare and Medicaid programs that reasonably assures that:

1. Residents will be transferred from the facility to the hospital and ensured of timely admission to the hospital when transfer is medically appropriate as determined by the attending physician.
2. Medical and other information needed for care and treatment of residents and—when the transferring facility deems it appropriate—for determining whether such residents can be adequately cared for in a less expensive setting than either the facility or hospital will be exchanged between the institutions.

The facility is considered to have a transfer agreement in effect if the facility has attempted in good faith to enter into an agreement with a hospital sufficiently close to the facility to make transfer feasible. See Exhibit 6–1 for an example of a transfer agreement.

## MEDICAL-SOCIAL SERVICE DEPARTMENT

The medical-social service function in the modern nursing facility is very broad. Services are provided to meet the medically related social and personal needs of the resident. Generally, the social service department or function makes provision for the following:

- **Personal Adjustment of the Resident to Nursing Facility Environment**—The social service department makes provisions for the writing of social histories on residents prior to or immediately after admission. The department obtains necessary information from various referral sources such as other social service agencies, residents, family members and physicians. The social history is then made available as part of the medical record to professional and paramedical personnel concerned with the resident; confidentiality of this record is

**Exhibit 6–1** Community-Wide Transfer Agreement

A sample community-wide transfer agreement as developed by the American Health Care Association is adapted as follows:

THIS AGREEMENT is made as of the _____ day of _____, 19 _____ by and between _____ a nonprofit corporation (herein called "Hospital") and _____ (herein called "Nursing Facility").

WHEREAS, both the Hospital and Nursing Facility desire, by means of this Agreement, to assist physicians and the parties hereto in the treatment of residents, (a) by facilitating the timely transfer of residents and medical and other information necessary or useful in the care and treatment of residents transferred, (b) and determining whether such residents can be otherwise adequately cared for than by either of the parties hereto, and (c) to ensure continuity of care and treatment appropriate to the needs of the residents in the Hospital and at the Nursing Facility, utilizing the knowledge and other resources of both facilities in a coordinated and cooperative manner to improve the professional health care of residents.

NOW THEREFORE, THIS AGREEMENT WITNESSETH: That in consideration of the potential advantages accruing to the (a) residents of each of the parties, (b) their physicians, and (c) the mutual advantages accruing to the parties hereto, the Hospital and Nursing Facility hereby covenant and agree with each other as follows:

1. In accordance with the policies and procedures to be established by the Liaison Committee, as hereinafter provided, upon the recommendation of an attending physician, who is a member of the medical staff of the Hospital, that such a transfer is medically appropriate, such residents shall, if the resident is at the
   a. Hospital, be admitted to the Nursing Facility, or
   b. Nursing Facility, be admitted to the Hospital as promptly as possible under the circumstances. Hospital and Nursing Facility mutually agree to exercise their best efforts to provide for prompt admission of residents provided that all usable and reasonable conditions of admission are met.

2. Hospital and Nursing Facility agreed to provide each other with full and adequate information concerning the other's resources so that either can determine whether the other can provide the care needed by a resident as prescribed by his or her physician.

3. Hospital and Nursing Facility agree:
   a. To arrange for appropriate and safe transportation of the resident,
   b. To arrange for the best possible care for the resident,
   c. To transfer the personal effects (including money and valuables) and information relating to the same and be responsible therefore until signed for by a representative of the party to whom transferred,
   d. That clinical records of a resident transferred shall contain evidence that the resident was transferred promptly and safely, and
   e. That transfer procedures shall be made known to the resident care personnel of each of the parties.

4. Hospital and Nursing Facility agree to transmit with each resident at the time of transfer, or in the case of an emergency, as promptly as possible thereafter, an abstract of pertinent medical treatment without interruption and to provide identifying and other information. Such medical and other information must include:
   a. Current medical findings,
   b. Diagnosis,
   c. Rehabilitation potential,
   d. A brief summary of the course of treatment followed in the Hospital or Nursing Facility,
   e. Dietary and nursing information useful in the care of the resident, and
   f. Administrative and pertinent social information.

5. If the services performed by the Hospital are not payable to the Hospital under the terms of any third-party insurance or other coverage and if requested by the Nursing Facility, the Hospital may bill the Nursing Facility directly, and the Nursing Facility assumes responsibility for the payment to the Hospital for the reasonable cost of any services, including emergency or outpatient services performed for the residents of the Nursing Facility. The Hospital assumes responsibility

*continues*

**Exhibit 6–1** continued

for payment to the Nursing Facility for services performed solely under identical circumstances.

All other bills incurred with respect to services performed by either Hospital or Nursing Facility for residents received from the other pursuant to the Agreement, shall be collected by the party rendering such services directly from the resident, third-party insurance coverage or other sources normally billed by the party, and neither Hospital nor Nursing Facility shall have any liability to the other for such charges.

6. Promptly upon the execution hereof, a Liaison Committee shall be formed to facilitate the general implementation of the Agreement. The Liaison Committee shall consist of the Administrators of the Hospital and Nursing Facility and such other members as each may designate. The Committee shall have the responsibility: to plan and supervise the initial implementation of the Agreement, establish and approve policies and procedures, consistently and conveniently conduct a periodic review of such procedures, consider and resolve problems arising under this Agreement, and recommend revisions thereto if and as the same become appropriate.

7. Any dispute that may arise under this Agreement shall first be discussed directly by the Departments of the parties that are directly involved. If the dispute cannot be resolved at this level, it shall be referred to the Liaison Committee for discussion and resolution.

8. The Board of Directors of the Hospital and the Board of Directors of the Nursing Facility shall have exclusive control of the policies, management, assets and affairs of their respective facilities. Neither party assumes any liability by virtue of this Agreement, for any debts or other obligations incurred by the other party to this Agreement.

9. Nothing in this Agreement shall be construed as limiting the rights of either party to affiliate or contract with any other Hospital or Nursing Facility on a limited or general basis while this Agreement is in effect.

10. Neither party shall use the name of the other in any promotional or advertising materials unless review and approval of the intended use shall first be obtained from the party whose name is used.

11. This Agreement shall be effective from the date of execution and shall continue in effect indefinitely except that either party may withdraw by giving 60 days notice in writing to the other party of its intention to withdraw from this Agreement. Withdrawal shall be effective at the expiration of the 60 days notice period. However, if either party shall have its license to operate revoked by the State or become ineligible as a provider of service under Title I, Part I of Public Law 89-97, this Agreement shall terminate on the date such revocation or ineligibility becomes effective.

This Agreement may be modified from time to time by mutual agreement of the parties, and any such modification or amendment shall be attached to and become part of this Agreement.

A confirmed copy of this Agreement with all amendments, if any, together with a copy of the current policies and procedures, referral forms and other documents adopted by the Liaison Committee to implement this Agreement shall be kept in the administrative file of the each of the parties for ready reference.

IN WITNESS WHEREOF, the parties hereto have executed this Agreement the day and year first above written.

ATTEST:

_____ By _____
                        for the Hospital

_____ By _____
                        for the Nursing Facility

**Individual Transfer Agreement**

Following is a sample of a transfer agreement between the nursing facility and an individual hospital:

_____ Hospital and _____ Nursing Facility, believing that the interests of the patient can best be served by assuring continuity of in- and post-hospital care, hereby agree to the following:

1. Nothing in this transfer agreement shall be construed as limiting the facility's exclusive control

*continues*

**Exhibit 6–1** continued

of its separate identity and integrity, such as: management, assets, debts and other obligations.

2. Neither institution shall be responsible or assume any responsibility for the moral or legal obligations of the other institution.

3. The name of the neither institution shall be used for any form of publicity or advertising by the other institution without the written consent of the institution whose name is to be used.

4. Each institution shall have the right to enter into transfer agreements with other institutions.

5. _____ Hospital shall admit residents from _____ Nursing Facility upon the request of the resident's physician.

6. _____ Nursing Facility shall retain a bed for the transferred resident and shall accept the resident as soon as the physician discharges the resident from the Hospital.

7. Residents transferred from _____ Nursing Facility to _____ Hospital, shall be considered on an emergency priority.

8. Transfer Record, Form # _____, shall be completed by the transferring institution and shall accompany the resident to the receiving institution.

9. The resident shall be held responsible for the inpatient and outpatient charges incurred in each institution. Neither institution shall be responsible for the resident charges.

10. The resident shall be held responsible for payment of all transferring charges (i.e., ambulance).

11. The two institutions shall adopt standardized medical record forms and policies.

12. Medical records kept in each institution should remain the property of that institution.

13. The medical staff organization of _____ Hospital shall establish a utilization review committee which shall supervise the medical audit and utilization review of the residents in the _____ Nursing Facility.

14. Disputes arising from this transfer agreement shall be resolved by the arbitration committee or persons selected by the two institutions.

15. This transfer agreement shall be terminated by either institution by notifying the other institution by registered letter 60 days prior to the termination date.

16. This agreement shall be terminated by either institution if license to operate is repealed, suspended or placed on probation by any governmental licensing agency.

This transfer agreement shall become effective on _____.

_____  _____
Date            For Hospital

_____  _____
Date            For Nursing Facility

_____  _____
Date            For Hospital Medical Staff

---

very important. The department will assist the resident to adjust to his or her new environment and help him or her to cope with the underlying problems relating to adjustment.

- **Helping the Resident To Get Along with Other Residents**—The social service department works daily with the other professional and paramedical personnel in the facility and the community in the planning and implementation of supportive and rehabilitative services for the residents during their stay in the nursing facility. Residents are encouraged to participate in group activities as indicated by their physical condition and to seek pastoral counseling and volunteer services as required by

the resident's condition. The department may consult with other nursing home personnel should they encounter social adjustment problems of the resident with other residents in the facility.

- **Helping the Resident To Get Along with Family**—The social service department maintains a relationship with the family of the resident and keeps them informed of the resident's adjustment and progress in the facility. This may include such activities as dealing with the attitudes of the family toward the resident and the nursing facility, and assisting both the family and resident regarding financial problems, emotional problems or other problems relating to the care of the resident.

- **Helping the Resident To Reach into Community Resources**—The resident is assisted in tapping into community resources and in satisfying particular social or psychological problems as they relate to medical conditions. The social service department evaluates each resident's need for continued care in the facility and assists in the determination as to whether the resident should remain or return to the community or family. This department helps the resident transferred to another facility if the need arises or in the event that the nursing facility cannot continue to provide the needed services for the resident's adjustment to his or her medical problems. The social service department also would help to find a suitable environment for the resident if he or she is dissatisfied with the facility, and this dissatisfaction cannot be resolved. Working also with the staff in the facility and with other social service agencies in the community, this department helps solve the particular problems of the resident in his or her home. Family service, a community agency, may participate in evaluating the need for a person to go to a nursing facility and relate to the family why a particular facility is adequate or inadequate to fulfill the physical, emotional and psychological requirements of the potential resident.

The medical-social service department maintains information on various social service agencies to which referrals may be made for the different types of social problems. The name, address, phone number and the person to contact regarding the particular services, for instance, should be made available to the administrator and kept current. This department encourages the establishment of community resources to fulfill the needs of the elderly in the community.

## Staffing and Responsibility of the Social Service Department

The social service department or the function—if not a separate department—ordinarily reports directly to the administrator. Ideally, the medical-social worker is a trained social worker with a master's degree in medical-social work. In parts of the country where resources for trained individuals are particularly short, a person with an associate bachelor's degree in sociology or with certification as a social service technician may be used. The following alternatives may be considered in the absence of a full-time trained social worker on the staff:

1. Arrange for a consulting social worker on a contractual basis employed by hospitals, family service bureaus or other social agencies on a regular hourly or daily basis.
2. Assign some of the facility personnel to hospitals or other qualified agencies to receive intensive inservice training and supervision or have an employee work under the direction and supervision of a trained social service worker.

## Records of the Social Service Department

Social data relating to the personal and family relations of residents is confidential and should be made available only to the attending physician, appropriate members of the nursing staff and other personnel who are directly involved in the care of the resident. Policies and procedures should be instituted to ensure the confidentiality of these records. Separate social work records very often are kept on each resident. Social service histories, summaries and progress notes should be maintained on all residents during the stay of the resident and upon discharge from the facility. Some health facilities keep the social service records separate from the medical record while the resident is in the facility; after discharge, they may be part of the medical record.

## Policies and Procedures Regarding the Social Service Department

Such policies and procedures ensure that the social worker:

1. Has office space that will allow him or her to conduct private interviews with the resident and/or relatives of the resident.
2. Maintains information on social services and assists the residents and families to use them.
3. Has full access to residents unless contradicted by the attending physician, the wishes of the family or the resident.
4. Makes certain that each resident has read and understands the resident's bill of rights.

5. Keeps in touch with residents and families regarding medical and social problems, participation in care and discharge planning, any financial or legal problems and community resource needs.
6. Compiles social service histories (including background, family resources and interests) on each resident. These are kept with the medical record or in a separate file in the social service department. Confidentiality of these records is ensured.
7. Works with other nursing facility personnel as a member of the interdisciplinary team responsible for resident assessment and care plans and is active in the training and orientation of all staff members to promote understanding of the social components in nursing facility care.
8. Arranges for adaptive equipment, clothing and other personal items residents may need.
9. Informs professional and paramedical personnel that if they feel that the resident could use the services of the social service department, a referral form is available that can be sent to the social service department.
10. As a key person in management of the facility, develops a good working relationship with other professional and paramedical personnel and uses consultants (psychiatrists, psychologists and other social service agencies) upon receiving approval from the attending physician.

## Social Services
### 42 CFR, Sec. 483.15 (G), Ch. IV (10-1-98)

Medicare and Medicaid require that certain conditions be met relating to social services. The facility must provide medically related social services to attain or maintain the highest practicable physical, mental or psychological well-being of each resident.

1. A facility with more than 120 beds must employ a qualified social worker on a full-time basis.
2. Qualifications of a social worker are:
   a. A bachelor's degree in social work, or
   b. A bachelor's degree in a human services field, including but not limited to sociology, special education, rehabilitation counseling and psychology, and
   c. One year of supervised social work experience in a health care setting, working directly with individuals.

## RESIDENT'S RIGHTS

The Department of Health, Education and Welfare first published the "Resident's Bill of Rights" in the *Federal Register* in October 1974. The rules contained in this bill of rights are guaranteed to all nursing facility residents under federal and state law.

The fact that a resident has been adjudicated incompetent, is medically incapable of understanding or exhibits a communication barrier will not absolve the nursing facility from advising a resident of his or her rights to the extent that the resident is able to understand them. In the case where the resident is incapable of understanding his or her rights, the facility will advise the guardian, next of kin or sponsor.

To implement this responsibility, the staff social worker and activity director shall arrange a meeting among all residents physically and mentally able to understand the provisions of these policies. The resident's bill of rights will be read to the group and discussed. Each resident will be provided with a copy and be asked to sign a statement that he or she has received it and that the contents have been read and explained. Exhibit 6–2 depicts a form that may be used to acknowledge receipt of this information.

The administrator will ensure that adequate in-service sessions are scheduled for staff to familiarize them with the contents of this policy. In the following text, actual rules and regulations are in italic type; interpretations are not.

---

**Exhibit 6–2** Acknowledgement Certificate

I, _____(Name of Resident or Legal Surrogate)_____, certify that I have received a copy of the **Resident's Bill of Rights** issued by _____(Name of Facility)_____. The contents have been explained to me and I understand my rights as set forth therein.

_____
Signature of Resident

_____
Witness

Dated this _____ day of _____, 19 _____.

### Resident's Bill of Rights
**42 CFR, Sec. 483.10.12, .13 and .15, Ch. IV (10-1-98)**

*The resident has a right to a dignified existence, self-determination and communication with and access to persons and services inside and outside the facility. A facility must protect and promote the rights of each resident.*

#### Privacy and Respect

Under this requirement, the *resident has a right* to:

1. *Personal privacy and confidentiality of his or her personal and clinical records.*

   *Personal privacy includes accommodations, medical treatment, written and telephone communications, personal care, visits, and meetings of family and resident groups. This does not mean that the facility must provide a private room for each resident.*

   Personal and clinical records include all types of records the facility might keep on a resident; they may be social, medical, financial, automated or other records. The resident has the right to keep the record and the information in these records private. A violation of this right may result in a law action in invasion of privacy against the facility.

2. *Approve or refuse release of personal and clinical records to any individual outside the facility.* A resident may refuse to release any information in any of the records the facility keeps on him or her.

   *The resident's right to refuse release of personal and clinical records does not apply when the resident is transferred to another health care institution, or when record release is required by law.*

3. *Reside and receive services in the facility with reasonable accommodation of individual needs and preferences except when the health and safety of the individual or other residents would be endangered.*

   "Reasonable accommodation of individual needs and preferences" means that the facility can adapt certain physical areas and staff behavior to help the resident to have independent functioning, dignity and well-being. It does not mean that interior design modifications are necessary for a resident's room (such as repainting walls and replacing carpeting or tile). Space may be created flexibly for various resident needs. For example, privacy for visitation or meetings may be arranged by using a dining area between meals, a vacant room or office, or a chapel.

   Covered also in the term "reasonable accommodation of needs" is the way the facility's physical environment is used to aid residents in maintaining unassisted functioning. This includes making it easier for the resident to move about; the use of furniture and equipment that gives proper support for residents to stand by themselves without assistance (such as arm supports or correct chair heights); and the use of proper equipment for disabled residents in going to the bathroom (such as grab bars or elevated toilet seats). The facility also must have in place measures to make it safe for confused residents who wander—allowing them to walk around unrestrained. The facility should have readable calendars and clocks displayed, wall hangings reflecting the lives of residents and other measures to encourage resident or resident-staff interaction.

4. *Receive notice before the resident's room or roommate in the facility is changed.*

   The issue of notice regarding change of room and/or roommate is more fully explained under the section concerning transfer or discharge of the resident.

   It is important under this right that the resident is informed in advance about a change in room or roommate and why the change is taking place. Another area of concern is whether the resident is moved when he or she asks to be moved.

5. *Refuse transfer to another room within the institution, if the purpose of the transfer is to relocate from the distinct part of the institution that is a SNF to a part of the institution that is not a SNF, or from a NF to a distinct part of the institution that is a SNF. The resident's exercise of this right does not affect his or her eligibility or entitlement to Medicaid benefits.*

6. *Exercise his or her right as a resident of the facility and as a citizen or resident of the United States.*

   Exercising rights means that the residents have autonomy and choice to the maximum extent possible about how they want to live their everyday lives and to receive care subject to the facility's rules affecting resident conduct and those regulations governing the protection of resident health and safety.

In determining the rights of residents, the resident's rights are weighed against those of society. If society or other residents in the facility may be harmed, the resident may stand to lose some of his or her rights.

Under this requirement, the *facility must:*

1. *Care for its residents in a manner and in an environment that promotes maintenance or enhancement of each resident's quality of life.*
2. *Promote care for residents in a manner and in an environment that maintains or enhances each resident's dignity and respect in full recognition of his or her individuality.*

    "Dignity" means that the staff of the facility in their work with residents shows an appreciation for and makes every attempt to promote each resident's self-worth. Areas in which the staff can enhance the resident's self-image and self-worth relate to grooming, helping to dress and respecting each resident's right to private space and property (i.e., not changing the radio or TV without the resident's permission). The staff also should respect each resident's social status by speaking respectfully, listening carefully and addressing each resident in the way he or she wishes.

3. *Inform the resident both orally and in writing in a language that the resident understands of his or her rights and of all rules and regulations governing resident conduct and responsibilities during the stay in the facility. Such notification must be made prior to or upon admission and during the resident's stay. Receipt of such information and any amendments to it must be acknowledged in writing.*

    "To inform the resident in a language that he or she understands" means that the passing on of information concerning rights and responsibilities must be both clear and understandable to the resident. If the resident cannot understand English, the rights must be explained in a foreign language familiar to the resident.

For foreign languages commonly used in a local area, the facility must have written translations of its statement of rights and responsibilities and should make available the services of an interpreter.

In the case of a foreign language not common in a given local area, a representative of the resident may sign that he or she has interpreted the statement of rights to the resident prior to the resident's acknowledgement of receipt.

For hearing-impaired residents who communicate by sign language, the facility is expected to provide an interpreter. *Large print texts* of the facility statement of resident's rights and responsibilities also should be available.

"Both orally and in writing" means that if a resident can read and understand written materials without assistance, an oral summary along with the written document is acceptable.

"During the resident's stay" means that if the rules and regulations governing resident conduct or rights change, the facility must update residents about these changes.

*If a resident is adjudged incompetent under the laws of a state by a court of competent jurisdiction, the rights of the resident are exercised by the person appointed under state law to act on the resident's behalf.*

*Any legal-surrogate designed in accordance with state law may exercise the resident's rights to the extent provided by state law where the resident has not been adjudged incompetent by a state court.*

4. *Promptly notify the resident and (if known) the resident's legal representative or interested family member when there is a change in room or roommate assignment.*
5. *Promptly notify the resident and (if known) the resident's legal representative or interested family member when a change occurs in resident's rights under federal or state law or regulation.*
6. *Record and periodically update the address and phone number of the resident's legal representative or interested family member.*

### Medical Care and Treatment

Under this requirement, the *resident has a right* to:

1. *Access all records pertaining to himself or herself, including clinical records, within 24 hours of an oral or written request by the resident or his or her legal representative. After receipt of his or her records, the resident has a right to purchase at cost (not to exceed the community standard) photocopies of the records or any portions of them upon request providing the facility receives two working days advance notice.*

   "Right to inspect" may apply either to the resident or to others based upon state law (i.e., guardian, conservator, holder of durable power of attorney). It is important when residents request to inspect their records that no unnecessary delays occurred in allowing them to do so.

   "Purchase" means that the resident may be charged for photocopy costs at the prevailing community charge. The information and content of the record is the resident's property, but the actual paper the record is written on is the property of the facility.

   "Two working days advance notice" means two business days, excluding holidays and weekends.

   Should a resident wish to see his or her medical record—contrary to the instructions of the attending physician—the nursing staff should contact the physician who may want to visit with the resident, family or legal guardian before complying with the request.

2. *Be fully informed in language that he or she can fully understand of his or her total health status, including but not limited to medical condition.*

   "Total health status" includes medical care, nursing care, dietary needs, rehabilitation and restorative potential, activities, mental status, dental-health status, psychosocial status, and sensory and physical impairments.

   The resident should be consulted and involved in his or her assessment and care planning process, including a discussion in a language that the resident can understand about his or her diagnosis, treatment choices, risks (if any) and prognosis.

3. *Refuse treatment, refuse to participate in experimental research and formulate an advance directive.*

   When a resident refuses treatment, it is important that the refusal is documented in the resident's record. If possible, the health and safety consequences of his or her refusal and any alternatives

to the refused treatment should be discussed with the resident. If a resident refuses all treatment, the only alternative for the facility is to discharge the resident on the grounds that the facility is incapable of meeting his or her health needs. (This is explained further under "Admission, Transfer and Discharge Rights" in this chapter.)

   "Experimental research" means using residents to develop and test clinical treatments (new drugs or therapy) involving treatment and control groups. If a resident is considered for participation in experimental research, he or she must be fully informed of the nature of the experiment and understand the possible consequences of participating. The resident or his or her legal representative must give written consent prior to participation. Experimental research also must respect the privacy of the resident; any direct observation requires the consent of the resident, his or her legal representative or family member. General resident statistics that do not identify individual residents may be used for studies without obtaining the resident's permission.

   It is important that the facility have an institutional review board or other committee that reviews and approves research protocol. (See "Advanced Directives" in this chapter for facility responsibilities in this area.)

4. *Choose a personal attending physician.*

   The right to choose a personal physician does not mean that the physician must or will serve a resident, or that a resident must designate a personal physician.

   If a resident does designate a personal physician and that physician fails to fulfill given requirements under Medicare and Medicaid law, the facility will have the right after informing the resident to seek alternative physician participation to assure the provision of appropriate and adequate care and treatment.

5. *Be fully informed in advance about care and treatment and of any changes in that care or treatment that may affect the resident's well-being.*

6. *Participate in planning care and treatment or changes in care and treatment unless adjudicated incompetent or otherwise found to be incapacitated under the laws of the state.*

"Informed in advance" means that the facility discusses with the resident or his or her legal representative, treatment options and alternatives. The resident selects and approves the specific plan of care before it is instituted. This requirement does not apply to emergency procedures in life-threatening situations unless advance directives are in effect.

7. *Self-administer drugs if the interdisciplinary team has determined that this practice is safe.*

The interdisciplinary team includes the attending physician, a registered nurse with responsibility for residents and other appropriate staff depending upon the resident's needs. Participation of the resident or legal representative is allowed to the extent practicable.

The interdisciplinary team must ask the resident during the assessment whether he or she wishes to self-administer drugs. If the resident says no, the resident has exercised his or her right and the responsibility then becomes that of the facility. If the resident says yes, the interdisciplinary team must assess the resident's understanding, and physical and visual ability to carry out this responsibility. If the interdisciplinary team determines that the resident is incapable to carry out this responsibility because of a danger to the resident or others, the team may withdraw this right.

It is the responsibility of the nursing staff to record self-administer doses in the resident's medication administration record.

Medication errors occurring with residents who self-administer drugs should not be counted in the facility's medication error rate. A number of medication errors by the resident should call into question the judgment made by the facility in allowing the resident to self-administer drugs.

Under this requirement, the *facility must:*

1. *Immediately inform the resident, consult with the resident's physician, and (if known) notify the resident's legal representative or interested family member when problems arise.*
   These include:
   a. *An accident involving the resident that results in injury and has the potential for requiring physician intervention.*

b. *A significant change in the resident's physical, mental or psychosocial status (i.e., a deterioration in health, mental or psychosocial status in either life-threatening conditions or clinical complications).*
   c. *A need to alter treatment significantly (i.e., a need to discontinue an existing form of treatment due to adverse consequences, or to commence a new form of treatment).*
   d. *A decision to transfer or discharge the resident from the facility.*

2. *Inform each resident of the name, specialty and way of contacting the physician responsible for his or her care.*

If the facility has a clinic or similar arrangement, they should supply residents with the name and contact information for the primary physician and/or central number for the clinic staff.

### Freedom from Abuse and Restraint

Under this requirement, the *resident has the right* to:

1. *Be free of interference, coercion, discrimination or reprisal from the facility in exercising his or her rights.*

The facility must not hamper, compel by force, treat differently or retaliate against a resident for exercising his or her rights.

The facility should support and encourage resident participation in meeting care planning goals as documented in the resident assessment and care plan. This is not interference or coercion.

Some examples of trying to limit the choice of the resident in exercising his or her rights are:
   a. Reducing the group activity time of a resident trying to organize a resident group.
   b. Requiring residents to seek prior approval to distribute information about the facility.
   c. Discouraging a resident from hanging a religious ornament above his or her bed.
   d. Isolating residents for prejudicial treatment.
   e. Assigning inexperienced aides to a resident with long-term care needs because the resident exercises his or her rights.

2. *Be free from any physical restraints imposed or psychoactive drug administered which are not required to treat the resident's medical symptoms for the purposes of discipline or convenience.*

"Physical restraints" are any manual methods, physical or mechanical devices, or material or equipment attached or adjacent to the resident's body in a way that the individual cannot remove the restraint easily, and the restraint restrains freedom of movement or normal access to the body by the resident. Some common examples of physical restraints are leg restraints, arm restraints, hand mittens, soft ties or vest, wheelchair safety bars and geriatric chairs.

"Psychoactive drugs" are drugs prescribed to control mood, mental status or behavior.

"Discipline" is any action taken by the facility for the purpose of punishing or penalizing residents.

"Convenience" is any action taken by the facility to control resident behavior or maintain residents with the least amount of effort by the facility. This occurs not in the best interest of the resident, but for the benefit of the facility.

"Less restrictive measures" than restraints (such as pillows, pads, removable lap trays) are often effective in achieving proper body positions, balance and alignment and in preventing contractions.

A facility must have evidence of a consultation with health professionals (such as occupational or physical therapists) in the use of less restrictive support devices prior to using physical restraints.

If after a trial of less restrictive measures, the facility decides that a physical restraint would enable and promote greater functional independence, the use of the restraining device must first be explained to the resident, family member or legal representative. If the resident, family member or legal representative agrees to the treatment alternative, the restraining device may be used for specific periods for which the restraint has been determined to help.

If medical symptoms appear life threatening (i.e., dehydration, electrolyte imbalance, urinary blockage), a restraint may be used temporarily to provide necessary life saving treatment. Physical restraints may be used for brief periods to allow medical treatment to proceed if documented evidence is available of resident, family or legal representative approval of the treatment.

One consideration in the use of restraints is staff consultation with the resident, family or legal representative in weighing the risks and benefits in using physical restraints.

There should be some evidence in the resident's care plan that the need for restraints is periodically reevaluated and that efforts to eliminate their use have been made.

3. *Be free from verbal, sexual, physical or mental abuse, corporal punishment and involuntary seclusion.*

Residents are not to be abused by anyone. This includes facility staff, other residents, consultants, volunteers, staff or other agencies serving the resident, family members, legal guardians, friends and other individuals.

"Verbal abuse" means any use of oral, written or gestured language including disparaging and derogatory terms in relation to residents or their families. Also prohibited is describing residents in a derogatory way within their hearing distance regardless of their age, ability to comprehend or disability.

"Sexual abuse" includes sexual harassment, coercion or assault.

"Physical abuse" includes hitting, slapping, punching, kicking and controlling behavior of the resident through corporal punishment.

"Involuntary seclusion" means separation of a resident from other residents or from his or her room against the resident's will or the will of the resident's legal representative.

"Temporary monitored separation" from other residents is not considered involuntary seclusion if used as therapeutic intervention to reduce agitation as determined by professional staff and consistent with the resident's plan of care.

"Mental abuse" includes humiliation, harassment, threats of punishment or deprivation.

Under this requirement, the *facility must:*

1. *Develop and implement written policies and procedures that prohibit mistreatment, neglect and abuse of residents, and misappropriation of resident's property.*

As part of the written policies and procedures developed by the facility under this section, a mechanism should be in place for the investigation of alleged violations of abuse or neglect. Any alleged violations of individual rights are thoroughly investigated and appropriate action taken and documented.

2. *Not use verbal, mental, sexual or physical abuse, including corporal punishment or involuntary seclusion.*

3. *Not employ individuals who have been found guilty by a court of law of abusing, neglecting or mistreating individuals.*

4. *Have a finding entered into the state nurse aide registry concerning abuse, neglect, mistreatment of residents or misappropriation of their property.*

5. *Report any knowledge of actions by a court of law against an employee that would indicate unfitness for services as a nurse aide or other NF staff to the state nurse aide registry or licensing authorities.*

6. *Ensure that all alleged violations involving mistreatment, neglect or abuse (including injuries of an unknown source), and misappropriation of a resident's property are reported immediately to the administrator of the facility and other officials in accordance with state law through established procedures.*

7. *Must have evidence that all alleged violations are thoroughly investigated and must prevent further potential abuse while the investigation is in progress.*

8. *Must report the results of all investigations to the administrator or his or her designated representative and other officials in accordance with state law within five working days of the incident; if the alleged violation is verified, appropriate corrective action must be taken.*

### Freedom of Association and Communication in Privacy

Under this requirement, the *resident has the right* to:

1. *Examine the results of the most recent survey of the facility conducted by federal or state surveyors and any plan of correction in effect with respect to the facility.*

    "Survey results" means the statement of deficiencies and plan of correction, if required.

    The posting of the results of a survey "in a place readily available to the residents" means at eye level in a central *public place* in the facility such as a lobby or in areas frequently visited by most residents.

2. *Receive information from agencies acting as client advocates and be afforded the opportunity to contact these agencies.*

3. *Have privacy in written communications, including the right to send and receive mail promptly that is unopened and have access to stationery, postage and writing implements at the resident's own expense.*

    "Promptly" as used in this section means delivery to the resident within 24 hours of arrival in the facility and delivery to the postal service within 24 hours except on weekends.

    Some of the things surveyors will look for include:

    a. Is the resident's mail sealed when he or she receives it?

    b. Does the resident have access to stationery, paper and writing materials?

4. *Receive visitors with the facility allowing access to the resident for such visitors at any reasonable hour.*

    "At any reasonable hour" means at least eight hours per day arranged in such a way that daytime, evening and weekend visitation times are available to meet most health practitioner and non-family visitor schedules. The resident retains the right to refuse to see a visitor.

5. *Immediate access to a variety of visitors. These include:*

    a. *Any representative of the secretary of HHS.*

    b. *Any representative of the state.*

    c. *The resident's individual physician.*

    d. *The state long-term care ombudsman.*

    e. *The agency responsible for the protection and advocacy system for developmentally disabled individuals.*

    f. *The agency responsible for the protection and advocacy system for mentally ill individuals.*

    g. *Immediate family or other relatives of the resident subject to the resident's right to deny or withdraw consent at any time.*

    h. *Others who are visiting with the consent of the resident which is subject to reasonable restrictions and the resident's right to deny or withdraw consent at any time.*

6. *Have reasonable access to the use of a telephone where calls can be made without being overheard.*

    "Private" means hearing privacy and, to the extent feasible, visual privacy.

Surveyors will look for telephone equipment that accommodates the hearing-impaired and wheelchair-bound resident. They will also inquire as to the means of residents to make private calls—whether the resident receives assistance when needed and whether the resident receives his or her messages.

7. *Share a room with his or her spouse when married residents live in the same facility and both spouses consent to the arrangement.*

   A request by both spouses to share a room must be honored, even if case-mix and other classification groups vary.

   Facilities are not required to grant room sharing rights to nonmarried consenting adults.

   The facility must explain their policies on room sharing request to prospective residents prior to admission.

   Facilities should attempt to accommodate residents' wishes and preferences in roommates whenever possible.

8. *Participate in social, religious and community activities that do not interfere with the rights of other residents in the facility.*

   The facility should accommodate, if possible, an individual's needs and choices for how he or she spends time inside and outside the facility.

9. *Organize and participate in resident groups in the facility.*

   This right does not require that residents must organize a family group. However, whenever residents or their families want to organize, facilities must allow such organizations to exist. The facility is required to provide the group with space, privacy for meetings and staff support. Normally, the designated staff person responsible for assistance and liaison between the group and facility administration would be the only staff person present during the resident or family group meetings—and only if the group requests assistance.

*In addition, the resident's family has the right to meet in the facility with the families of other residents in the facility.*

A resident or family group means a group that meets on a regular basis to discuss and offer suggestions about facility policies and procedures affecting the residents' care, treatment and quality of life; to plan resident and family activities; to participate in individual activities; and for any other purpose.

Under this requirement, the *facility must:*

1. *Post the results of the most recent survey in a place readily accessible to residents.*
2. *Provide reasonable access to any resident by any entity or individual that provides health, social, legal or other services to the resident (subject to the resident's right to deny or withdraw consent at any time).*
3. *Allow representatives of the state ombudsman to examine a resident's clinical records with the permission of the resident or the resident's legal representative.*
4. *Provide a resident or family group (if one exists) with private space.*
5. *Provide a designated staff person responsible for providing assistance and responding to written requests that result from group meetings.*
6. *Listen to the views and act upon the grievances and recommendations of residents and families concerning proposed policy and operational decisions affecting resident care and life in the facility.*

### Activities

Under this requirement, the *resident has the right* to:

1. *Choose activities, schedules and health care consistent with his or her interests, assessments and plans of care.*
2. *Interact with members of the community both inside and outside the facility.*
3. *Make choices about aspects of his or her life in the facility that are significant to the resident.*

Under this requirement, the *facility must:*

1. *Provide medically related social services and ongoing programs of activities to attain or maintain the highest practicable physical, mental or psychosocial well-being of each resident.*

   The surveyor may inquire whether or not the resident can make free choices regarding:
   a. *Getting up in the morning or retiring in the evening.*

b. *Eating of meals other than at scheduled meal-times.*
c. *Eating with residents of his or her choice.*
d. *Leaving the facility for short periods of time.*
e. *Planning of his or her own daily activities.*

## Work

Under this requirement, the *resident has the right* to:

1. *Refuse to perform services for the facility.*
2. *Perform services for the facility if he or she chooses, when:*
   a. *The facility has documented the need or desire for work in the plan of care.*
   b. *The plan specifies the nature of the services performed and whether the services are voluntary or paid.*
   c. *Compensation paid for services is at or above prevailing rates.*
   d. *The resident agrees to the work arrangement described in the plan of care.*

"Prevailing rate" means the wage paid to nondisabled workers in the community surrounding the facility for the same type, quality and quantity of work requiring comparable skills.

All resident's work, whether voluntary or paid, must be part of his or her plan of care. A resident's desire to work is subject to medical consideration. If the work is a part of a resident's plan of care, the therapeutic assignment must be formally agreed to by the resident. The resident has the right to refuse such treatment at any time.

## Personal Possessions

Under this agreement, the *resident has the right* to:

1. Retain and use personal possessions, including some furnishings and appropriate clothing as space permits, unless to do so would infringe upon the rights or health and safety of other residents.

All of the resident's possessions—regardless of their value to others—must be treated with respect for what they are and for what they represent to the resident. This right assures the resident that his or her personal possessions are important. The right to retain and use them creates a homelike environment.

The facility may be held liable for negligently handling the private possessions of residents. Therefore, the facility should use every reasonable effort to advise the resident of the risks of having valuable items in the facility. The facility should encourage labeling of all resident personal possessions kept in the facility. It is the facility's responsibility to investigate promptly incidence of loss or damage to property.

Many of the property right disputes might be handled through the resident and family groups.

## Grievances and Complaints

Under this requirement, the *resident has the right* to:

1. *Voice grievances without discrimination or reprisals. Such grievances include those with respect to treatment that has been furnished, as well as that which has not been furnished; and*
2. *Prompt efforts by the facility to resolve grievances the resident may have, including those with respect to behavior of other residents.*

Under this requirement, the *facility must:*
*Furnish a written description of the legal rights including:*
   a. *The manner of protecting the personal funds; and*
   b. *The resident's right to file a complaint with the state survey and certification agency concerning resident abuse, neglect and misappropriation of resident property in the facility.*

## Financial Affairs

Under this requirement, the *resident has the right* to:
*Manage his or her financial affairs.*
*The facility may not require residents to deposit their personal funds with the facility.*

Unless the resident has been determined incompetent by a court under state law, the resident has a right to manage his or her own financial affairs and is under no moral or legal obligation to deposit personal funds with the facility. If the resident chooses, he or she may ask the facility to manage his or her funds. In that case, the facility must manage the funds. The facility must keep the resident's funds in an account or accounts that are separate from any facility operating funds or funds of any person other than another resident (pooled resident's funds are permitted).

Whether the account is individual or pooled, the facility must maintain a system that assures a full, complete and separate accounting of each resident's assets and earnings. In the case of a pooled account, an individual resident's share of earnings must be protected on a regular basis. The facility must afford the resident or legal representative reasonable access to the record.

Under this requirement, the *facility:*

1. *Must inform each resident who is entitled to Medicaid benefits about charges that may be incurred. This request must be made in writing at the time of admission to the nursing facility or when the resident becomes eligible for Medicaid of:*
   a. *The items and services that are included in nursing facility services under the state plan and for which the resident may not be charged.*
   b. *Those other items and services that the facility offers and for which the resident may be charged and the amount of charges for the services.*
2. *Must inform the resident before or at the time of admission and periodically during the resident's stay of services available in the facility and of the charges for those services (including any charges for services not covered under Medicare or by the facility's per diem rate).*

   "Periodically" in this section means as often as the facility changes its services or the charges for these services.

   If upon admission or during the stay of a resident, a Medicare SNF provider believes that Medicare will not pay for skilled nursing or specialized rehabilitation services, the facility must inform the resident or his or her legal representative in writing why these specific services may not be covered. The provider must keep a copy of this letter on file.

   If the resident requests that the bill be submitted for the intermediary or coverage carrier for a Medicare decision, evidence that this submission has occurred should appear in the resident's record.

   Advance notice to the resident of changes in services or charges is not required. Whenever possible, however, advance notice should be given in order to be consistent with the intent of the law which is to allow residents to be fully informed of

what they owe the facility. The burden of proof is a good faith effort to inform the resident fully of services and charges and related changes.

3. *Must furnish a written description of legal rights. This includes:*
   a. *A description of the manner of protecting personal funds.*
   b. *A description of the requirements and procedures for establishing eligibility for Medicaid, including the right to request assessment that determines the extent of a couple's nonexempt resources at the time of institutionalization. It also attributes to the community spouse an equitable share of resources that cannot be considered available toward the cost of the institutionalized spouse's medical care in his or her process of spending down to Medicaid eligibility levels.*
   c. *A posting of names, addresses and telephone numbers of all pertinent state client advocacy groups, such as the state survey and certification agency, state licensure office, state ombudsman program, the protection and advocacy network, and Medicaid fraud control unit.*
   d. *A statement that the resident may file a complaint with the state survey and certification agency concerning resident abuse, neglect and misappropriation of resident property.*
4. *Must display prominently in the facility written information and provide to residents and potential residents oral and written information about how to apply for and use Medicare and Medicaid benefits and how to receive funds for previous payments covered by such benefits.*
5. *Must upon written authorization of a resident, hold, safeguard, manage and account for the personal funds of the resident deposited with the facility. Also the facility must:*
   a. *Deposit any resident's personal funds in excess of $50 in an interest-bearing account (or accounts) that is separate from any of the facility's operating accounts. It must credit all interest earned on the resident's account to his or her account.*
   b. *Maintain a resident's personal funds that do not exceed $50 in a noninterest-bearing account or petty cash fund.*
6. *Must establish and maintain a system that assures full, complete and separate accounting, accord-*

ing to generally accepted accounting principles, of each resident's personal funds that are entrusted to the facility on the resident's behalf.

  a. In addition, the system must preclude any commingling of resident funds with facility funds or with the funds of any person other than another resident.

  b. The individual financial record must be available through quarterly statement on request to the resident or his or her legal representative.

7. Must notify each resident who receives Medicaid benefits.

  a. When the amount in the resident's account reaches $200 less than the Social Security Insurance (SSI) resource limit for one person.

  b. If the amount in the account, in addition to the value of the resident's other nonexempt resources, reaches the SSI resource limit for one person, the resident may lose eligibility for Medicaid or SSI.

8. Must convey within 30 days the resident's funds, and a final accounting of those funds, to the individual or probate jurisdiction administering the resident's estate upon the death of a resident with a personal fund deposited with the facility.

9. Must purchase a surety bond, or otherwise provide assurance satisfactory to the secretary, to assure the security of all personal funds of the residents deposited with the facility.

10. May not impose a charge against the personal funds of a resident for any item or service for which payment is made under Medicare or Medicaid (except for applicable deductible, copayments and coinsurance amounts). The facility may charge the resident for requested services that are more expensive or in excess of covered services.

  a. During the course of a covered Medicare or Medicaid stay, the facility may not charge for the following categories of items and services: nursing services, dietary services, activity programs as required and certain routine personal hygiene items and services required to meet the needs of residents.

  b. The general categories and examples of items and services that the facility may charge to the resident's funds if they are requested by the resident are: telephone; personal comfort items, clothing, reading matter, flowers and plants; social events and entertainment outside activ-

ity programs; noncovered special services (i.e., privately hired aides and nurses); private room (except if therapeutically required); and specially prepared or alternative food requested.

11. Must not charge a resident for any item or service not requested by the resident.

  a. The facility must inform the resident requesting an item or service, for which a charge will be made, that there will be a charge and what the charge will be.

### Admission, Transfer and Discharge Rights

Admissions Policy. Under this agreement, the facility:

1. Must not require a third-party guarantee of payment to the facility as a condition of admission, expedited admission or continued stay in the facility.

2. Must not charge, solicit, accept or receive in addition to any amount otherwise required to be paid under the state plan, any gift, money, donation or other consideration as a precondition of admission, expedited admission or continued stay in the facility in the case of a person eligible for Medicaid.

3. Must not require residents or potential residents to waive their rights to Medicare or Medicaid.

4. Must not require oral or written assurance that residents or potential residents are not eligible for, or will not apply for, Medicare benefits.

5. May require an individual who has legal access to a resident's income or resources available to pay for care, to sign a contract (without incurring personal financial liability) to provide the facility payment liability from resident's income or resources.

6. Must not require a resident to request any item or service as a condition of admission or continued stay.

7. May charge a resident who is eligible for Medicaid for items and services the resident has requested and received and that are not specified in the state plan as included in the term "nursing facility services." The facility may charge provided it gives proper notice of the availability and cost of these services to residents and does not condition the resident's admission or continued

stay on the request for and receipt of such additional services.

8. *May solicit, accept or receive a charitable, religious or philanthropic contribution from an organization or from a person unrelated to a Medicaid eligible resident or potential resident. However, this may be done only to the extent that the contribution is not a condition of admission, expedited admission or continued stay in the facility for a Medicaid eligible resident.*

*States or political subdivisions may apply stricter admissions standards under state or local laws than those mentioned above to prohibit discrimination against individuals entitled to Medicaid benefits.*

*Equal Access to Quality Care.* Under this *requirement:*

1. *The facility must establish and maintain identical policies and practices regarding transfer, discharge and provision of services under the state plan for all individuals regardless of source of payment.*
2. *The facility may charge any amount for services furnished non-Medicaid residents consistent with the notice requirements; the facility must describe the charges.*
3. *The state is not required to offer additional services on behalf of a resident other than services provided in the state plan.*

*Bed-Hold Policy.* Under this requirement, the *facility must:*

1. *Provide written information to the resident and a family member or legal representative before transferring a resident to a hospital or allowing a resident to go on a therapeutic leave. It specifies:*
   a. *The duration of the bed-hold policy under the state plan (if any) during which the resident is permitted to return and resume residence in the facility; and*
   b. *The facility's policies regarding bed-hold periods permitting a resident to return.*
2. *Provide written notice to the resident and a family member or legal representative at the time of transfer of a resident to a hospital or for therapeu-*

tic leave which specifies the duration of the state and facility bed-hold policies.

3. *Must establish and follow a written policy under which a resident whose hospitalization or therapeutic leave exceeds the bed-hold period under the state plan is readmitted to the facility immediately upon the first availability of a bed in a semiprivate room, if the resident*
   a. *Requires the services provided by the facility, and*
   b. *Is eligible for Medicaid nursing facility services.*

*Transfer and Discharge.* Transfer and discharge includes the movement of a resident to a bed outside of the certified facility whether the bed is in the same physical plant or not. Transfer and discharge does not refer to movement of a resident to a bed within the same certified facility.

Under this requirement, the *facility must:*

1. *Permit each resident to remain in the facility and not transfer or discharge the resident from the facility unless:*
   a. *The transfer or discharge is necessary for the resident's welfare and needs that cannot be met in the facility.*
   b. *The transfer or discharge is appropriate because the resident's health has improved sufficiently so the resident no longer needs the services provided by the facility.*
   c. *The safety of the individuals in the facility is endangered.*
   d. *The health of individuals in the facility would otherwise be endangered.*
   e. *The resident has failed after reasonable and appropriate notice to pay for (or to have paid under Medicare or Medicaid) a stay at the facility. (For a resident who becomes eligible for Medicaid after admission, the facility may charge the resident only allowable charges under Medicaid.)*
   f. *The facility ceases to operate.*

In each case for transfer under (a) through (e), the basis for the transfer or discharge must be documented in the resident's clinical record by the resident's physician and the interdisciplinary care planning team.

The facility has the burden of demonstrating that appropriate remedial efforts have been made and have failed before discharging a resident because of his or her behavior.

The facility must provide the resident proper notification before moving him or her to a different room.

The relocation of a resident upon discharge should be a planned event. The facility staff should handle the transfer or discharge in a way that minimizes resident and family anxiety.

Sufficient preparation by the facility may include trial visits by the resident to a new location, working with the family in helping to assure personal possessions are not left or lost, orienting the facility staff to resident's daily patterns and reviewing with the facility staff routines for handling transfers and discharges to minimize transfer trauma.

2. *See that the resident's clinical record is documented when the facility transfers or discharges a resident under any of the above circumstances. This is done by:*
   a. *The resident's physician when transfer or discharge is necessary to meet the resident's needs or she or he no longer needs the facility's services; and*
   b. *A physician when transfer or discharge is necessary where the health of individuals in the facility would be otherwise endangered.*
3. *Provide sufficient preparation and orientation to residents to ensure safe and orderly transfer or discharge from the facility.*
4. *Do before transfer or discharge:*
   a. *Notify the resident and (if known) a family member or legal representative of the resident of the transfer or discharge and the reasons for the move in writing and in a language and manner they can understand at least 30 days beforehand (except as noted below).*
   b. *Record the reasons in the resident's clinical record.*
   c. *Include the items the resident has failed to pay for.*
5. *May notice as soon as practicable before transfer or discharge when:*
   a. *The safety of individuals in the facility would be endangered.*

b. *The health of individuals in the facility would be endangered.*
   c. *The resident's health improves to allow a more immediate transfer.*
   d. *An immediate transfer or discharge is required by the resident's urgent medical needs.*
   e. *A resident has not resided in the facility for 30 days.*
6. *Include the following in the content of the notice transfer or discharge:*
   a. *The reason for discharge or transfer.*
   b. *The effective date of transfer or discharge.*
   c. *The location to which the resident is transferred or discharged.*
   d. *A statement that the resident has the right to appeal the action to the state.*
   e. *The name, address and telephone number of the state long-term care ombudsman.*
   f. *For residents with developmental disabilities, the mailing address and telephone number of the agency responsible for the protection and advocacy of developmentally disabled individuals.*
   g. *For mentally ill residents, the mailing address and telephone number of the agency responsible for the protection and advocacy of mentally ill individuals.*

(See "Transfer of Residents" in this chapter for facility transfer agreement requirements.)

## NURSING SERVICE DEPARTMENT

### Role and Function

The nursing service in a facility organizationally reports to the administrator regarding the operation of that department. The degree of nursing coverage required in a facility depends upon the type of facility. The depth of professional nurses in a skilled nursing facility is greater than in a domiciliary home for the aged. The key to staffing in a facility depends upon the nursing needs as indicated in the resident care plans of the residents in the facility.

One of the important functions of the nursing service department is to provide supervision for each shift in the nursing facility. The facility must designate a registered nurse to serve as a full-time director of nurses. To provide the necessary supervision, a delegation of responsibilities and adequate supervision must be available for the activities taking place. Some facilities have listed and continue to list the director of nurses as being responsible for the care in the facility for 24 hours a day. From a practical viewpoint it is next to impossible to have one director of nurses available 24 hours a day to adequately supervise the nursing department. There should be assistants to the director of nurses to actually take charge of the 3 p.m. to 11 p.m. shift and the 11 p.m. to 7 a.m. shift. These assistants should prepare reports, supervise the activities of resident care and make assignment of duties to personnel on the floor.

## Policy Manual in the Nursing Department

A policy manual should be prepared for the health care facility taking into consideration the peculiar organizational structure and setup of the individual facility. Some of the policies to be included in the manual for the nursing department are:

1. Admission routine.
2. Transfer of residents.
3. Valuables of residents.
4. Incident reports regarding areas such as residents and visitors.
5. Death—Policy regarding notification of next of kin, post-mortem requests.
6. Discharge procedure and the role of the business office.
7. Physicians' orders such as telephone orders, standing orders, verbal orders and narcotic orders.
8. Medications—Policies for requisitioning and return of drugs credit on returned drugs.
9. Personnel policies.
10. Private duty nursing.
11. Daily reports.

## Procedure Manual

The manual is an explanation of a detailed procedure to implement a particular policy. For example, the policy for valuables may be that all valuables must be checked at the business office. To carry out the intent of the policy, certain steps must be taken:

1. Go to business office.
2. List the valuables.
3. Sign a receipt.
4. Return the receipt.

## Nursing Services
### 42 CFR, Sec. 483.30, Ch. IV (10-1-98)

Medicare or Medicaid law requires that the following requirements are compiled with relating to the functions of the nursing services.

### Sufficient Staff

The facility must have sufficient nursing staff to provide nursing and related services to attain or maintain the highest practicable physical, mental and psychosocial well-being of each resident, as determined by the resident assessments and individual plans of care.

The facility must provide services by sufficient numbers of each of the following types of personnel on a 24-hour basis to provide nursing care to all residents in accordance with resident care plans:

1. Licensed nurses, except when waived, and
2. Other nursing personnel.

The facility must designate a licensed nurse to serve as a charge nurse on each tour of duty, except when waived.

### Registered Nurse

The facility must use the services of a registered nurse for at least 8 consecutive hours a day, 7 days a week, except when waived. The facility must designate a registered nurse to serve as the director of nursing on a full-time basis, except when waived. The director of nursing may serve as a charge nurse only when the facility has an average daily occupancy of 60 or fewer residents.

### Nursing Facility Waiver of Requirement to Provide Licensed Nurses on a 24-Hour Basis

A facility may request a waiver for the requirement that it provide a registered nurse for at least 8 consecutive hours a day, 7 days a week or the requirement that it provide licensed nurses on a 24-hour basis (including a charge nurse), if the following conditions are met:

1. The facility demonstrates to the satisfaction of the state that it has been unable—despite diligent efforts including offering wages at the community prevailing rate for nursing facilities—to recruit appropriate personnel.
2. The state determines that a waiver of the requirements will not endanger the health or safety of individuals staying in the facility.
3. The state finds that for any periods in which licensed nursing services are not available, a registered nurse or physician is obligated to respond immediately to telephone calls from the facility.
4. A waiver granted under these conditions is subject to annual state review.
5. In granting or renewing a waiver, a facility may be required by the state to use other qualified licensed personnel.
6. The state agency granting a waiver of such requirements provides notice of the waiver to the state long-term care ombudsman and the protection and advocacy system in the state for the mentally ill and mentally retarded.
7. A nursing facility granted a waiver by the state notifies the residents of the facility (or, where appropriate, the guardians or legal representatives of such residents) and members of their immediate families of the waiver.

### SNFs Waiver of the Requirement to Provide Services of a Registered Nurse for More than 40 Hours a Week

The HHS secretary may waive the requirement that a SNF provide the services of a registered nurse for more than 40 hours a week (including a director of nursing), if the secretary finds that the facility:

1. Is located in a rural area and the supply of skilled nursing facility services in the area is not sufficient to meet the needs of individuals residing in the area.
2. Has one full-time registered nurse who is regularly on duty at the facility 40 hours a week.
3. Either:
   a. Has only residents whose physicians have indicated (through orders or admission notes)

that they do not require the services of a registered nurse or physician for a 48-hour period, or
   b. Has made arrangements for a registered nurse or a physician to spend time at the facility as determined necessary by the physician to provide necessary skilled nursing services on days when the regular full-time registered nurse is not on duty.
4. The HHS secretary provides notice of the waiver to the state long-term care ombudsman and the protection and advocacy system in the state for the mentally ill and mentally retarded.
5. The facility granted the waiver notifies the residents of the facility (or, where appropriate, the guardians or legal representatives of such residents) and members of their immediate families of the waiver.

A waiver of the registered nurse requirement is subject to annual review by the HHS secretary.

## Director of Nursing Service

The director of nursing service has dual responsibilities in the health care facility. She or he is responsible to administration for assisting and developing nursing service objectives and acceptable standards of nursing practice, for developing nursing procedural manuals and job descriptions for each level of nursing personnel and for participating in the department's budgetary aspects.

The director of nursing service should meet with the administrator and discuss realistic staffing and recommend the number of personnel that should be hired. She or he has responsibility in the recruitment of nursing personnel, for planning of nursing orientation and in-service training programs, and for assignment and proper supervision of nursing personnel in the health care facility. She or he also makes recommendations relative to termination of nursing personnel.

The director of nursing service should see that a proper nursing care plan is implemented in the facility and that the plan is revised and modified to meet the demands and requirements of modern day nursing. A **nursing care plan** is a written care plan for the resident based, on the nature of the resident's illness, the treatment prescribed, and so on. It is designed for use by nursing personnel and indicates what nursing care is needed, how it can best be implemented, and what modifications are needed for the best care of the resident.

She or he is a key person in the development and implementation of resident care policies and a member of the quality assessment and assurance committee. She or he is responsible for coordinating nursing activities with the other activities in the health care facility, such as the dietary department, housekeeping department and physical therapy, in **comprehensive care plans** involving the total needs of each resident.

## Nursing Personnel

### Nursing Supervisor

The nursing supervisor should be a trained professional nurse. In larger facilities a nursing supervisor may be assigned for the various clinical areas (such as medical, surgical or fracture). She or he should make daily rounds of all nursing units as a part of her or his duties. While doing this she or he should review the staff assignments to make sure that qualified personnel are functioning in their areas and review the clinical records—paying special attention to the adequacy of the nurses' notes and the recording of drugs and distribution of medications to the residents. If possible, she or he should accompany the physicians making rounds.

### Charge Nurse or Head Nurse

This person should be qualified as a professional registered nurse (RN) or a qualified licensed practical nurse (LPN). The head nurse is responsible for a resident unit and usually supervises staff nurses, restorative nurse assistants, nurses' aides and orderlies. Graduate nurses generally work under the charge nurse's supervision. She or he should have some training in the basic areas of nursing administration and supervision and should be able to recognize significant changes in the condition of residents and to take immediate action when necessary.

### Staff Nurse

The staff nurse is responsible for the care given to a number of designated residents. If the facility uses a team approach to nursing, she or he usually is the captain of the team. The staff nurse should be very familiar with each resident's medical and nursing needs and aware of the plan of care outlined by the physician for both physical and emotional needs of each resident. She or he is generally responsible for the distribution of medications and in this area carries a very serious legal responsibility. Some of the less technical procedures regarding the care of the resident may be delegated to auxiliary nursing personnel (including nurses' aides, orderlies and student nurses).

## Auxiliary Nursing Personnel

The director of nursing service must be responsible ultimately for the assignment of tasks in the nursing department. In doing this, she or he exercises professional judgment. Because the nursing facility generally hires many auxiliary personnel, this job takes on an additional importance.

Each health care facility should have sufficient nursing personnel available to assure that the resident gets:

1. Proper treatments, medications and diet as prescribed by the attending physician in accordance with care plans.
2. Proper care to prevent bed sores and is kept well groomed and clean.
3. Protection from accident and injury while in the health care facility.

### Nurse Assistant/Certified Nurse Assistant

A nurse aide is trained to assist the RN and the LPN. She or he has the most contact with residents during the day. OBRA 1987 requires that nurse aides receive 75 hours of state-approved initial training, pass a competency exam and have continuing in-service education. She or he performs specific duties but should not be expected to assume responsibilities involving nursing judgment. A nurse assistant may observe the resident but is obligated to report observations to professional nurses in charge. She or he may perform certain routine activities such as taking temperatures and recording pulse rates.

A few institutions permit nurse assistants to administer drugs and to take blood pressures. Unless some understanding exists on the nature of the procedure that is being performed, it is meaningless to give these functions to the auxiliary nursing personnel. Some serious legal implications also may arise should there be a question of liability.

The American Nurses Administration has provided a list of functions that it considers to be within the realm of good nurse assistant practice. These functions are:

1. Assist with:
   a. Admission, transfer and discharge of residents.
   b. Dressing and undressing of residents.
   c. Weighing of residents.
   d. Feeding of residents.
   e. Resident's bath.
   f. Measuring fluid intake and output of residents and recording on appropriate forms.
2. Answer the call system, responding to the needs of the resident in conformance with the delegated tasks given and notifying the registered nurse of any observations.
3. Take temperatures.
4. Direct visitors.

Orderlies are male nurse assistants employed primarily to assist in the care of male residents. They also perform such duties as moving, lifting and transporting residents, and using heavy equipment on the floor. The orderly usually reports directly to the head nurse.

### Required Training of Nurse Aides
### 42 CFR, Sec. 483.75(e), Ch. IV (10-1-98)

Medicare and Medicaid law mandates that the following requirements are complied with relating to the training of nurse aides:

- **General Rule**—A facility must not use any individual working in the facility as a nurse aide for more than four months on a full-time or other basis unless:
  1. That individual has completed a training and competency evaluation program or a competency evaluation program approved by the state, or
  2. That individual has been determined competent by the state, and
  3. That individual is competent to provide nursing and nursing related services.

- **Rule for Nonpermanent Employees** — A facility may not use an individual as a nurse aide on a temporary, per diem, leased or any basis other than a permanent employee unless the employee meets the requirements of this section.

- **Competency**—A facility may use an individual who has worked there less than four months as a nurse aide only when:
  1. The individual is a full-time employee in a training or competency evaluation program approved by the state,
  2. The individual has demonstrated competence by completion of the above-mentioned program, and
  3. The facility has asked and not yet evaluated a reply from the state registry for information concerning the individual. (The facility must follow up to see that such an individual actually becomes registered.)

- **Multistate Registry Verification**—A facility must check with all state nurse aide registries that it has reason to believe contains information on an individual before using that individual as a nurse aide.

- **Required Retraining**—When an individual has not performed paid nursing or nursing-related services for a continuous period of 24 consecutive months since the most recent completion of a training and competency evaluation program, the facility must require the individual to complete a new retraining and competency evaluation program.

- **Regular In-service Education**—The facility must provide regular performance review (at least every 12 months) and regular in-service education to ensure that individuals used as nurse aides are competent to perform services as nurse aides. In-service education must include at least 12 hours per year of training for nurse aides and address areas of weakness determined in the reviews and special needs (including care of the cognitively impaired) of the residents in the facility.

- **Nurse Aide**—Means an individual providing nursing or nursing-related services to residents in a facility. This definition does not include an individual who volunteers to provide such services without pay, who is a registered dietitian, or who is a licensed health professional.

- **Licensed Health Professional**—Means physician; physician assistant; nurse practioner; physical, speech or occupational therapy assistant; registered professional nurse; licensed practical nurse; or licensed or certified social worker.
- **Proficiency of Nurse Aides**—The facility must ensure that nurse aides are able to demonstrate competency in skills and techniques necessary to care for residents' needs as identified through resident assessments and described in the plan of care.

### Restorative Nurse Assistants

A restorative nurse assistant assists residents with required therapies and must have an understanding of the aging process, the aged and related assessment skills. Specialized in-service training is required.

### Ward Clerks

These are clerical positions carried out with regard to non-nursing functions. Ward clerks may do such things as answer the phone, relate messages and assist in the clerical paperwork involved in operating a nursing unit.

### Practical Nurses

What can a practical nurse do? Most state laws concerned with nursing practices provide little assistance to help administrators in developing a sound program for assignments of tasks to practical nurses. Under the theory of *Respondeat Superior*, the health care facility or administrator may be held responsible for certain acts of the practical nurse.

The assignment of duties to all nursing personnel, including LPNs, nurse aides and orderlies, is based upon the training and experience of the individual involved.

### Orientation and Training of Personnel

A plan used in the orientation and training of personnel should include:

1. The objectives of the facility.
2. A statement concerning understanding the aged resident.

3. An outline of changes relating to psychological and physiological aspects of aging.
4. A section pertaining to the special needs of aging.
5. A section mentioning the problems of aging.
6. An outline of the care of underactive, overactive and maladjusted residents.

### Objectives of the Facility

A simple statement of the aims and objectives of the nursing facility would read: "The aim or objective of the Prairieweed Nursing Home is to treat each resident with respect as a human being. Many of the residents in the facility have infirmities and other disabilities, requiring dependence upon the services that we render. However, as a general rule, the aging person continues to have the needs of people in any age group."

### Understanding the Aged

If life is made interesting and stimulating for residents, they will be less inclined to live in the past. The aging resident, like any other person, needs to look forward to something each day. It is important to remember that these individuals have been independent for a good portion of their lives. With the aging process, independence and self-assurance becomes somewhat diminished, causing a threat to security. Thus, assisting with the adjustment from family to nursing facility life is an important role for the staff. It chiefly involves helping the aging person to help himself or herself by encouragement, persuasion or polite requests that things be done. The most successful approach with older (as with younger) people is to ask rather than demand.

Common problems of the aged concern:

1. Financial insecurity.
2. Social insecurity relating to the loss of loved ones and friends.
3. Decreasing mental efficiency.

Psychological changes relating to the aged include:

1. Energy and initiative are decreased.
2. The ability to concentrate is lessened.
3. The acceptance of new concepts and ideas is very often slower.
4. Very often old times are thought about and stories about the past are related.

5.  The memory span becomes shortened for present events.

Physiological changes relating to the aged include:

1.  Hearing ability very often diminished.
2.  Eyesight impaired.
3.  Tiring easily.
4.  Changes in the muscles, bone and joint structure.
5.  More diseases because of impairment of circulation.
6.  Usually graying or loss of hair.
7.  Taste buds decease; food may be enjoyed less.

Needs of the aged include some of the following:

*   **Spiritual Fulfillment**—The religious aspect takes on an added meaning for those who are growing older. Many are aware there are not too many more years to live and wish to be prepared for whatever life there is after death. Some who may not have been spiritually or religiously inclined during younger years may take on a whole new pattern of life becoming more religious as they grow older.
*   **Need to Be Loved and to Love**—This need is tied up with the need to feel useful and be wanted. The aging process does not diminish in any way the desire for love and acceptance by friends, family and acquaintances in the daily living environment. Staff assist by acknowledging the individual's dignity and desire for respect. Knowing that someone is there who cares helps build security and comfort.
*   **Companionship**—One of the basic and most difficult problems in adjustment to older life is loneliness. Companionship received from fellow residents will play an important role in filling this need. Staff can help residents to meet those with common relationships and encourage contacts with family and friends so that they will feel less cut off from the outside community.
*   **Recognition**—A person needs to be recognized as an individual and for the actions and accomplishments that help give him or her a role and meaning to life. Staff can assist here by acknowledging residents as individuals and commenting sincerely and positively on their achievements.
*   **Personal Achievement**—It is very important that the older person feel and derive satisfaction from

his or her actions. Respect needs to be given for what residents have done throughout their lives and for present accomplishments and contributions.
*   **Security**—Because of the dependency that develops with aging, the assurance of security is very important to the older person. Residents need to know that their needs will be met and that they will not be abandoned. Independence, privacy and social interaction will help build the confidence and identification with the facility, which in turn enhances security.

### General Care of Residents

The **underactive resident** is one who is physically and mentally impaired, often appears to be in a state of depression and rejection, and exhibits feelings of inferiority and guilt. This resident exists in his or her surroundings without involvement and may refuse to participate in former activities. Sleep patterns may change and food intake decrease.

Causes include arteriosclerosis, epilepsy or senility.

**Resident Care Plan:**

1.  Cultivate the resident's understanding and perseverance.
2.  Do not argue with the resident about any delusions.
3.  Appreciate the fact that any positive reactions to efforts on resident's behalf may take a long time.

**Nursing Care Plan:**

1.  Stimulate the resident's interests; provide a variety of activities.
2.  Maintain body nutrition and supervise meals.
3.  Maintain a regular schedule and daily routine for the resident to follow to help develop interest in surroundings and reduce confusion.
4.  Administer medication as ordered by the physician.
5.  Make sure there is close supervision of the resident to prevent injury.

The **maladjusted resident** is one who has difficulty adjusting to the particular environment and manifests to an abnormal degree any of the following symptoms: fatigue, fear, anxiety, insomnia, irritability, gastrointestinal disturbances, palpitations or nervousness. This can occur upon admission or after a significant social, physiological or environmental change.

### Resident Care Plan:

1. Give guidance and support.
2. Help the resident to develop insight and recognition of his or her personality.

### Nursing Care Plan:

1. Make every effort to establish a good rapport with the resident.
2. Reassure and encourage the resident to improve.
3. Offer support and guidance; validate his or her concerns to avoid confusion.
4. Make certain that the resident gets a minimum of bed rest and participates in activities of facility.
5. Help the resident react to stress and strain without his or her security being threatened.
6. Plan a specific program of occupational therapy to fit the resident's particular needs; encourage display of items from the past and discuss them with the resident.

An **overactive resident** has periods of euphoria out of proportion to the actual stimulation in the environment. He or she appears to have a great deal of energy, is mentally and physically overactive, is emotionally unstable and has a great deal of self-confidence.

Causes include alcoholism, arteriosclerosis, brain tumor, acute and chronic encephalitis, epilepsy, brain injury or general paresis.

### Resident Care Plan:

1. Observe the resident carefully and accurately; record important observations of conversations or behavior.
2. Try to understand in a general way the cause of the resident's behavior and to react as objectively as possible.
3. Do not register anger, irritation or amusement at the resident's behavior, and be firm, tolerant and considerate.

### Nursing Care Plan:

1. Help the resident maintain body nutrition by supervising meals.
2. Help the resident develop regular habits of elimination; supervise bathroom visits.
3. Emphasize cleanliness, ensuring that the resident keeps neat and clean.
4. Remove all harmful objects from his or her environment.
5. Provide physical, recreational and occupational therapy.
6. Give medication as prescribed by a physician.
7. Make sure that the resident has adequate supervision around the clock (spot checks).
8. Monitor behavior for discussion with interdisciplinary care team.

## PHYSICAL AND OCCUPATIONAL THERAPY AND REHABILITATIVE SERVICES

Regulations are written to ensure that residents receive the necessary specialized rehabilitation services as determined by the comprehensive assessment and care plan to prevent avoidable physical and mental deterioration. A licensed therapist develops a specific plan of care according to the individual's physician.

The federal regulations and interpretive guidelines spell out that the resident's health should not deteriorate except when clinical conditions make this decline inevitable. The resident is expected to make progress in the activities of daily living, such as bathing, dressing, grooming, transferring and ambulating, toileting, eating and communicating (CFR 483.25). The federal regulations require that the staff be proactive in dealing with disability. The administrator should make sure that the staff members have documented any problems that a resident may have and what the staff has done to help the resident overcome them.

### Provision of Services
### 42 CFR, Sec. 483.45, Ch. IV (10-1-98)

If specialized rehabilitative services (such as physical therapy, speech-language pathology, occupational therapy and health rehabilitative services for mental illness and retardation) are required in the resident's comprehensive plan of care, the facility must:

1. Provide the required services, or
2. Obtain the required services from an outside resource.

Specialized services must be provided under the written order of a physician by qualified personnel.

### Establishing a Therapy Department

The delivery of rehabilitation therapies has been shifting from the hospitals to SNFs. This results in an increase in residents requiring rehabilitation services and improvement of skills. Generally, the purpose of physical therapy is to prevent and treat disease and impaired motion to improve and/or maintain current functional levels. For nursing facility residents, this endeavors to improve the quality of life and morale by keeping individuals independent as long as possible by providing treatment as ordered by the physician in such areas as performance of activities of daily living (ADLs) and adjustment to handicaps, alleviating pain, avoiding or correcting deformity, and maintaining mobility. Many facilities will organize physical therapy in-house and contract with outside providers for other needed therapy services. These programs are ongoing and require active facility involvement to ensure quality of care, community awareness and financial feasibility.

Before making the decision on the type and intensity of rehabilitation services to be offered, the facility needs to consider a variety of factors including:

1. Review of each resident's comprehensive plan of care to determine the type of rehabilitative services needed.
2. Utilization review and summarization of statistics for each therapy discipline as a base for identifying any erratic patterns and forecasting use.
3. The available providers of rehabilitative services and supplies, their reliability, holiday and emergency back-up support, clinical management skills and quality assurance.
4. Development of in-house programs for the facility and what will be offered such as outpatient rehabilitation clinics (types and intensity), specialized skilled nursing, subacute rehabilitation,

speech-language pathology and occupational therapy.
5. Whether or not various rehabilitative services and/or consultations will be offered to other facilities in the community.
6. Staff needs, multidisciplinary cooperation, management needs, and whether or not the physical therapist will be responsible for conducting educational services (i.e., lifting or turning) to staff members, volunteers and/or family members.
7. Costs and availability of necessary space, equipment, certification and any admission and discharge procedures.
8. Financial management of the programs, including per diem revenues from allocation to ancillary therapy programs, arrangements with agents and outside providers, and reimbursement from Medicare Parts A or B.

The nursing facility will need to set aside appropriate space for physical therapy and related activities. This area should be pleasant and possibly have an FM radio available for background music. Sufficient space should be available for an office, hydrotherapy and other equipment needs such as hydroculator packs, aqua-k pads, overhead pulleys, chair bicycle, exercise mat and mat table, treatment table with shelf, mobile tilt table, portable parallel bars, six-foot wall mirror, weights of various sizes, lap boards, and safety walking belts. The selection of the equipment to be used in the physical therapy department usually is made by the administrator in consultation with the physical therapist.

The ownership and administrator, upon a study committee's recommendation, would determine the extent of the program and the role of the therapist considering such functions as consultant to the rehabilitation services policy, resident care planning and quality assessment and assurance committees, conduct of in-service and training to physical therapy aides and/or other personnel, and provision of treatments. If a full-time therapist is hired, a clause to the effect that he or she will devote full-time to the facility and not treat residents on a private basis should be included in the employment contract. If a part-time or a consulting physical therapist is hired, the fees for direct treatments, in-service education, program planning, supervision of professional and assistant personnel, and committee work should be determined either on an hourly rate, per-resident rate or flat contractual sum. The hourly rate may encourage generalized consultation services that reach all residents of the facility and would be more conducive to teaching simple and effective rehabilitation techniques.

## MEDICAL RECORDS DEPARTMENT

### Purposes of the Health Records

In addition to meeting state law requirements, several reasons exist for health care facilities to maintain health (clinical) records on residents. These records are basic to ensuring that each resident receives ongoing care by providing the caregivers with current information as to individual progress, care plan and emerging needs. The care given by each member of the health team and the response of the individual are reflected and provide a base for necessary medical decisions and possible in-service personnel training needs. The records are an overall measurement of the kind of work being carried out in the facility and assist in the evaluation of that care. They provide documentary evidence of the quality of care being given in order to have third-party payers properly pay insurance claims and for legal proceedings such as administrative hearings and lawsuits. Health records also are used in scientific study. A medical records practitioner or full-time employee under the supervision of a medical records practitioner should keep these records up to date and safeguarded.

### Clinical Records
### 42 CFR, Sec. 483.75 (L), Ch. IV (10-1-98)

If the facility wishes to participate in Title XVIII (Medicare) or Title XIX (Medicaid), adherence to the following standards relative to health records is required.

The facility must maintain clinical records on each resident in accordance with accepted professional standards and practices, that are:

1. Complete.
2. Accurately documented.
3. Readily accessible.
4. Systematically organized.

Clinical records must be retained for:

1. The period of time required by state law.
2. Five years from the date of discharge when there is no requirement in state law.
3. For a minor, three years after a resident reaches legal age under state law.

The facility must safeguard clinical record information against loss, destruction or unauthorized use.

The facility must keep confidential all information contained in the resident's record regardless of the form or storage method of the records, except when release is required by:

1. Transfer to another health care institution.
2. Law.
3. Third-party payment contract.
4. The resident.
   (Note: Residents have a right to access their clinical records. See "Resident's Rights" in this chapter for more detail.)

The clinical record must contain:

1. Sufficient information to idenytify the resident.
2. A record of the resident's assessments.
3. The plan of care and services provided.
4. The results of any preadmission screening conducted by the state.
5. Progress notes.

### Responsibility for Health Records

Ultimately the ownership of the nursing facility is responsible for the quality of care that is rendered in the facility. The responsibility for the determination and rendering of high-quality care should be delegated to the medical staff or medical consultants. The attending or consulting physician is primarily responsible for such entries as history, physical examination, doctors' orders, diagnosis and progress notes in the health record. The administrator is responsible for providing an adequate and clearly defined health record system, designating personnel to carry out this system, establishing job descriptions and policies pertinent to the keeping of health records, and providing specialized equipment (such as fire resistant files) to store the records. The nurse is responsible for that portion of the health record including the patient record (TPR), nurse's notes, nurse's daily progress reports and charting of medications.

The attending or consulting physician is responsible for seeing that all opinions concerning the health record and the treatment of the resident are documented and that no information is missing. Each record should contain sufficient data to give a complete picture of the diagnosis, the course of treatment and the prognosis of each resident. Each entry requiring a physician's signature should be signed in ink with his or her complete legal signature. A physician using rubber signature stamps must sign a statement that says he or she is the only one possessing and using the stamp. The statement is kept in the administrative offices. Electronic signatures are accepted in computerized medical records; a list of computer codes and signatures also is kept under safeguards in the administrative office.

A **qualitative analysis** is the rendering of an opinion as to the quality of care that is being given in the nursing facility. The organized medical staff (or medical consultant if there is no medical staff organization) is responsible for the quality of health records. A regular analysis of the health records must be made by a professional staff committee that includes the attending physician or medical consultant, the record librarian, a representative from nursing service, and other persons who contributed to the care of the resident.

A **quantitative analysis** is a review of the record by a medical records practitioner or trained technician to see that all required reports and forms are included and signed.

No format or time period is specified for **documentation** of the actual experience and progress toward achievement of the behavioral and functional goals of each resident in the facility. This documentation is separate from comprehensive (annual), periodic (resident status changes) and monitoring (quarterly) assessments. This is done on an individual basis, ensuring that the staff has current and sufficient information to manage, conduct and review each care program.

## The Health Record

The Health Care Financing Administration (HCFA) has mandated automation of the minimum data sheet (MDS) backed by an ongoing state specified resident assessment instrument (RAI) to ensure continued clinical relevance. This information system is to feed into records developed and maintained by HCFA and/or the state. HCFA has developed MDS 2.0, and required that all states transition to this new form as of January 1, 1996, unless the state has been granted an extension from HCFA.

Effective automated medical records provide time-efficient information collection and dissemination, customized data reports and current information to caregivers. Computerization of records can take time-consuming routine tasks off of nursing professionals and allow more time for direct resident care. It helps to provide and coordinate considerable information from all disciplines involved in a resident's assessment and care plan into a conveniently accessible comprehensive resident history. Staff nursing, aides and other caregivers will be more knowledgeable about individual care needs, enabling provision of quality care in compliance with state and federal regulations. Care is improved where computerization eases completion of the required documentation in medical records and helps eliminate omissions and duplication of efforts. The latest physicians' orders and up-to-date care plans are readily accessed and use consistent standardized language, content, practice and statistics with improved legibility.

Generally, the health record is composed of two major sections—the informational and personal section and the medical section. The health record should contain sufficient information to identify each resident clearly, to justify the diagnosis and treatment, and to document the results. All health records, as a minimum, should contain the following items.

### Informational and Personal Section

*Identification.* The identification data sheet should record the following information on the resident:

1. Name.
2. Nursing facility number.
3. Address.
4. Telephone number of the resident or relative.
5. Age.
6. Date of birth.
7. Place of birth.
8. Citizenship.
9. Sex.
10. Marital status.
11. Next of kin or responsible representative.

12. Address and telephone number of the next of kin or responsible representative.
13. Father's name (if a minor).
14. Mother's name (if a minor).
15. Occupation or former occupation.
16. Religious preference of the resident.
17. Name and address of the clergy.
18. Social Security number.
19. Any necessary insurance data.
20. Date of admission to the nursing facility.
21. Time of admission to the nursing facility.
22. Place from which admitted.
23. Referred by (name of person or facility the resident was referred by).
24. Name, address and phone number of the attending physician.

*History of the Resident.* This record should include such items as:

- **Chief Complaint** containing a concise statement of when the complaint began, how long it lasted and the details of the present illness.

  An **inventory of the various systems** of the resident is as follows:
  1. General, any sensitivity to drugs.
  2. Skin.
  3. Head (ears, eyes, nose and throat).
  4. Cardiovascular system.
  5. Respiratory system.
  6. Gastrointestinal system.
  7. Genitourinary system.
  8. Gynecological system (female).
  9. Musculoskeletal system.
  10. Neurological system.
  11. Psychiatric system.
- **Past history** of the resident covering such items as childhood diseases, adult diseases with the dates of each disease, operations and injuries.
- **Social history** containing a description of the social and environmental aspects of the resident and answering such questions as: where did the resident live, what are some of his or her social habits, what kind of work did the resident perform, and what is the relationship of the resident with his or her family and friends.
- **Family history** includes the health of parents, brothers, sisters and children; an indication of the

cause of death of any deceased relatives; and any significant family diseases. The taking of the family history should be objective and should not reflect the personal opinions of the interviewer.

### Medical Section

*Report of Physical Examination.* This report should contain all pertinent findings resulting from an assessment of all systems of the body. If a complete history has been recorded and a physical exam performed within 30 days prior to admission to the nursing facility, a legible copy of each of these reports may be used if these reports were recorded by a duly qualified member of the medical profession. If the facility does use reports supplied by other physicians, an internal admission note should be made stating the fact.

*Diagnostic and Therapeutic Orders.* These orders should include any written orders by individuals who have medical practice privileges in the facility. Telephone orders by a physician should be accepted and written only by a licensed nurse and used only in urgent circumstances. Such orders should be signed by the responsible attending or consulting physician 48 hours after they were given.

*Observations.* These reports should include progress notes by the attending physician, consultation reports by specialists, nurses' notes and entries by allied health personnel (such as physical therapist or social worker). Progress notes by the attending physician should give a chronological problem-oriented report of the resident's course of treatment and action. Opinions requiring medical judgment should be written only by medical staff members.

*Report of Findings and Actions.* These should include such items as pathology reports, laboratory and radiology examinations, medical and surgical treatments, and diagnostic and therapeutic procedures.

*Orders.* The physician should write and sign his or her orders covering any medications, tests to be performed, treatments and special diets. Orders should include the data on which they are written and the full signature of the physician; they are to be reviewed at least every 30 days by the physician. Drugs should be ordered by the physician with a specific period of time written as part of the order. Physicians may fax their orders (except for controlled substances) if the original copy is signed by the physician and available on request. Because some fax copies may fade in time, the original may be sent to the facility or the fax may be photocopied to be kept in the medical record. Safeguards are needed to protect this system from abuse.

*Automatic stop orders.* Automatic stop orders on dangerous medications are a routine procedure and will go into effect in all cases. Under this system all medications such as narcotics, sedatives, stimulants, antibiotics, tranquilizers and anticoagulants must be discontinued after seven days unless ordered specifically for a longer time by the attending physician or as otherwise required by law. When this automatic stop order goes into effect, the staff needs to notify the physician that the drugs are being discontinued. No prescription should be refilled without the written authority of the attending or consulting physician.

*Progress Notes.* During the resident's stay in the nursing facility, the following individuals who are employed or work with the facility may record or make entries in his or her health record: consulting physicians, attending physicians, dentists, nurses, therapists, laboratory and X-ray personnel, any professional or technical consultants, and dietitians. These notes are customarily kept separate in the health record. The nurses' progress notes should commence with an admitting note outlining the general condition of the resident upon admission and end with a discharge note stipulating the condition of the resident at the time of release and how he or she left (stretcher, wheelchair, etc.). The nurses' notes should contain meaningful observations (these notes may be admitted into evidence in the courts) and be properly dated and signed by the person making the observation. It is important from a legal viewpoint that any reaction to drugs, apparent change in the condition of the resident and any accident that occurs during the time that the resident is in the facility is duly recorded.

Special medical records health forms generally are used for recording of the vital signs (TRP), blood pressure, intake and output of fluids, medications, and treatments given. Incident reports are used to document any unusual incidents. Other special forms or reports that might be included particularly in an SNF are laboratory and X-ray reports and physical and occupational therapy records.

*Conclusions.* These should include the admitting diagnosis, the primary and secondary final diagnosis, the clinical summary, and any postmortem reports. The provisional diagnosis should reflect the physician's evaluation of the resident's condition upon entry to the nursing facility. All relevant discharge diagnoses should be properly and duly recorded. The clinical resume should briefly summarize the significant findings and events of the resident's admission, his or her condition on discharge, and recommendations for future care. A copy of the clinical resume should be sent to the attending physician or person(s) responsible for subsequent care of the resident.

*Other Forms.* The nursing facility should have the following forms:

1. Any legal papers pertaining to commitment, guardianship and powers of attorney concerning the resident.
2. Release forms signed by a responsible person or the resident relative to leaving the premises of the facility, the responsibility for discharge against medical advice and the release of information.
3. Death certificate and any autopsy reports.

### Filing Systems and Statistics

*Completion of Health Records.* Health records should be written within 48 hours and kept current. The health records of discharged and deceased residents should be completed promptly (within 30 days, generally) and properly filed. In the case of a deceased resident, the completed health record should contain evidence of disposition and a death certificate signed by the mortician or person duly authorized by the state to sign these certificates.

If the management of a health care facility changes hands, all resident records remain as the property of the facility and are transferred to the new owner. Generally, the resident owns the content of the medical record and the facility owns the medical record itself.

*Filing Systems.* In order to properly identify a resident's record, various filing systems have been devised by record librarians. The most prevalent systems in use are the:

• **Alphabetical System**—This is a system whereby the names of the residents are placed by the last name, first name and middle initial. The alphabetical system is feasible for smaller facilities or those having little resident turnover.

- **Numerical System**—The numerical systems currently used are the numerical unit system or numerical serial system or a combination of both:
  1. **Numerical Unit System**—This system assigns a number to each resident in sequence upon admission to the facility and the resident keeps that number in all subsequent admissions. This kind of system is more prevalent in an SNF where there is a turnover of residents. Under this system, all records on a given resident will have the same number and will be filed together in one place.
  2. **Numerical Serial System**—Under this system, a new number is given to the resident every time he or she is admitted to the facility. Thus the records of that resident could be filed in several different places.
  3. **Unit-Serial System**—Some health care facilities use a combination of the numerical unit and serial systems. Under the unit-serial system a new number is given to the resident upon every admission, but all previous health records of the resident are under the latest number assigned with a note attached that the record has been moved to the latest number.

*Statistics.* Records to be maintained in this area are:

- **Residents' Index File**—An alphabetical name file of every resident admitted to the nursing facility. A card is kept for each resident, filed alphabetically by the resident's last name and includes such basic information as the resident's name, address, telephone number, date of birth, dates of admission and discharge, and file number. These cards should be kept as a perpetual master index.
- **Resident's Admission and Discharge Record**—This record is kept in a single bound volume. The admission section of the volume includes the name of the nursing facility or hospital number, date of birth, name of the resident, date of admission and referral form. The discharge section includes the resident's number, name, date of discharge, name of the facility or person(s) discharged to, and the final diagnosis.
- **Disease Index**—An index where the resident's records are filed by the condition or disease that the resident has and is being treated for. This kind of index is maintained by those health care facilities that must report residents by a diagnostic or disease code to the welfare and/or other regulatory agencies and where any research is being conducted.
- **Resident Discharges**—Provides the number of residents who have been formally released from the nursing facility.
- **Resident Census**—Indicates the number of residents occupying beds at a given time.
- **Resident Days of Care**—A unit of measurement indicating the care available and rendered to one resident for a particular time.
- **Discharged Resident Days**—A statistic indicating the total number of days each discharged resident has spent in the health care facility.
- **Average Daily Census**—The average number of residents in the facility each day for a given period of time. This is computed by taking the total number of resident days of care throughout a particular period and dividing by the total number of days in that period. If there are 300 resident days and 304 days in a particular period, divide the 300 resident days by 30 and come out with the average daily census of 10 residents per day.
- **Percentage of Occupancy**—The ratio of actual days to maximum resident days as determined by the bed complement. The percentage of occupancy is computed by dividing the actual number of resident days of care rendered by the bed complement. If there is a bed complement of 60 beds and 30 of those beds are occupied, divide the 60 into 30 which gives 50% occupancy.
- **Bed Turnover Rate**—The number of times the bed complement of a facility changes residents during a given period of time. This is determined by dividing the average occupied beds by the total discharges for the same period of time.
- **Average Length of Stay**—The average number of days of service rendered to each resident discharged during a given period. This is computed by dividing the total number of resident days of care rendered to residents discharged during a period of time by the total number of residents discharged during that period. If there are 10,000 resident days of care for a period and the total number of residents discharged is 300, divide the 10,000 by 300 to arrive at a 30 day average length of stay.

- **Gross Death Rate**—The ratio of deaths in the health care facility during a period of time to the total number of discharges for that period of time. If there are 30 deaths and 300 discharges, the gross death rate is 10%.

## DIETARY DEPARTMENT

### Purpose of the Dietary Department

The dietary department of a health care facility plays a major role in the operation of the facility. The major function is to provide the nutritional and related therapeutic aspects of the resident care plan. The importance of therapeutic diets in modern medicine has emphasized the need for trained personnel in this department. Another essential function of this department is to help maintain resident morale and overall life satisfaction by serving well-prepared meals in a pleasant environment. Going to the dining room for meals provides a time for leaving one's room, enjoying a good meal and visiting. Separate eating places are usually provided for those residents with eating problems.

General goals of the dietary department are to:

1. Provide food meeting the nutritional and special diet needs of each resident.
2. Provide hot and attractively prepared food to residents.
3. Educate the resident regarding any special and therapeutic diet he or she requires.
4. Participate in budget planning to carry out these goals with maximum cost efficiency.

### Organization of the Department

The dietitian is the administrative head of the dietary department and should report directly to the administrator or assistant administrator in larger facilities. A clear delineation of functions should be made between the dietary and nursing departments. Generally, the passing of resident trays is a dietary function and the picking up of trays is a nursing function.

### The Dietitian—Role and Function

The dietitian is hired by the administrator and is responsible for the food service operation of the health care facility. She or he is considered to be a department head and has a direct line of communication to the administrator. If the person is not a professionally qualified dietitian (i.e., a member of the American Dietetic Association [ADA]), regularly scheduled consultation with an ADA dietitian or other properly trained person is mandatory. This consultant may be a qualified dietitian from another health care facility. Reports to the administrator include such items as date, time and duration of visits from the dietary consultant; tasks (resident visits, menus reviewed or food preparation); problems and solutions; and personnel matters. The cost of food reported includes the number of meals served (resident, staff, visitors) and raw food costs (total and per resident day).

The dietitian is responsible for assignment of tasks, orientation and training of food service personnel, and working closely with the administrator in the formulation of personnel policies relative to the food service department. The dietitian should be knowledgeable about purchasing foods; the purchasing department usually handles the purchase of staples and the dietitian the purchase of meat, although the dietitian may perform both functions. She or he is responsible for menu preparation for well-balanced and therapeutic diets.

### Food Service Supervisors

Because of the shortage of trained professional dietitians, a trend has emerged toward the use of food service supervisors. These food service supervisors are generally responsible for the routine operation of the department such as the preparation of meals, the supervision and scheduling of work hours, and the distribution of food to the residents.

### Food Services

The work of the dietary department must be organized so that food is served on a routine basis with adequate staffing for implementation.

Accrediting agencies (i.e., Joint Commission on Accreditation of Healthcare Organizations and Medicare and Medicaid) indicate that the following guidelines be effectuated regarding the dietary department:

1. An organized department directed by a qualified person.

2. Facilities and equipment that meet the local sanitary codes for the storage, preparation (including special diets) and distribution of food.
3. A systematic record of diets.
4. Interdepartmental conferences on a regular basis.

### Pattern of Food Services

Facilities may utilize a centralized or a decentralized system to serve food:

- **Decentralized Service**—This is one of the oldest methods of serving food. Food is prepared and sent to the floor kitchens from a central kitchen. The trays are served from the floor kitchen, which has a refrigerator, a hot plate, a toaster, a dishwasher and other appliances. The trays are delivered to the resident by dietary personnel. Soiled trays are returned to the central kitchen for washing.

  Advantages of the decentralized service allow a more flexible system to accommodate last minute changes and to provide more personalized resident service and hotter food because of the proximity of the decentralized kitchen to the resident.

  Disadvantages include more noise and odors penetrating into the resident areas, expensive duplication of items such as refrigerators, steam tables or tray stands, and staff and a possible lack of supervision of dietary aides in each kitchen.

- **Centralized Food Service**—This is a system where all sub-floor kitchens are eliminated. The central service area is generally located near the main kitchen, which enhances the flow process of cooked food to the distribution area. Many modern health care facilities are constructed so that assembly line tray service is feasible.

  With a low percentage of special diets, the assembly line system works very well. A special diet system requires a longer assembly line where the completed tray is distributed to the resident areas by dumbwaiter (in vertical construction), conveyer belt (in horizontal construction) and tray carts using steam or hot pallets. Soiled trays are returned to a dishwashing unit near the service area.

  The greatest disadvantage of a centralized tray service is getting the tray from the central area to the resident.

With the advent of convenience foods (individual frozen packets of food and ultrasonic heating systems), the whole pattern of food service may change dramatically in the next decade.

### Menu Planning

Because meal satisfaction often becomes a central focus, it is an important morale factor. Ethnic group food preferences and socioeconomic backgrounds should be considered in the menu planning. Recommended daily requirements of the basic types and quantities of food per the Food and Nutrition Board of the National Research Council are: meat (4 oz.), fruit and vegetables (2 cups), bread and cereal (4 servings) and milk (2 cups). Although these will provide the recommended daily allowances of minerals and vitamins to maintain health, variations occur according to age, health, activity levels and size factors. Such variations may be addressed by therapeutic diets ordered by the physician and approved by the dietitian which are designed to correct and/or prevent nutrition related problems. There should be alternative menus and therapeutic diets to satisfy each resident's nutritional needs and tastes. Daily menus should be rotated to provide variety.

### Food Storage

All food should be stored on clean surfaces above the floor in accordance with time and temperature controls to prevent the growth of bacteria and toxigenic micro-organisms. Potentially hazardous foods (animal products, eggs, fish, meat, poultry, fruit and vegetables, synthetic food ingredients or specialty foods) must be stored at 45° F or below and frozen foods at 0° F or below.

### Food Preparation

Food must not be exposed to light too long, overcooked in large quantities of water, overcooked to attain a soft texture, or have baking soda added. Food of both plant and animal origin must be cooked and maintained at proper internal temperatures: hot foods—140° F or above, cold foods—48° F or below, and frozen foods—0° F or below.

### Nourishment

So that residents do not become malnourished, note should be taken of such factors as seasonings in the food, denture use, individual food preferences and quantity of meal eaten; corrective measures need to be taken as required. Special equipment and utensils must be provided to help residents with problems of eating independently. These include enlarged handles (for impaired coordination), postural supports (for arm, head or trunk), and sectional plates (for visual handicaps). Those who cannot eat alone must be fed by someone else as long as this is feasible. Residents need to be monitored as to the percentage of food eaten at mealtimes and for significant or unusual weight loss.

### Therapeutic Diets

Some common diets used to meet residents' special nutritional needs are soft diets low in fiber with soft texture and mild flavor; mechanical soft diets where food is easier to chew (chopped, pureed, ground); strict full-liquid diets where food is liquid at body temperature; high-fiber diets providing bulk with hard-to-digest foods (such as fruits, vegetables or whole grain bread); and high-calorie, high-protein diets providing additional sources of protein (such as meat, milk, shakes).

## Dietary Services
### 42 CFR Sec. 483.35, Ch. IV (10-1-98)

Medicare and Medicaid law requires compliance with the following requirements relating to the dietary and food service department.

The facility must provide each resident with a nourishing, palatable, well-balanced diet that meets the daily nutritional and special dietary needs of each resident.

### Staffing

The facility must employ a qualified dietitian, either full-time, part-time or on a consultant basis. If a qualified dietitian is not employed full-time, the facility must designate a person to serve as the director of food service who receives frequently scheduled consultation from a qualified dietitian.

A dietitian is qualified upon:

1. Registration by the Commission on Dietetic Registration of the ADA, or
2. On the basis of education, training or experience in identification of dietary needs, planning and implementation of dietary programs.

### Sufficient Staff

The facility must employ sufficient support personnel competent to carry out the functions of the dietary service.

### Menus and Nutritional Adequacy

Menus must:

1. Meet the nutritional needs of residents in accordance with the recommended dietary allowances of the Food and Nutrition Board of the National Research Council, National Academy of Sciences.
2. Be prepared in advance.
3. Be followed.

### Food

Each resident receives and the facility provides:

1. Food prepared by methods that conserve nutrition value, flavor and appearance.
2. Food that is palatable, attractive and at the proper temperature.
3. Food prepared in a form designed to meet individual needs.
4. Substitutes offered of a similar nutritive value to residents who refuse food service.

### Therapeutic Diets

Therapeutic diets must be prescribed by the attending physician.

### Frequency of Meals

Each resident receives and the facility provides at least three meals daily at regular times comparable to normal mealtimes in the community.

1. The facility must offer snacks at bedtime daily.
2. There must be no more than 14 hours between a substantial evening meal (three or more menu items, including meat, fish, eggs or cheese) and breakfast the following day except when a nourishing snack is provided at bedtime. Up to 16 hours may elapse between a substantial evening meal and breakfast the following day, if a resident

group agrees to this meal span and a nourishing snack is served.

### Assistive Devices

The facility must provide special eating equipment and utensils for residents who need them.

### Sanitary Condition

The facility must:

1. Procure food from sources approved or considered satisfactory by federal, state or local authorities.
2. Store, prepare, distribute and serve food under sanitary conditions.
3. Dispose of garbage and refuse properly.

## PHARMACY DEPARTMENT

### Role and Function of the Pharmacist

Pharmacy service may be provided to a nursing facility by a retail pharmacist, a full-time pharmacist employed by the facility or a part-time hospital pharmacist in the community. Although the nursing facility pharmacist is a cross between the hospital and the community drug store pharmacists, his or her role is more similar to that of the hospital pharmacist as medications and drugs given to the residents usually are controlled by the professional nurse except when self-administration of medication by the resident is permitted. In the typical drugstore or retail pharmacy situation, the drug is given to the resident directly who administers it to himself or herself.

A determination must be made as to the scope of the pharmacist's duties in the facility. Will she or he provide services outside the realm of routine duties or be available on a consulting basis in conjunction with routine duties? Will the pharmacist use the drug inventory already available in the nursing facility, thereby providing only the necessary professional supervision or the pharmacy service, or utilize the drug inventory of his or her own hospital or community drug store?

Another consideration is whether the pharmacist will be hired on a full-time or a part-time basis. The pharmacist may be retained on a continuing basis for as many hours as necessary to establish written policies and procedures for handling drugs that are in accord with all federal, state and local regulations. A part-time pharmacist also should be retained as a consultant who is available for overall supervision of the pharmacy service.

The minimum duties and responsibilities of a pharmacist (full-time or part-time) include:

1. Working closely with the consulting physician to establish written policies and guidelines.
2. Monthly inspection visits to the drug room and preparation of an evaluation report of the drug room and the pharmacist's activities.
3. Provision of drug information service to the medical and the nursing staff concerning dosage, side effects, contraindications, cost and chemical data.
4. Assisting with development of safe procedures for handling drugs.
5. Provision of required drug supplies upon receipt of a proper order form.

### Drug Administraiton

Some of the newer methods of drug administration utilize the following:

- **Unit Dosage Packing**—Innovative approaches to the packing of medications for nursing facilities assure the resident a clean sterile medication in a single dose.
- **Mobile Medication Cart**—This allows the nurse to pour, distribute, count and chart medications at the resident's bedside—carrying the unit dose system of distribution a step further. Some of the advantages of the mobile medication cart are:
  1. Ensuring correct identification of the drug at the bedside of the resident.
  2. Increasing the efficiency of the charting procedure.
  3. Eliminating the need for medication dosage cards because the nurse may refer directly to the medication cardex (rather than making up a medication card and dispensing from that).
  4. Increasing efficiency as nursing personnel are closer to the resident without having to go back and forth between the nursing station and residents rooms.

## Pharmacy Policy and Procedures

To support related federal, state and local regulations, skilled and nursing facilities must have a current policy manual that:

1. Includes policies and procedures, defining the functions and responsibilities relating to the pharmacy service.
2. Is reviewed annually to keep abreast of current developments.
3. Has a formulary system approved by a responsible physician and pharmacist.

Some of the areas the pharmacy policy manual should cover are:

1. Automatic stop orders with regard to drugs.
2. Appropriate control systems for narcotics, alcohol, barbiturates, amphetamines and any stimulant or depressant medications controlled by the Food and Drug Administration (FDA).
3. Control of investigational drugs.
4. Handling of physician's medication samples.
5. Use of medications at the resident's bedside.
6. The availability of an emergency drug kit, contents of the drug kit and the inspection procedure.
7. Periodic inspections of the nursing station medication centers.
8. Labeling medications and changing containers.
9. Removal of medications from the pharmacy in the absence of a pharmacist.
10. Procedure on medications to be taken home by the resident.
11. Reporting adverse drug reactions for all health care personnel to the FDA or the American Medical Association (AMA).
12. Reporting medication errors and incident reports on any serious injury to residents.
13. Pharmacy inventory control system.
14. Adding items to parenterals.
15. Creation of a pharmacy and drug therapeutic committee that meets at least quarterly; minutes are kept of the proceedings of this committee.
16. Initiation and maintenance of a formulary or drug list.
17. The qualifications of the pharmacist.
18. Record keeping.
19. Poison control center communications and who to contact in case of an emergency.
20. Audit of narcotics and other controlled drugs at the nursing station.
21. An official list of medical abbreviations that are used in the administration and dispensing of drugs.
22. Procedure in relation to the writing and signing of medication orders.

Supporting these areas of general policy, pharmacy procedures should ensure that:

1. A contractual arrangement is made with the community pharmacist or a full-time pharmacist; he or she must be licensed in the state and meet all other legal qualifications pertaining to a licensed pharmacist. In this contractual arrangement, the appropriate method and procedure for obtaining, dispensing and administering drugs and biologicals, and coverage during absences is outlined.
2. An emergency drug kit is required in an SNF. The pharmacy committee develops and approves the contents. The kit is sealed or locked and readily available. If a registered nurse finds a seal broken or unlocked, she or he must notify the pharmacist immediately.
3. Periodic inspections of the nursing station and medication carts should ascertain the following procedures:
   a. External medications are kept apart from internal drugs.
   b. The biological refrigerator has a thermometer with a range of 35° to 50°. Biologicals may be stored in a separate section in a regular refrigerator for general use.
   c. There are not outdated medications being used.
   d. The medication cabinets are kept locked at all times.
   e. A method, conversion or metric to English weight table is available at each nursing station.
   f. Text references on drug uses and side effects of drugs are available to personnel administering drugs. *Physicians' Desk Reference* is recommended.
4. All medications administered to residents are ordered in writing by his or her physician. Oral orders are given only to a licensed registered nurse

and reduced to writing as soon as possible, signed by the nurse and countersigned by the physician within 48 hours.

5. Medications not specifically limited as to the time or dosage should be on the automatic stop-order system in accordance with written policy that has been approved by the physicians advising the facility on medical-administrative matters. The resident's attending physician should be notified of stop-order policies and contacted promptly for renewal of such orders so there is a continuity of the resident's therapeutic regimen as far as drugs are concerned.

6. The nurse and the attending physician should review monthly each resident's medications.

7. Medications are administered by licensed medical or nursing personnel, or unlicensed personnel under the supervision of a licensed nurse, in accordance with the state medical and nursing practice act.

8. Self-administration of medications by residents is permitted unless the interdisciplinary team has determined for each resident that this is unsafe.

9. All medications are released with residents on discharge only on written authority of the attending physician. The resident should acknowledge by signature that she or he has received them. A registered nurse may place only one dose in a new container.

10. Each nurse is responsible for items being readily available for the proper administration of medications.

11. When administering medications, medication cards are used and checked against physician's orders.

12. Medications prescribed for one resident are not administered to any other residents.

13. Any drugs or medications removed from the pharmacy in the absence of the pharmacist must be in the manufacturer's labeled container or in a pre-packaged labeled container prepared under the direct supervision of the pharmacist.

14. Drug containers may be labeled only by the pharmacist. The label should contain the resident's full name, the physician's name, strength and quantity of the drug, any precautionary statements, expiration date, pharmacist and date dispensed. Any containers with marred or illegible labels must be returned to the issuing pharmacist for relabeling or disposal. Containers that have no labels should

be destroyed in accordance with state and federal laws.

15. The medications of each resident are kept stored in their originally received containers and transferring between containers is forbidden. Drugs must be put in locked storage with internal and external drugs separated.

16. Controlled drugs listed in Schedule 2 of the Comprehensive Drug Abuse Act of 1970 (including narcotics, barbiturates or amphetamines) and other dangerous drugs are separately locked under double lock and key in securely fastened boxes or drawers. Locked compartments, trays and carts should not be left unattended.

17. Medications requiring refrigeration are generally kept in a separate locked box within the refrigerator in the nursing station.

18. Poisons and medications for external use are kept separate from other medications.

19. Medications no longer in use are disposed of or destroyed in accordance with federal and state regulations. Discontinued controlled drugs are destroyed by the pharmacist. Noncontrolled drugs are destroyed by a responsible person from the facility.

20. A narcotic record must be maintained. It should list on separate sheets for each narcotic drug such information as the date, time the drug was administered, the name of the resident, the dosage, the physician's name, the signature of the person administering the drug and a figure indicating the number of pills remaining. The general statute of limitations with regard to the keeping of pharmacy records is 5 years.

21. The pharmacy inventory control system includes the dating and organized placing on shelves of all stock.

**Pharmacy Services**
**42 CFR, Sec. 483.60, Ch. IV (10-1-98)**

Medicare and Medicaid law requires that the following requirements relating to the pharmacy department are complied with.

The facility must provide routine and emergency drugs and biologicals to its residents, or obtain them under an agreement with outside resources. The facility may permit unlicensed personnel to administer drugs if state law permits, but only under the general supervision of a licensed nurse.

### Procedures

A facility must provide pharmaceutical services (including procedures that assure accurate acquiring, receiving, dispensing and administering of all drugs and biologicals) to meet the needs of each resident.

### Service Consultation

The facility must employ or obtain the services of a licensed pharmacist who:

1. Provides consultation on all aspects of the provision of pharmacy services in the facility.
2. Establishes a system of records of receipt and disposition of all controlled drugs in sufficient detail to enable an accurate reconciliation.
3. Determines that drug records are in order and that an accounting of all drugs is maintained and periodically reconciled.

### Drug Regimen Review

The drug regimen of each resident must be reviewed at least once a month by a licensed pharmacist. The pharmacist must report any irregularities to the attending physician and the director of nursing, and these reports must be acted upon.

### Labeling Drugs and Biologics

The facility must label drugs and biologics in accordance with currently accepted professional principles and include the appropriate accessory and cautionary instructions and the expiration date when applicable.

### Storage of Drugs and Biologics

In accordance with state and federal laws, the facility must store all drugs and biologicals in locked compartments under proper temperature controls and permit only authorized personnel to have access to the keys. The facility must provide separately locked, permanently affixed compartments for storage of controlled drugs listed in Schedule II of the Comprehensive Drug Abuse Act of 1970 and other drugs subject to abuse.

Exceptions are made when the facility uses single unit package distribution systems in which the quantity stored is minimal and a missing dose can be readily detected.

### Comprehensive Drug Abuse Prevention and Control Act of 1970

A licensed administrator should be acquainted with this act because the pharmacy program must comply under the Code of Federal Regulations, 21 CFR 1308. The purpose of the act is to classify and set standards for use of substances that have abuse potential. It establishes five schedules of drugs:

- **Schedule I Substances**—Drugs with no accepted medical use in the United States and with a high abuse potential. Examples include heroin and other opium derivatives, LSD and marijuana. To sell, possess or use these drugs is a criminal offense.
- **Schedule II Substances**—Drugs with a high abuse potential and with severe psychic or physical dependence. These drugs require a written prescription from a physician. These prescriptions may not be refilled or transferred to a person other than the resident for whom originally prescribed.
  There are three classes of Schedule II substances:
  1. Narcotics (examples are morphine, codeine, cocaine).
  2. Stimulants (examples are amphetamines and Ritalin).
  3. Depressants (examples are Seconal and Nembutal).
- **Schedule III Substances**—Drugs having less abuse potential than Schedule II drugs and containing limited quantities of certain narcotics. These require prescription by a physician and may be refilled up to five times in a six-month period. After six months, a new prescription is required. Examples include Empirin with codeine and Paregoric.
- **Schedule IV Substances**—Drugs with less abuse potential than Schedule III substances. These are dispensed on the same basis as Schedule III drugs. Examples are Librium, Valium, Equanil and Dalmane.
- **Schedule V Substances**—Drugs with less abuse potential than Schedule IV substances. These con-

tain limited quantities of certain narcotics designed for use generally as antitussive and antidiarrheal preparations. Examples are Robitussin AC and Parepectolin.

## ACTIVITIES DEPARTMENT

Recreation is a person-centered activity and in a nursing facility must be adapted to the needs, abilities and particular interests of the individual in accordance with the care plan. The concept of recreational activities is that the experience must involve the individual and that the individual must choose to participate. Generally, the purpose of recreation is to give satisfaction and to present challenges that are meaningful. A director of activities coordinates the activity program, working with the nursing and other appropriate staffs. He or she will recruit and supervise volunteers, acquainting them with the job duties and responsibilities and maintaining records of hours spent, services recognized and materials needed.

The nursing facility resident has certain limitations upon his or her activities because of physical or psychological problems. Because a facility recreational program can give an individual motivation to develop to his or her greatest potential capacity, it has a therapeutic effect on personal well-being. A great deal of recreation for nursing facility residents involves the proper development of attitudes and the learning of skills and habits. The shorter work week and the fact that many people retire at an earlier age has dramatically increased leisure time. Many persons in our society simply have not prepared themselves in younger years for retirement and leisure activities. Many older persons have devoted most of their lives to working activities and have not developed skills relative to leisure.

One of the residents' basic needs is satisfaction through recreational experiences to release any tensions and strains that may have built up during the day. These activites should create balance and give opportunities to attain each individual's best potential. It is one of the responsibilities of the administrator to see that such activities are available in a recreation program and that residents are able to participate to the best of their ability. Staff needs to know required technical aspects of the activities and how to work with the elderly and infirm in a positive manner. Certain administrative problems may be created by the establishment of the recreational department and related activities. These may be resolved when both the administrator and involved staff are convinced that the program is there to promote the well-being of the residents.

Generally, good activity programs encompass and satisfy the following basic needs of the resident:

- **Companionship**—As human beings, experiences are more meaningful when shared with others and especially with those of similar age and in similar situations. The satisfaction and pleasure derived from an event is not merely the experience but the sharing of it. We often invite people to chat with us to exchange ideas. Sharing of similar experiences and discussing them with others can alleviate frustration and help gain insight into common problems. Older persons enjoy reminiscing; groups discussing "Who am I?" and "Where have I been?" can help develop new friendships and renew old ones. Group activities provide this opportunity for companionship and the mechanism for sharing feelings and accomplishments with others.
- **Feeling Important**—Individuals have a feeling of accomplishment when something is completed of which one is proud. Setting a goal and achieving it gives pride; recognition and appreciation of human efforts by others increase senses of accomplishment, significance and importance. Learning a new hobby or reviving crafts from the past may help the resident develop this sense of accomplishment, particularly if other residents express approval for a job well done.
- **Identification with a Group**—The need for identification and acceptance by a group is basic to our society. Efforts identified with a group are accepted as meaningful, and increase status or prestige within that group. Group acceptance and recognition leads to more self-assurance. Residents must identify with the peer group to establish an identity and develop self-confidence. The establishment of resident councils, advisory groups and committees that have effective function in the facility life is one way to give the resident this opportunity for self-identification and acceptance.
- **Feeling Needed**—How often has it been heard that once a certain magical age is achieved, our society by mandatory retirement arbitrarily puts the individual out to pasture. It is not strange that residents may have feelings of futility, being set aside and

uselessness. However, older persons are needed and a part of our society. Activity programs can help residents feel cared for and needed when individual talents are recognized and promoted, when others benefit by their actions and when various projects are successful.

## Program Needs

Once the administrator (along with the medical director, director of nurses and activities director) has determined the type of program activities best suited to the facility residents and whether to use a full-time, part-time or shared recreational leader, he or she must determine what equipment, space, personnel and budget are needed for setting up such a program. The recreational programs may be started on a small scale to provide what is needed to meet the residents' needs and be publicized and scheduled at a convenient time. In obtaining equipment for the recreational department, should the equipment be owned by the nursing facility or purchased by the resident? Equipment such as table games, cards, puzzles and outside active games can be purchased by the facility whereas equipment for use in crafts programs often is owned individually. There is a possibility also that some of the equipment could be borrowed through various sources in the community such as recreation and parks departments, schools or libraries.

As part of the recreational activity, other community resources may be available to the residents including lectures at the library, concerts, community theaters and classes at the university. Visitations into the community and participation in such events can draw the resident into the community and help maintain and develop outside contacts. Of course, this type of activity would not be feasible for those who are bedridden or cannot get out for other reasons.

## Budgetary Considerations

The recreational program is considered a part of the total operation of the facility and should be included in the budgetary aspects. Considerations in the budget relative to the establishment and operation of a recreational program will involve basically the cost of personnel, equipment, supplies and facilities. The person-

nel cost will vary depending upon the number of full-time, part-time and volunteer staff required to implement and carry out the program.

The cost of equipment and supplies depends upon what portion of these are bought by the facility or the individual participants, or shared cooperatively with other facilities or organizations. Renovation costs would include such items as rewiring, plumbing, storage and display cases. Any transportation costs involving use of community resources in this area could be shared with social services.

## Activity Programming

In determining the kinds of activities in the recreational program, it is important to know the resident needs to be met and to provide opportunities for choice. Activities should help enhance the well-being of the participant, providing greater potential to respond to treatments, socialize, become involved and develop a self-worth. Projects can provide a chance to learn new or build on life-time skills within individual capabilities. Instruction and materials may be provided along the way progressively to avoid confusion. Recognition (through displays, thanks or sales) enhances the sense of accomplishment. Participatory activities include arts and crafts programs, collecting activities, dancing, bingo, games, sports and other physical activities, playing a musical instrument and singing, and outing activities in the community. Passive activities include listening to music, attending dramas or plays, attending music festivities, and watching programs on television.

Arts and crafts are considered a valuable tool for working with older residents and can fill in a great deal of time for those who might be bored with the routine of the nursing facility. A volunteer worker in this area must be an effective teacher and know the skills of the art or craft being taught. Some facilities sell the products made during arts and crafts; others put on displays and shows. A nonprofit corporation should be careful about selling items at a profit because this might interfere with the nonprofit setup. Arts and crafts should create a finished and useful product within the capabilities of the individual resident.

Getting residents together as a group enhances their social compatibility, and helps to create special friendships and to develop interests. Some general group activities for the residents include dancing, drama, flower arranging, guest speakers talking about current or other interesting events, special workshops and classes, discussion groups, music, motion pictures and parties for special occasions. Some other activities involving volunteer participation are making posters, collecting magazines, providing treats for holidays and/or afternoon tea, and working in the area of public relations.

## Kinds of Activities in a Recreational Program

### Exercise

Both physical and mental exercise should be provided and can help residents to become more independent physically. It is wise to obtain a physician's approval before the resident participates in strenuous physical exercise. Exercise activities may include:

- **Supervised Activities**—Pick a time, preferably in the morning, and place for a short exercise program. These programs may be conducted by a trained staff member. Set up a room with proper equipment for gym exercises and have available items such as jump ropes, nerf balls and elastic ropes.
- **Bicycle Riding**—During good weather, this may be a good source of exercise for those residents able to participate.
- **Purpose or Goal Walks**—Conduct walks outlining a purpose. Some suggestions would be rock hunts, looking for leaves to decorate a room, or other similar projects. It is mind refreshing to get outside. One sleeps and eats better.
- **Games**—Balloon volley ball, bean bag toss and croquet are all types of games older persons can enjoy. Arrange for use of a neighborhood bowling alley; many will give special discount rates to senior citizens through golden age clubs, for instance.
- **Swimming**—After obtaining medical advice, organize and arrange to have those residents who can participate go to a swimming pool upon agreement with a local health club, YWCA or YMCA.
- **Mental Gymnastics**—Puzzles, problem solving, board games and educational activities will help stimulate the mind.

### Social Interaction

An activity program should have among its goals sociability, fun and interaction with fellow residents both inside and outside of the facility. Residents can remain in touch with and become part of the larger community both by community members coming into the facility and by resident outings. Such activities give residents something to look forward to, some meaning and some purpose, and promote caring and self-worth. This program can help the resident psychologically to feel wanted and can help precipitate desire to continue to live. Resident councils can be active in several of these areas. A secondary benefit may be improved public relations and community relationships for the facility as a whole. Social activities might include:

- **Dances**—A phonograph, a pianist or an accordian player may provide the music for dancing. Dancing is good exercise and encourages social interaction. Residents may help plan, decorate and entertain.
- **Community Clubs**—Men's and women's service clubs, church groups, senior citizen centers, and so on, may be invited to the facility to conduct or sponsor activities for the residents.
- **Tours**—Plan trips to points of interest in the immediate area (such as to the mall, for a luncheon, to a play, a hatchery or a picnic) for ambulatory residents. Renting a bus for an overnight trip to a nearby tourist area has proven successful.
- **Friendly Visiting**—Have the social service department work with local agencies to arrange for visitation to people in the community who are disabled or lonely.
- **Correspondence Clubs**—Encourage exchange of ideas by having residents write to other elderly people in another state or country.
- **House Organ or Internal Newspaper**—A nursing facility newspaper can be published inexpensively on a quarterly or monthly basis. Appoint a committee to establish it, select reporters, artists, and so on. Send the newspaper to community-minded groups in the town.
- **Family Day**—A special day or days can be set aside to invite the families of the residents to the facility. Potlucks encourage the family to bring the resident's favorite dish. Old friends and interested community members also can attend.

- **Birthday Parties**—Keep a record of the birthdays of all the residents. Once a month have a birthday party for all the residents born in that particular month, respecting those who do not want this recognition.

### Recreational Activities

Programs of a major nature may be tied into the various seasons of the year (such as a Christmas party, Mardi Gras or a winter festival). Other activities, which can take place within or outside the facility, could include:

- **Games**—Have a variety of games (such as pool or bingo) available that can be played individually or with a group. Teach the residents how to play them and encourage practice with families or friends.
- **Music Appreciation**—Provide a listening room where the resident can be alone or with friends to listen to a variety of music. Arrange for attendance at community and school concerts or parades. Perhaps a music discussion group could be organized to discuss different types of music.
- **Free Choice Time**—Do not over-schedule activities for residents. There should be opportunity to just meet spontaneously. Have a list of events prepared for residents wishing to participate in them.
- **Hobby Shows**—Hold hobby shows for the residents and the community as a way of encouraging hobbies.
- **Sports Activities**—Arrange transportation for those residents who are interested in sports activities (school games, fishing, sport shows). Discuss the possibility of a reduced rate for such events with their sponsoring groups.

### Service Activities

Service activities also can build the resident's self-confidence and feelings of self-worth, and foster socialization. These may include:

- **Volunteer Work**—Encourage residents to serve as volunteers for such programs as hospital visitation or the American Red Cross.

- **Sales Outlet Store**—If there is an outlet to sell items that residents have made, residents can help with the displays, sales and clerical work connected with the activities of the store.
- **Gardening**—Encourage residents to do some gardening. Container gardening or portions of gardening beds are ideal for growing both flowers and vegetables; these can be used for decoration and food in the facility. Prizes could be awarded to the resident raising the nicest flowers or vegetables.
- **Traveling Entertainment**—Residents who are musically or dramatically talented can be encouraged to organize as a group and give performances at hospitals, schools or other community functions.

### Spiritual Activities

Administrators should realize the significance of religious habits in the lives of the residents and be familiar with the basic concepts of various faiths in a general way. Usually as a person grows older, he or she tends to participate more fully in programs of a spiritual nature. It is, therefore, important to provide opportunities to share in religious activities. Chapel services and visitation of clergy of all faiths can be arranged on a regular basis. A few guidelines to consider in religious programming are:

- **Bible Reading and Prayer**—Set aside a certain time of the day for devotional reading. Bible classes and/or discussion groups may be held for those interested.
- **Chapel**—An area should be set aside for a chapel or other devotional activities with adequate space for ambulatory and nonambulatory persons.
- **Sabbath Services**—Provisions may be made for parishioners in community churches to transport ambulatory residents to services of their choice.
- **Speakers**—The local ministerial society can provide programs of interest to the residents on various aspects of religious beliefs. Establish good relationships with this society. Encourage visitation to individuals in the facility; make available nonconfidential related information.
- **Wall Hangings**—Murals and pictures of a religious nature painted by the residents could be displayed.

- **Reading Material**—Reading material of several denominations should be available for any residents interested in reading them.

### *Educational Activities*

Some of the following could provide interesting information to residents and help keep broad interests and minds active:

- **Short Courses**—Qualified individuals can present courses on such topics as creative thinking, economics, medicine, and so on.
- **Travelogues**—Encourage residents who have been in other countries or in other parts of this country to tell about travel experiences.
- **Speakers Bureau**—You may obtain lecturers on current events or other areas of interest to residents from the community speakers bureau.
- **Library**—Provide a reading room with varied reading material such as magazines and newspapers.
- **Correspondence Courses**—Investigate the possibility of correspondence courses in areas of possible resident interest.

## Activities
### 42 CFR, Sec. 483.15 (F), Ch. IV (10-1-98)

Medicare and Medicaid require that certain provisions are met relating to activities.

The facility must provide an ongoing program of activities designed to meet in accordance with the comprehensive assessment, the interests and the physical, mental and psychosocial well-being of each resident.

The activities program must be directed by a professional who must fulfill one of these qualifications:

1. Is a qualified therapeutic recreation specialist or an activities professional who is:
   a. Licensed or registered, if applicable, by the state where practicing, and
   b. Eligible for certification as a therapeutic recreation specialist or an activities professional by a recognized accrediting body on October 1, 1990.
2. Has 2 years of experience in a social or recreational program within the last 5 years, 1 of which

was full-time in a resident activities program in a health care setting.
3. Is a qualified occupational therapist or occupational therapy assistant.
4. Has completed a training course approved by the state.

## VOLUNTEER SERVICES

It has been determined beyond a reasonable doubt that the emotional, psychological and sociological needs of the elderly are basically the same as those of younger persons. The feelings of love, the desire to be loved, approval, acceptance and self-esteem are basic to all individuals. The volunteer service should help meet these needs with some of the following goals to:

1. Help the resident to make the most of his or her current abilities, to restore those abilities temporarily lost and to minimize the handicaps that he or she may have.
2. Give the resident something to look forward to and to believe in.
3. Help the resident to develop an interest in life.
4. Stimulate the resident's interest in the outside world.
5. Encourage participation in creative activities of an intellectual and/or recreational nature to help the resident become more independent.
6. Stimulate the resident's physical and mental health and to prevent regression.
7. Assure the resident that he or she is a member of society and the community and is not forgotten.
8. Help the resident attain a feeling of self-confidence and achievement.

### Volunteer Programs

The two types of volunteer programs use adults and younger people. The adult volunteer workers carry on such programs as reading, writing, visiting, organization of study groups and recreational activities. The second general category is staffed by younger people and very often is associated with schools, clubs of a technical nature (Future Farmers, Future Nurses, American Red Cross or church youth groups). The scope of activities conducted by the younger people are usually more limited than those conducted by the adults and are usually confined to the nursing facility proper, requiring greater supervision. Some psychiatrists and medical authorities indicate that many of our young people find it quite easy to relate to the aged. Younger people in the nursing facility really give a psychological lift to the resident.

## Role of the Volunteer

The role of the volunteer entails that of a person coming in from the community who is not personally involved in the stresses, strains and problems of the resident and whose only purpose is to build a constructive relationship with the resident. If the volunteer understands the process of aging and the psychological and sociological needs of aging residents, he or she can develop a lasting relationship with several residents in the facility. The volunteer also can work in group activities involving residents in constructive activities and maintaining their interests in the community. Volunteers can help enhance the quality of residents' lives by showing that they are individuals, are worthwhile, are part of the community and are cared about. New faces, ideas, talents and friendships are brought in to help make facility life as good as possible in declining years.

## Recruitment of Volunteer Workers

The following traits should be sought when recruiting volunteer workers:

1. Sufficient time and willingness to learn the interests of the residents.
2. Sense of responsibility and dependability.
3. Sincere interest in older people, appreciation of the worth of an individual and ability to accept the ways of the aging, their interests and variant moods.
4. Capacity to establish relationships with the elderly easily.
5. Ability to use good judgment and be an attentive listener.
6. Willingness to work under supervision, take direction and accept the rules and regulations of the facility.

## Orientation and Training of the Volunteer Worker

A differentiation should be made between the roles of the volunteer worker and the women's auxiliary member in the nursing facility. The women's auxiliary basically conducts fund-raising activities and helps bridge the gap between the facility and the community. The volunteer worker provides activities and services to the resident within the nursing facility walls.

Because the volunteer works directly with the residents within the facility, it is important that the volunteer worker be properly trained and oriented. There is a potential that liability for the acts of volunteers who are negligent will be imputed to the institution under the theory of *Respondeat Superior*.

A good orientation program for volunteer workers will include the facility's objectives, rules, regulations, ethical conduct and programs. Training sessions held for the volunteers should make sure that they understand the psychological and emotional problems involved in the nature of the residents with whom they will be working. This includes the concept of regression, the need for personal identity, the effect of motivation and the concurrent problems of disease. The orientation also will cover the importance of confidentiality of residents' personal information and respect of individual religious beliefs.

## Friendly Visiting

A friendly visitor is a volunteer who visits the resident on a continuing basis and develops a one-to-one relationship. This person spends time listening to the resident, finding out his or her background and interests, and becoming a friend. She or he can help the individual to keep in touch with both the facility and outside communities. The volunteer may:

1. Engage the resident in discussion about everyday current events.
2. Pay attention to the physical aspects of the resident by noticing when the resident, for instance, has a new dress or shirt.
3. Read the newspaper aloud to the resident.
4. Encourage the resident to participate in various hobbies.

5. Play games of a constructive nature with the resident.
6. Encourage the resident to become acquainted with other residents.
7. Assist the resident with personal grooming.

---

## BIBLIOGRAPHY

Allen, J.E. 1992. *Nursing home administration*, 2nd ed. New York, NY: Springer Publishing.

Code of Federal Regulations, Title 42, Parts 430 to end.

Davis, W. 1994. *Introduction to health care administration*. Bossier City, LA: Professional Printing & Publishing.

Lane, L.F. 1991. Rehabilitation services enhance resident care and marketability. *Provider*. December, 1991.

Department of Health and Human Services, Health Care Financing Administration. 1992. *Interpretive Guidelines: State Operations Manual* #250. Baltimore, MD.

Sullivan, W. 1994. High tech. *Provider*. March, 1994.

Tishman, E. 1981. Entering the age of computers. *Provider*. March, 1991.

# CHAPTER 7

# Resident Care Management: Principles of Medical Care

## CHRONIC ILLNESS AND DISEASE PROCESS

The majority of residents in long-term care facilities are there because of some chronic physiological disorder. Some also may be recovering from accidents or acute illnesses; others may have chronic infections, inflammations, chronic neurosis or psychosis. In many residents, combinations of acute illnesses complicate diagnosis and therapy.

The aging process, while continuous, is not physically or psychologically identical in any two individuals. Aging is undirectional and varies in rates of deterioration. Normal physical effects of aging include losses of physical stamina, vision, hearing, smell and taste. Pathological physical aging includes chronic disease (such as arthritis or heart disorders) brought on or hastened by increased age. Normal psychological aging may entail slow memory retrieval and difficulty in relating and adjusting to new concepts or change, whereas pathological psychological aging may entail marked memory loss, dementia and delusions. Confusion caused by medication and certain illnesses is generally not considered part of the aging process.

The onset of chronic diseases occurs without the individual clearly recognizing that anything is wrong. Very little relationship can exist between the symptoms and the severity of the existing disease because initial symptoms may present such small deviations from normal behavior that the resident and family are not aware that anything is wrong. Chronic diseases extend over months or even years, whereas most acute diseases involve sudden onset with subsequent complete recovery. Often disability and handicaps occur with chronic problems. Common misconceptions in our society with regard to chronic diseases are that they cannot be treated effectively and are not painful; therefore, persons with such diseases do not require the attention of top physicians and can receive good care and treatment in lesser facilities at a lower cost than the care and treatment required by acute disease.

The nursing facility administrator should be familiar with the nature of chronic illness relating to the geriatric resident to better understand both physical and psychological problems of residents in the facility. He or she should understand the basic terms used by health care personnel in order to make sound decisions when conferring with the staff. The administrator also should be familiar with commonly used drugs and their therapeutic actions and with medical abbreviations used in nurses' notes and physicians' orders. The nursing staff must understand problems of the residents in order to determine the level of care and amount of supervision needed for each resident. Development of medical programs should take into consideration the importance of health maintenance and restorative nursing.

Chronic illnesses may be generally divided into four categories. They are diseases concerning the circulatory and respiratory systems (see descriptions under Disease Recognition in this chapter), the musculoskeletal system, tumors (neoplastic diseases) and the metabolic system. Following is a review and brief discussion of the various physiological systems and their relation to the aging residents.

## Circulatory System

One of the first systems to encounter the effect of aging is the cardiovascular system including the heart and the blood vessels. As an individual grows older, the heart becomes less capable of responding to the demands of heavy work.

### Arteriosclerosis

Arteriosclerosis, which is commonly known as hardening of the arteries, is the major cause of cardiovascular disease. It is a slowly developing process whereby the blood vessels lose their elasticity and may become narrowed as the linings become thickened with deposits of fats and plaque. This process can occur all over the body (general arteriosclerosis) or only in certain areas of the body (local arteriosclerosis) and results in lack of oxygen and other nourishments to vital organs. Increased resistance to the flow of the blood causes the heart to become larger and pump faster to compensate and maintain the necessary blood flow.

Complications of this disease include:

- **Angina pectoris** is where lack of oxygen shows itself as a severe suffocating pain under the breastbone that radiates to the left arm. This pain may become very traumatic but generally subsides at rest.
- **Cerebrovascular accident** (CVA or stroke) is caused by hemorrhage or a blood clot in the arteries of the brain. With a lessening of the blood supply, the nerve cells die causing a decrease in efficiency of the motor and accessory activities of the brain. Stroke can produce a paralysis on the side opposite to the site of the clot. The resident usually survives a stroke if it is not massive but may have difficulty in speech and/or in the use of an arm or leg.
- **Congestive heart failure** (CHF) is where the heart cannot pump enough oxygen to body tissues; abnormal amount of blood in circulatory system causes fluids to leak into tissues (water accumulation in legs) and organs (lungs).
- **Coronary thrombosis** (heart attack) occurs when a blood clot in the general coronary artery causes an obstruction. This may kill its victim within a few minutes or cause a collapse allowing the victim to survive long enough to go to the hospital.

- **Increase in blood pressure or hypertension** is where the arteries of the kidney are affected, resulting in associated diseases of other organs.

Residents coming into the facility with cardiovascular disorders should be identified by a notation on their health records so that the entire staff is aware of the problem. From a viewpoint of care, it is important that the resident receive adequate medical supervision, a closely supervised diet and the proper amount of physical exercise. Many permanent disabilities, including psychological and emotional changes, result from cerebral thrombosis and may be avoided if vigorous rehabilitative programs are implemented that take into consideration aspects of depression, hostility, anxiety, personal habits and stressful family situations.

In writing resident care policies, it may be wise to obtain standing orders from the attending or consulting physician should the cardiovascular patient undergo an acute coronary thrombosis. The resident care plan should be reviewed monthly and the staff made aware of the basic things to do when a resident has a sudden heart attack. The resident should not be turned or moved until seen by a physician. Nonprofessionals must immediately report the situation to a professional nurse. The resident care policies should take into consideration that making the resident's bed or bathing the resident is not recommended until at least 48 hours after the cardiovascular attack to avoid dislodging a blood clot and possibly causing immediate death.

After a severe heart attack, the resident should be educated as to why certain procedures are taken. Try to minimize the fear and tension that is attendant with such an attack. The resident should realize that he or she will get smaller meals, tire very easily and must avoid any overexertion. However, it should be explained that as the physical condition progresses, more moderate activity can be added. Bowel hygiene and adequate elimination is important as abdominal distension may stimulate acute episodes. The cardiac resident should not be placed in stressful situations. It is important that a roommate does not become a source of tension.

### Thrombophlebitis

This condition is associated with circulatory problems and often occurs after prolonged bedrest; early ambulation has lessened this complication to a considerable degree. Many older residents experience internal hemorrhages which result in blood clots. If these become dislodged from the wall of a vessel and block oxygen to a vital organ, serious consequences may occur. Changes in blood pressure, which can cause blood clots to dislodge, are associated with emotional stress. One of the important roles of the administrator is to keep the residents as free from anxiety as possible. Activity programs properly suited to the resident will avoid mental and physical deterioration. As mentioned in the section on activity planning, past occupations, hobbies and present interests of each resident should be considered in planning his or her activity program.

## Musculoskeletal System

As one becomes older, the body undergoes a change whereby the muscle and bone structure may cause a stooped posture or a limitation in mobility. These changes tend to impair such important activities as breathing, urination and defecation. Lack of exercise often leads to degenerative breakdown or atrophy of the muscles and joints. Therefore, the elderly person should be encouraged to participate in the facility exercise programs and be physically active within individual capacities. Arthritis is one of the most prevalent chronic diseases among the elderly.

### Rheumatoid Arthritis

Rehumatoid arthritis is generalized inflammatory disease of the body primarily manifested in the joints and involves wide systematic involvement. This disease may be considered to be an affliction of the young that occurs usually between ages 20 and 35. Its onset may be sudden and acute but is usually insidious. Rheumatoid arthritis most often affects the joints of the hands, wrists, knees and feet; the typical situation involves both hands or both knees. These inflammatory changes in joints and related structures lead to crippling joint deformities.

### Degenerative Arthritis

Degenerative arthritis or osteoarthritis more commonly occurs in the middle and later years of life, affecting approximately 10% of those over age 60. The basic process of osteoarthritic changes are growth of bone spurs and thinning and eventual disappearance of the cartilage which forms the smooth gliding surface of the weight-bearing joints; such changes are detectable by X-ray. The symptoms are stiffness and aching pain caused when "bare bones" move against each other with higher levels of pain at night or after excessive activity. This pain can become quite severe and disabling and may be relieved by rest, physical therapy, heat and/or analgesics.

## Neoplastic Diseases

A neoplasm may be defined as a new and abnormal formation of tissue. Tumors fall into this category.

### Tumors

A tumor is a swelling or any new or unnecessary pathological growth forming an abnormal mass and serving no useful function. Tumors may occur throughout the body. They may grow locally and not spread to other parts of the body (benign) or they may invade neighboring tissues and/or metastasize and spread throughout the entire body (malignant, cancerous). Tumors are generally noninflammatory and develop independently of normal laws of growth. Tumors occur in the:

1. Stomach. Benign tumors are relatively rare.
2. Breast, uterus, intestinal tract, skin and tongue. Carcinomas are common.
3. Muscle, bone tissue. Sarcomas are cancers occurring here.
4. Duodenum. Tumors are rare and generally involve surgical removal.
5. Liver. Most common tumor is hepatoma, a benign tumor occurring in patients with chronic cirrhosis or chronic infection. Cancer of the liver is relatively rare.
6. Gall bladder. Tumors generally involve polyps or small growths projecting from the wall of the gall bladder into its cavity. Cancer may occur in patients who have had gall stones or chronic inflammation for many years.
7. Pancreas. Tumors are rare and less than 10% malignant. The prognosis is very poor for cancer of the pancreas and may be manifested by jaundice particularly in older males.

8. Small bowel. Tumors are rare and usually benign. Symptoms are obstructions and detectible by X-ray when large enough.
9. Colon. Benign tumors projecting into the canal of the colon are termed polyps; these vary in size from a quarter inch to several inches in diameter. A symptom of larger polyps is blood in the stool. Symptoms of a malignant tumor vary; a cancerous growth on the right side of the colon is indicated by diarrhea because it interferes with the absorption of water from fecal material and on the left side by constipation because part of the passage is blocked off by the growth.

## Metabolic Diseases

Metabolism is the absorption and conversion of nutrients by chemical reaction throughout the body to produce energy and ensure the various body functions. Metabolic disease interferes with metabolism and occurs when a loss of balance occurs between food intake and the body's use of these nutrients to provide energy, elimination and maintenance, and a variety of disorders results.

### Gastrointestinal System

An elderly person becomes more preoccupied with food, eating habits and elimination of food. Eating patterns are manifested by less fluid intake and a craving for sweets. At the same time the body requires less calories due to a decrease in metabolic rate. The elderly usually experience a decrease in smell and taste, reduced motility of the stomach and intestines, and a decrease in the ability of the body to produce digestive juices in the stomach. As a result of these physical factors, the resident often becomes constipated, which can lead to bowel incontinence and hemorrhoids.

Eating habits also play an important psychological role. The ingestion of food very often is tied into emotional aspects such as affection and security. The social environment or the lack of companionship may affect the elderly person relative to eating habits. Some will neglect their meals; others will overeat as compensation for their loneliness. As a result, many older people develop poor eating habits which can lead to obesity or to malnutrition and have such harmful consequences as an increase in the risk of heart disease, stroke, diabetes or arthritis.

### Diabetes Mellitus

This disease can develop at any age, but with the modern drugs and treatments a person with diabetes can live a normal life. Diabetes mellitus occurs with the disfunctioning of the pancreas where insulin is secreted. It interferes with the carbohydrate metabolism and manifests itself in a rise in the blood sugar and the presence of sugar in the urine. The exact cause is not known but the disease is considered to be inherited or congenital. The pancreas (a large gland lying beneath the stomach) may not make available enough insulin to burn these foods as energy or store them for future uses; certain ductless glands in the brain or other parts of the body may be at fault. Diabetes mellitus can be fatal if not controlled.

A diabetic must have a special diet. Serious consequences can occur if a staff member inadvertently gives a diabetic a wrong diet. A positive educational program should be conducted with the resident to encourage his or her cooperation with the nurses, staff and physician; the diabetic resident must be familiar with his or her condition and with the symptoms that indicate the beginning of insulin shock. The teaching program should include such things as dietary needs, how to administer insulin, care of the feet and skin, and complications that may occur. The diabetic resident should have an identification tag, noting that the individual is a diabetic, his or her type of insulin, the insulin dosage and whom to notify in the case of an attack.

### Pernicious Anemia

Pernicious anemia results from the failure of red blood cells to develop and mature in a normal way due to a lack of vitamin B12 production by the body. These red cells (termed macrocytes) are enlarged and appear to be overloaded with hemoglobin while the total red cell count is decreased. Muscular weakness and gastrointestinal and neural disturbances occur. The disease is quite common among individuals in their fifties and sixties, but rare before the age of 30.

### Obesity

Obesity is an excessive proportion of fat in the body (20-30% over normal weight) determined usually in relation to one's age, sex and height. It has been determined that obesity shortens the outlook for a long life and may contribute to problems with gall bladder, diabetes mellitus, high blood pressure, osteoarthritis (knees), and some types of cancer.

## Special Problems of the Handicapped Aged

In the typical long-term care facility, a mix of residents are found relative to their ability to participate in various activities. They range from those who are completely bedridden to those who are ambulatory and able to take part in most mental and physical activities. Included are those with problems relating to handicaps. Some handicaps of the elderly are discussed below:

### Defective Vision

A resident who is declared visually impaired must receive the understanding and assistance of those in the facility responsible for the particular care required to maintain self-sufficiency. However, the staff should be cautioned not to do so much for the visually impaired resident that dependency might be encouraged and self-confidence discouraged. Reassurance is an important aspect of this care. The resident should keep personal belongings in the same place all the time so that he or she can locate what is wanted; furniture in the room should be placed so there is no obstruction when moving about the room. Residents should be able to feed themselves and at their own pace after a staff member points out the selection and location of the food on the tray.

Blindness may create some emotional reactions; foremost are withdrawal from the world, stress and depression. Staff should encourage and help the resident to realize that by participating in activities, working with his or her hands on crafts and showing interest in what others are doing will improve the quality of life. Trained occupational and recreational therapists can help with specialized activities. Because of stress, psychiatric problems may occur in the blind resident requiring treatment by a qualified psychiatrist; depression should be watched very carefully. Try to have a radio available for visually impaired residents for entertainment and keeping in touch with community and world happenings.

### Defective Hearing

Lack of response to questions may be an indication that a resident is suffering from hearing loss. This resident may appear nervous and under tension while trying to read lips. Loud speech also could be an indication of a hearing loss because the speaker is unable to hear his or her own voice. Many emotional problems are associated with a hearing loss. The person with a hearing loss reacts defensively in relationships with others, sometimes manifesting symptoms of paranoidal nature, feeling that people are talking about him or her. It is important to develop good working relationships and communication with these residents. Experts make the following suggestions on communicating with people who have hearing impairments:

1. Look directly at the individual.
2. Speak distinctly.
3. Avoid shouting.
4. Speak slowly.
5. Write down names or complicated ideas.

Encourage residents with hearing difficulties to become involved in creative or group activities and to work with his or her hands and mind. Self-assurance will return with communication and understanding with the other residents and staff. Patience and understanding are a must among the staff.

When a person is suspected of being hearing impaired, he or she should be referred to an otiologist who will give a hearing test to determine the degree of loss and the source (nerve damage or sound not being sent to the inner ear). A hearing aid can be the solution if the resident can interpret the sounds being relayed to the brain; recommendation for this purchase should come by referral from the physician.

### Fractures

When a resident sustains a fracture, a physician (preferably an orthopedic physician) must be notified to properly set the fracture. Afterward, the roles of the nurse and the physical therapist become very important in helping the resident regain maximum movement at the site of the fracture. If the resident has a fractured leg, the progress toward walking will be slow and taken in several steps: to a wheelchair, from the wheelchair to a walker, from the walker to crutches, and from the crutches to ambulating without them. The degree of recovery depends upon several factors: the severity of fracture, the healing power of the resident, the need for surgery, the mental attitude, and his or her ability to understand and cooperate with the rehabilitative efforts.

### Bedsores

The prevention of bedsores is an important aspect of the care of the bedridden elderly person who remains in one position. Bedsores occur in bony areas thinly covered with flesh (such as the end of the spine, buttocks, heels, elbows and shoulder blades). Considerations include the maintenance of circulation and avoidance of pressure on the various parts of the body.

Basic recommendations for prevention are keeping the bed clean and dry, frequent turning and changing of the resident's position in the bed to enhance circulation, and gentle massage to pressure areas to help prevent breaks in the skin. Any breakdown or irritation in the skin observed by the staff must be reported to the supervisors or professional nurses. Incontinent residents are very prone to decubitus ulcers (bedsores) because urea and ammonia compounds in the urine tend to break down the tissue of the body. It is important that wet beds be changed promptly; sheepskin, air or flotation beds may be needed. Any pressure area should receive immediate medical attention, and policies and procedures should include a standing order relative to the situation when a pressure site is noted.

### Amputated Appendages

Amputations usually stem from an accident or medical disease such as diabetes (which must be brought under control). Amputation very often results in serious emotional problems, sometimes requiring psychiatric consultation. The nurse, the physical therapist and the attending physician will play an important role in motivating the amputee to want to leave the wheelchair and use an artificial limb. Use of an artificial leg comes in steps: first the resident will be encouraged to move about in a wheelchair, then to crutches, and then the artificial limb will be fitted and the amputee helped to walk until he or she feels at ease.

### Paraplegia

Paraplegia is usually a result of damage to the spinal cord, resulting in paralysis of lower portions of the body and both legs. Care and rehabilitation include maintaining normal body functions (bowel activity, circulation and proper fluid balance). Thus, nutrition and the prevention of complications play an important role. Complications to be watched for include lung congestion, pneumonia, bedsores, contractures (such as foot dropsy due to improper position of a bed patient's foot) and bladder infections due to interference with contraction of the muscles in the bladder wall. Recovery is slow, requiring the services of a therapist. The supervision of a urologist is necessary during the phase where urinary drainage needs to be observed. Communication with the paraplegic resident is usually very good because there is no brain damage.

### Hemiplegia

Paralysis on one side of the body due to brain damage from a stroke or cerebral vascular accident is referred to as hemiplegia. Care and rehabilitation include the maintenance of normal body functions, adequate nutrition and prevention of complications (lung congestion, pneumonia, decubitus ulcer and contractures). The hemiplegic resident will require the services of a physical therapist to restore the use of his or her affected limb. Such therapy equipment as a hydrotherapy unit, exercise room, and devices for muscular stimulation and daily range of motion exercises will be needed. The regimen of therapy also will include the services of a trained speech therapist.

Very often emotional and personality changes occur. Hemiplegia is difficult to work with because of possible attendant brain damage. The resident often finds it difficult to communicate with and to be understood by those trying to give therapy. This leads to frustration, apprehension and fright. Reassurance and proper motivation in getting this resident interested in activities of daily living and setting realistic goals are important. The prognosis may be very slow and requires much patience on the part of the staff. Again the move toward rehabilitation will be a step-by-step situation, and encouragement is needed to complete recovery.

## DISEASE RECOGNITION

Administration should be aware of the common diseases of aging that afflict residents and of the facility's ability to address the basic care demands related to these diseases. A wide range of conditions are frequently encountered.

**Anemia** is a chronic condition in which there is a lowered number of red blood cells and/or hemoglobin to meet oxygen needs of the body.

**Cause:** A chronic blood loss, loss of bone marrow, bacterial toxins, iron deficiency or other chemical agents.

**Signs and Symptoms:**

1. Pallor of the skin, mucous membranes and nail beds.
2. Low hemoglobin.
3. Palpitation, angina pectoris.
4. Drowsiness.
5. Vertigo, faintness, weakness, general malaise.

**Resident Care Plan:**

1. The diet should be rich in proteins and other blood-building materials.
2. The resident should receive sufficient rest.
3. Mouthwashes and sponge stick if needed for mouth lesions.
4. Prevent infection.
5. Blood transfusions to restore blood volume and medication as ordered by the physician.

**Arteriosclerosis** is a chronic disease characterized by thickening, hardening and loss of elasticity in the artery walls. Blood clot formation may result in cerebrovascular accidents. This disease is considered to be indirectly one of the most common causes of death among older persons.

**Cause:** Unknown. Risk factors include: age, lack of exercise, high blood pressure, high cholesterol, obesity.

**Signs and Symptoms:**

1. Mental confusion.
2. Headache, dizziness.
3. Memory defects.
4. Fast pulse.

**Resident Care Plan:**

1. Tobacco (cigarette or other) use may have a highly vasospastic action and should be avoided if the resident has arteriosclerosis. These spasms may become serious enough to shut down the flow of the arterial blood to various vital tissues in the body.

2. Vasodilators and anticoagulant therapy may be prescribed by the physician to prevent spasms of the vessels and formation of blood clots.
3. Diets low in cholesterol and salt and high in fiber.
4. Regular exercise and physical therapy.
5. Avoid stress.
6. Therapy for any related treatable disease.

**Arthritis** is the inflammation of the joint or joints.

**Cause:** May result from or be associated with infections or various conditions including rhuematic fever, colitis, trauma, degenerative joint disease and gout.

**Signs and Symptoms:**

1. Irritability, fatigure.
2. Pain, swelling, redness and gradual deformity of joints.
3. Tenderness.
4. High temperature.
5. Reduced mobility.

**Resident Care Plan:**

1. Prevent contractions (by splinting), medication and treatments as ordered by physician.
2. Reduce or relieve pain.
3. Complete mental and physical rest.
4. High caloric diet to help build the resistance in the body.
5. Occupational and physical therapy such as moderate exercise and massage.
6. Warm baths or soaks before range of motion therapy.

**Bronchitis** is an inflammation of the mucous membranes of the bronchial tubes and is often a long-term problem.

**Cause:** Infectious agents (such as viruses, influenza or staphlycoccus) often preceded by common cold, chilling, fatigue, malnutrition, or inhalation of dusts or fumes.

**Signs and Symptoms:**

1. Cough.
2. Malaise and diffuse muscle pain.
3. Fever.
4. Headache.

**Resident Care Plan:**

1. Give the medications prescribed by physician.

2. Provide nourishing well-balanced diet.
3. Increase intake of fluids.
4. Bed rest until the fever disappears.
5. Emotional support and reassurance.

**Cancers** have the properties of uncontrolled growth of cells from the cells of normal tissue that can kill the host cells locally or be spread to other parts of the body. Cancers include carcinomas, sarcomas and leukemias.

**Cause:** This unregulated disorganized growth of cells may be stimulated by various chemicals, use of cytotoxic agents (tobacco), viruses and physical agents (radiation, ultraviolet light). High dietary fat and low fiber intake may be important factors in development of cancers.

**Signs and Symptoms:**

1. Any sore that does not heal.
2. Lump or thickening in the breast or elsewhere.
3. Any unusual external or internal bleeding or discharge.
4. Persistent indigestion or difficulty in swallowing.
5. Persistent cough or hoarseness.
6. Any dramatic change in bowel or bladder habits.
7. Change in size, shape or appearance of wart or mole.
8. Unexplained loss of weight.

**Resident Care Plan:**

1. Education to resident and family as to disease process and its progress, treatment, realistic pain control and outcome.
2. Emotional and coping support to resident and family; encourage verbalization of feelings and fears, especially in relation to death and dying.
3. Maintain fluids and nutritional status.
4. Give particular care to the resident as to hygiene and cleanliness, keeping resident as comfortable as possible and decreasing the effects of immobilization.
5. Medication and treatments as prescribed by a physician.

**Cerebrovascular accident** is a stroke, apoplexy or brain hemorrhage.

**Cause:** Rupture of a blood vessel or blockage of an artery by blood clot in the brain. Associated with high blood pressure and/or arterosclerotic disease.

**Signs and Symptoms:**

1. Emotional and personality changes.
2. Sudden loss of consciousness.
3. Paralysis on one side of usually the face, arm or leg.
4. Anxiety.

**Resident Care Plan:**

1. Psychological assessment.
2. Give treatment and medications as prescribed by physician.
3. Therapies (including speech, physical or occupational) and positive reinforcement.
4. Quiet rest periods.
5. Provide good hygienic care and encourage independence of activities of daily living (ADLs).
6. Evaluate, monitor and maintain feeding and bowel and bladder functions.
7. Prevent complications of immobility (bedsores or incorrect body alignment).
8. Educate resident and family as to therapeutic regimen and realistic goals.

**Congestive heart failure** is a syndrome caused by fluid congestion in pulmonary or systemic circulation.

**Cause:** Arteriosclerosis, heart attack, uncontrolled high blood pressure, coronary artery disease, heart failure.

**Signs and Symptoms:**

1. Difficult breathing upon exertion.
2. Edema of the lower extremities.
3. Decreased urinary output.
4. Pain over the heart and stomach area.
5. Cough and expectoration due to the congestion.
6. Blueness of the lips and nail beds.

**Resident Care Plan:**

1. Low salt and high potassium diet of foods that are easily digestible.
2. Sedatives as ordered by the physician to ensure that the resident is relaxed and rests.
3. Other medications and treatments as prescribed by the physician.
4. Oxygen therapy.

5. A regimen of regular weighing and measurement of the intake of fluids and output of urine to check gain or loss of fluids.

**Constipation** is abnormal infrequency or difficult defecation.

**Cause:** No regular bowel habits, sedentary life, improper diet, tumor, intestinal obstructions, anxiety, fear.

**Signs and Symptoms:**

1. Headaches.
2. Abdominal cramps.
3. Sluggish feeling.

**Resident Care Plan:**

1. Establish regular bowel habits.
2. Nonconstipating diet (fruits, vegetables and cereal fiber).
3. Medication as prescribed by the physician.
4. Increase fluid intakes.
5. Increase walking and activity.
6. Discuss any change in bowel habits with physician.

**Diabetes Mellitus** is a chronic disorder of the carbohydrate metabolism.

**Cause:** Not entirely known. Usually a result of a genetic disorder where the pancreas fails to produce necessary amount of insulin.

**Signs and Symptoms:**

1. Disturbed vision.
2. Excessive urine; sugar in urine.
3. Elevated blood sugar.
4. Increased appetite.
5. Excessive thirst.

**Resident Care Plan:**

1. Provide therapeutic diet and help the resident adjust to it.
2. Report any break in skin on resident to attending physician.
3. Test urine and blood sugar; check input and output of fluid at regular intervals.
4. Watch for insulin shock.
5. Encourage the resident to accept and understand the disease and to wear a Medic Alert bracelet.
6. Administer insulin as ordered by the physician.

7. Provide a consistent level of daily exercise.
8. Provide good hygienic and foot care, and consultation with podiatrist if needed.

**Epilepsy** is a chronic disease of the nervous system characterized by attacks of altered consciousness, motor activity or sensory phenomena with or without accompanying convulsions.

**Cause:** Not established. May be a chemical or a mechanical irritation of the brain.

**Signs and Symptoms:**

1. A cry and a fall. Individual may fall to the ground or droop over chair.
2. Imperceptible to dramatic loss of consciousness.
3. Convulsive movements of all extremities.
4. Incontinence.

**Resident Care Plan:**

1. Give medication as prescribed by physician.
2. Prevent injury but do not restrain movement.
3. Turn individual to side, allowing tongue to fall away from air passage and to drain saliva.
4. Loosen restrictive clothing.
5. Report the time, the length of the epileptic seizure and the resident's reactions.
6. Do not leave the resident alone.
7. Counseling regarding self-image, fear or anxiety.

**Gastritis** is an acute inflammation of the mucosa or lining of the stomach.

**Cause:** Generally unknown. Excessive ingestion of alcohol or sharp spicy food is a factor.

**Signs and Symptoms:**

1. A coated tongue.
2. Moderate fever.
3. Nausea, vomiting and thirst.
4. Acute pain and tenderness in the pit of the stomach.

**Resident Care Plan:**

1. Medication as ordered by the physician.
2. Withhold solid and semi-solid foods.
3. Bed rest.

**Nephritis** is inflammation of the kidney.

**Cause:** Bacteria or their toxins, streptococcal infections, diptheria, toxic drugs (such as arsenic) or alcohol.

**Signs and Symptoms:**

1. Blood in the urine.
2. Elevated blood count.
3. Swelling of the face.
4. Pain in the small of the back.
5. Dizziness, nausea and vomiting.
6. Fever accompanied by chills.

**Resident Care Plan:**

1. Make sure that the resident receives plenty of physical and mental rest.
2. Report signs of renal failure (lowered volume of urine, increase nitrogenous compounds and acids).
3. Medications as prescribed by physician.
4. Monitor blood pressure, hemoglobin and electrolytes (sodium, potassium). Observe, record and report blood in urine.

**Neuritis** is an inflammation of the nerve fiber associated with degeneration.
**Cause:** Infections, toxic or metabolic agents, trauma.
**Signs and Symptoms:**

1. Affected muscles and nerves become very tender.
2. Paralysis; muscular atrophy of part supplied by affected nerve.
3. Weakness increases.
4. Loss of sensation; lack of reflexes.
5. Numbness, tingling, prickling, burning.

**Resident Care Plan:**

1. Give treatment (such as massage, electrostimulation and exercise) and medication as prescribed by physician.
2. Absolute physical and emotional rest.
3. Remove the cause.
4. Monitor changes in motor and sensory functions.

**Parkinson's disease** is a slowly progressive disease of the brain characterized by muscular weakness and tremors. Does not affect the mental capacity.
**Cause:** Not always known. May be due to damage to small areas of the brain.

**Signs and Symptoms:**

1. Slow, measured speech.
2. Immobile, staring, masklike facial expression.
3. A tendency to lean forward with head bowed.
4. Trembling in the extremities.
5. Muscular rigidity and weakness.
6. Peculiar gait (such as faster pace or body leans forward).

**Resident Care Plan:**

1. Physical and occupational therapy.
2. Stress and fatigue must be avoided.
3. Help the resident to plan daily activities and to adjust to the disability.
4. Medications as prescribed by the physician.

**Phlebitis** is the inflammation of the veins.
**Cause:** Unknown. May occur in acute or chronic infections or following operations.
**Signs and Symptoms:**

1. Discoloration of skin.
2. Inflammatory swelling and edema below obstruction.
3. Painful tender areas along the veins in the legs; pain in joints
4. Some elevation of temperature.

**Resident Care Plan:**

1. Medications (including anticoagulants and analegsics) as prescribed by physician.
2. Use of elastic stockings.
3. Rest in bed; elevation of affected limb.
4. Avoidance of long periods of sitting or standing and crossing of legs.

**Varicose veins** are superficial veins which have become enlarged and twisted. Usually in lower extremities and the esophagus.
**Cause:** Hereditary weakness in the vein structure.
**Signs and Symptoms:**

1. Cramps in the legs.
2. Pain in feet and ankles.
3. Swelling and noticeable enlarged veins in the legs.
4. Ulcers on the skin.

**Resident Care Plan:**

1. Legs should be elevated whenever possible.
2. Circular garters, crossing of the legs and long periods of sitting and standing should be avoided to prevent formation of leg ulcerations.
3. Elastic bandages should be worn while performing routine activities to prevent pooling of the blood in the enlarged vessels.
4. Diet to lose weight, if necessary.
5. Watch for development of thrombophlebitis.

## RESIDENT CARE

Under the Code of Federal Regulations (CFR), a nursing facility must provide each resident equally with the necessary nursing, medical and medically related social services to attain his or her highest practicable physical, mental and psychosocial well-being as determined by his or her comprehensive assessment and plan of care. This care must be provided in a manner and environment enhancing each resident's quality of life. (See "Resident's Rights," Chapter 6.)

### Rehabilitation and Restorative Care

Omnibus Budget Reconciliation Act (OBRA) 1987 broadened the focus of resident care from comfort to restorative programs that are an integral part of all aspects of long-term care. These programs reduce restraints and emphasize the assistance to the resident to improve and/or maintain maximum functional levels toward a better quality of life. If this program is effective, residents function more independently, are less dependent on nurse assistance and are better oriented to their surroundings. Staff members gain satisfaction in doing and accomplishing something good for the resident and spend less time giving remedial care (feeding, dressing or toileting). Residents gain self-esteem, more independence in ADLs, better circulation and fewer bedsores, more socialization, mental alertness, better sleep and feelings that they still have goals to accomplish.

Rehabilitative programs involve a strict regimen toward maintenance and restoration of lost functions provided by trained professionals in physical, occupational and speech therapies. On the other hand, restorative care is ongoing and depends on interdisciplinary interaction among the nursing, dietary, social service, therapists and activities. Most hands-on care is provided by trained restorative nurse assistants.

Ongoing communications among staff members, constant input and assessment from several disciplines as each resident's needs and abilities change, re-establishment of goals, and resident willingness to be involved are vital aspects of the restorative nursing program. This program includes such activities as an exercise room (weight-bearing abilities, range of motion, circulation, muscle tone, standing and walking), use of self-feeding assistive devices, bowel and bladder training, and memory stimulation. This care looks beyond maintenance of health and functioning to achieve the highest possible level of self-care, independence, satisfaction with life and accomplishment of goals—whether it be a matter of several minutes of assisted standing each day, feeding and grooming oneself, using exercise equipment, playing games, or walking through the facility.

Restorative nursing objectives are established by the administrator and staff from the nursing, activities, dietary, social services and therapy departments. It starts with the screening and assessment by department heads and the attending physician within 14 days of admission. Goals are set, daily flowcharts of progress maintained and the success of each component of a resident's restorative care is evaluated at least every three months.

The nursing department plays an essential role in implementing the program. A registered nurse (RN) oversees and conducts resident assessments and may require special training in this area. Floor charge nurses supervise the restorative nurse assistants, documentation and residents' functioning abilities.

Treatment is started early and considers the individual's history, preferences, willingness and comprehension of the role of therapy in his or her care. ADLs, feeding and continence training; resident-to-resident interactions; walking, physical activity and muscle strengthening; and memory stimulation are essentials of most restorative care programs. Documentation (e.g., daily flowcharts) includes the progress and ability to perform of each resident. Some programs are informal extensions of nursing services; others set more formal policies of assessment and continued involvement.

Restorative nursing techniques are to be included in orientation and staff development programs. Daily routine rehabilitative and restorative nursing measures include:

1. Maintaining good body alignment and positioning in beds and wheelchairs.
2. Encouraging and assisting bed patients to change position every two hours to stimulate circulation and prevent bedsores, contractions and deformities.
3. Keeping medically able residents out of bed for reasonable periods of time, encouraging self-care and ambulatory activities unless contraindicated by physician's orders.
4. Assisting resident to adjust to disabilities, use prosthetic devices, and to redirect interest if necessary.
5. Assisting resident to carry out prescribed therapy and routine range of motion exercises.
6. Retraining bowel and bladder for the incontinent.

For more information on subacute care, see Chapter 2.

## Ethics Committee

The nursing facility is faced with complex ethical issues and decisions. Medical technology is able to prolong life for long periods of time, bringing difficult questions in the areas of heroic measures, life or death decisions and quality of life. Nursing abides by duties of protecting the ill and frail, ensuring privacy, maintaining competency and considering the needs of the aged in their care. OBRA supports ethical considerations by requiring respect for the individual, the right to self-determination, the right to privacy and quality care in resident care management. In actuality, problems arise in practice when the ethical issues become clouded. Workloads and physical settings can interfere with the provisions of privacy; full consent can become time consuming and impractical.

Individual assessments of needs, auditing of each resident's care management and auditing the outcomes of resident services help support ethical considerations in resident care.

Ethics committees help provide a systematic and principled approach to complex medical ethical issues, especially in the areas of life-sustaining treatment and the exercise of the right to refuse or withdraw such treatment. Families may seek help with the dilemmas and options brought on by aging or serious illness. An ethics committee provides education on the rights and responsibilities involved in life-sustaining treatment, a forum for supportive discussion of specific problems and recommendations for the formulation of written policies in this area.

Members from both the facility and the community (including clergy, lawyers, physicians, social workers, directors of nursing and admissions, registered nurses and lay persons) serve on this committee.

## Admissions

Residents are admitted to the facility only on a physician's order, which includes an admission diagnosis and an order for immediate care of the resident. A resident may be admitted on an emergency basis, but must have selected (or have selected for him or her) a physician who orders the immediate care and recommends continued stay.

The charge nurse will inform the physician when the resident to be admitted arrives. She or he will receive emergency orders until the physician arrives to give written orders. Each resident admitted is under the continuing care of a nurse or aides under the nurse's supervision. All nurses have a duty to comply with the orders of the physician and with the policies and procedures of the facility to achieve good resident care.

Each resident admitted is under the continuing supervision of the physician of his or her choice or one selected by his or her sponsor. This physician must comply with the policies and procedures of the facility regarding admission, treatment, discharge, medical records, emergency care and other matters necessary for achieving good resident care.

## Resident Assessment and Care Plans

The attending physician records the results of a physical examination done within 48 hours of admission or one that was performed within five days prior to admission. Under OBRA and the CFR, a comprehensive assessment and plan of care are required for each resident to assure that abilities and conditions diminished only under unavoidable clinical conditions. The comprehensive assessment must be conducted within 14 calendar days of admission and include direct observation and communication with the resident and both licensed and unlicensed staff who give direct care to the resident on all shifts. There are automated data processing requirements for encoding and transmitting this data to the state. Within 7 days of the resident's comprehensive assessment, the comprehensive care plan must be developed by an interdisciplinary team, including the physician, registered nurse, staff in appropriate disciplines, and the family or legal representatives. (For additional detail, see the following information under Resident Assessment, 42 CFR, Sec. 483.20, 10-1-98.)

## Medical Director

The medical director supervises the medical services and sees that related standards are maintained. He or she advises the facility's governing body, administrator and director of nursing on policy concerning medical care in such areas as admissions, discharge and transfer, infection control, nonphysician workers, policy and procedure, physician practice, accidents, services (including laboratory, radiology, pharmacy or rehabilitation) and utilization review. The medical director will assist the facility to ensure that physician visits are timely, progress notes signed, necessary entries are made in medical records and orders are issued.

## Resident Care Services

### Physician Services

The purpose of physician services is to achieve for each resident the highest level of good health possible for the individual in his or her circumstances by establishing an accurate diagnosis and by instituting, supervising and assisting in other planning to promote his or her social welfare. A physician is a doctor of medicine, doctor of osteopathy or doctor of dental surgery (or equivalent dental degree) who is licensed to practice in the state. An attending physician is one who has been accorded the privilege of admitting and treating residents in the facility.

The facility directly or through the medical director informs physicians of its policies concerning medical care and of any substantial changes. OBRA 1987 requires that the facility notify the attending physician if a significant change occurs in a resident's physical or psychosocial condition, if he or she is injured and may require physician's care, and what medical coverage must be provided in emergencies when the resident's personal physician is not available.

Facilities ultimately are responsible for the physicians' compliance with state and federal requirements. The facilities are not responsible for communication of these regulations to the physician, medical records departments through the medical director or with the attending physician directly, follow-up by reminders concerning rounds, signing of progress notes, and orders (including possible reduction of physical restraints and antipsychotic drugs) so as not to receive deficiencies during surveys.

### Nursing Services

The purpose of nursing services is to achieve for each resident the highest level of good health possible and to keep the resident comfortable and happy. An RN is licensed in the state where he or she is nursing and is responsible for the resident's care as ordered by the physician and the policies of the facility. When in doubt, the administrator or the attending physician always should be consulted.

### Diagnostic Services

The nursing facility makes arrangements with a hospital to provide required clinical laboratory, X-ray and other diagnostic services including the transportation of the residents to and from the hospital. All diagnostic services are provided only on the request of a physician who will be notified promptly of the test results. Simple tests (i.e., those customarily done by nursing personnel for diabetic residents) may be done in the facility. All reports are included in the clinical record.

### Dental Service

The nursing facility assists residents to obtain regular and emergency dental care. An advisory dentist provides consultation, helps with in-service education, recommends policies concerning oral hygiene and is available in emergencies. Whenever necessary, the facility will make every effort to inform the relatives of the dental attention a resident might need and arrange for transportation to a dentist's office. Nursing personnel assist the residents in carrying out the dentist's recommendations.

### Treatment, Medication and Supervision

Orders for treatment and medication are recorded in the medical record and must be signed by the attending physician. Such orders are in effect for the number of days specified by the physician, but no longer than 30 days without reordering in writing by the physician.

Nursing personnel must see that all prescribed medications are available in the facility; no drugs are administered unless ordered by a physician. Any drug reaction is reported to the physician. A physician's order must be secured before any physical restraint device is used. This order also requires that the resident under restraint be seen by a nurse or attendant at least every 30 minutes. Only a licensed nurse may accept an attending physician's telephone order, which is repeated to the physician after it is entered and signed in the resident's record. The physician must countersign such an entry within 48 hours.

The attending physician reviews the resident's total care program as necessary, and enters the result of the review and orders for any indicated revision of a plan of care in the resident's clinical record.

The attending physician visits his or her residents at least once every 30 days, or more often as necessary, and will enter appropriate progress notes in the clinical record. The attending physician also arranges for the physician care of his or her residents when not available for an emergency or when he or she expects to be absent. The physicians enters on the face sheet of the clinical record the name, address and telephone number of the physician to be called.

Consultation with another qualified physician is required when the diagnosis is obscure or when there is doubt on the most appropriate therapeutic measures. A satisfactory consultation includes examination of the resident and record, and a written opinion entered in the record and signed by the consultant.

The nurse makes rounds daily—or more often if needed—and enters appropriate notes in the nurses' notes or the resident's records. She or he receives the resident's total care program at appropriate intervals and reports to the physician.

The nurse also supervises all resident care personnel, makes work schedules and interviews new personnel with the cooperation of the administrator.

### Emergency

The skilled care facility provides that one or more physicians furnish necessary medical care in case of emergency if the physician responsible for the care of the resident is not immediately available. A schedule listing the names and telephone numbers of these physicians and the specific days each is on call is posted in each nursing station. Procedures have been established to be followed in an emergency that address immediate care of the resident, persons to be notified and reports to be prepared. General procedures are:

1. Examine the resident thoroughly.
2. Treat in this order immediately:
   a. Serious bleeding,
   b. Stoppage of breath,
   c. Poisoning, and
   d. Shock.
3. Send for help. Get a doctor. Alert the hospital, if necessary.
4. Give nothing to eat or drink to an unconscious person or person with internal injuries.
5. Make the resident comfortable. Don't let him or her see the injury. Be calm, cheerful. Keep onlookers away.
6. Move the resident only when absolutely necessary.
7. Notify nearest kin or other designated persons immediately.

In the event the attending physician's plan for emergency care fails to produce the necessary physician's service, the administrator or the nurse on duty will call a member of the emergency-call physicians in accordance with the schedule. The physician responding to an emergency call will make and sign an appropriate entry in the resident's clinical record. The physician will communicate any findings and any necessary changes in treatment to the attending physician. The emergency physician's name and the resident's name are recorded in the nursing notes. The nurse will report to the attending physician as soon as he or she is available.

### Communicable Disease

Residents who have a communicable disease, including tuberculosis, may not be admitted. The admitting physician shall certify the absence of such conditions at the time of admission.

When a physician discovers the presence of a communicable disease subsequent to admission, he or she must notify the administrator immediately. The physician must assist in making necessary arrangements to protect the health of the other residents by isolation with attendant safeguards or by transfer to a hospital. The nurse shall report the occurrences of infections, communicable diseases and food poisoning to the attending physician.

Provision should be made for isolating infectious residents and well-ventilated single rooms with separate toilet and bathing facilities. Such facilities also are available for the special care of residents who develop acute illnesses while in the facility and for residents who are in terminal phases of illness.

The attending physician is responsible for reporting to the appropriate health authorities the occurrence of infections, communicable diseases and food poisoning in accordance with the state and local public health requirements.

## Critically Ill

In case of serious illness or accident, medical care should be secured at once and the nearest kin or other designated person should be notified immediately. In case of death, both the physician and next of kin or other designated person should be notified promptly. Procedures to be followed in regard to serious illness are:

1. Check temperature, pulse and respiration, and blood pressure. Note resident's color, responses and any unusual symptoms that should be reported to the doctor when he or she is called.
2. Use oxygen as necessary.
3. Keep the resident warm and comfortable until the doctor arrives.

## Mentally Disturbed

The facility requires that the health care of every resident is under the supervision of a physician. In case of mental disturbance, the procedure is as follows:

1. Use humane restraints.
2. Call physician for orders.
3. Isolate the resident with those staff members most capable of understanding.
4. Arrange transfer to an institution equipped to care for this type of resident.

## Incident/Accident Reports

Questionable occurrences and any damaged or faulty equipment are reported to the administrator by the nurse.

## Medical Records

Medical records are the property of the facility and shall not be removed without the permission of the administrator. Generally, the information in the medical record is the private property of the individual; the medical record (sheets of paper) itself is the property of the nursing facility. Release of information requires the permission of the resident. All professional personnel providing care directly to the resident have access to his or her medical record. Access to medical records is afforded to staff physicians in good standing for bona fide study and research, consistent with preserving confidentiality of the residents' personal information.

## Supplies

Provision of resident care supplies and their ordering in cooperation with the administrator is the responsibility of the charge nurse.

## Resident Activities

Activities suited to the needs and interests of residents are provided as an important adjunct to the active treatment program and to encourage restoration to self-care and resumption of normal activities. The following policies are instituted toward these ends:

1. The individual in charge of resident activities has experience and/or training in directing group ac-

tivity, or has available consultation from a qualified recreational therapist or group activity leader.

2. The activity leader uses community social and recreational opportunities to the fullest possible extent.

3. Residents are encouraged but not forced to participate in such activities. Suitable activities are provided for those residents who are unable to leave their rooms. The facility makes available a variety of supplies and equipment adequate to satisfy the individual interests of residents such as books and magazines, daily newspapers, games, stationery, radio and television, and so on.

4. The resident's requests to see clergy are honored, and space is provided for privacy during visits. Those who are able and wish to are assisted to attend religious services.

5. Visiting hours are flexible and posted to permit and encourage visiting by friends and relatives.

## Discharge

When the attending physician deems that the resident's physical or mental needs can be met in the individual's own home or in a boarding type home, the physician will recommend discharge in accordance with a plan for care. Residents are discharged only on the written order of the attending physician. At the time of discharge, the attending physician completes the physician's part of the clinical record, states the final diagnosis and prognosis and signs the record. When the attending physician has discharged a resident, the nurse will report to the administrator. It is the nurse's responsibility to see that the resident's record is completed upon discharge.

## Resident Assessment
### 42 CFR, Sec. 483.20, Ch. IV (10-1-98)

The CFR requires that the following requirements relating to the medical care of residents be complied with.

The facility must conduct initially and periodically a comprehensive, accurate, standardized, reproducible assessment of each resident's functional capacity.

### Admission Orders

At the time each resident is admitted, the facility must have physician orders for the resident's immediate care.

### Comprehensive Assessments

The facility must make a comprehensive assessment of a resident's needs, using the resident assessment instrument (RAI) specified by the state.

The assessment must include the following as minimum:

1. Identification and demographic information.
2. Customer routine.
3. Cognitive patterns.
4. Communication.
5. Vision.
6. Mood and behavior patterns.
7. Psychosocial well-being.
8. Physical functioning and structural problems.
9. Continence.
10. Disease diagnoses and health conditions.
11. Dental and nutritional status.
12. Skin condition.
13. Activity pursuit.
14. Medications.
15. Special treatments and procedures.
16. Discharge potential.
17. Documentation of summary information regarding the additional assessment performed through the resident assessment protocols.
18. Documentation of participation in assessment.

The assessment process must include direct observation and communication with the resident, and licensed and nonlicensed direct care staff members on all shifts.

- **When Required**—The facility must conduct a comprehensive assessment of a resident as follows:
  1. Within 14 calendar days after admission, excluding readmissions in which there is no significant change in the resident's physical or mental condition. Readmission is defined as a return to the facility after a temporary absence for hospitalization or for therapeutic leave.
  2. Within 14 calendar days after the facility determines (or should have determined) that there has been a significant change in the resident's physical or mental condition. A significant change means a major decline or improvement in the resident's status that will not normally resolve itself without further intervention by the

staff or by implementing disease-related clinical interventions, that has an impact on more than one area of the resident's health status, and that requires interdisciplinary review and/or revision of the care plan.

3. Not less than once every 12 months.

- **Quarterly Review Assessment**—The facility must assess a resident using the quarterly review instrument specified by the state and approved by the Health Care Financing Administration (HCFA) not less frequently than once every 3 months.

- **Use**—The facility must maintain all resident assessments completed within the previous 15 months in the resident's active record, and use the results of the assessment to develop, review and revise the resident's comprehensive plan of care.

- **Coordination**—The facility must coordinate assessments with the preadmission screening and resident review program under Medicaid to the maximum extent practicable to avoid duplicative testing and effort.

- **Automated Data Processing Requirements**
  1. *Encoding Data*—Within seven days after the facility completes a resident's assessment, it must encode the following information for each resident in the facility:
     a. Admission assessment
     b. Annual assessment updates
     c. Significant change in status assessments
     d. Quarterly review assessment
     e. A subset of items upon a resident's transfer, re-entry, discharge and death
     f. Background (face sheet) information if there is no admission assessment.
  2. *Transmitting Data*—Within seven days after the facility completes a resident's assessment, the facility must be capable of transmitting to the state information for each resident contained in the minimum data set (MDS) in a format that conforms to standard record layouts and data dictionaries, and that passes standardized edits defined by HCFA and the state.
  3. *Monthly Transmittal Requirements*—The facility must electronically transmit, at least monthly, encoded, accurate, complete MDS data to the state for all assessments conducted during the previous month, including the following:
     a. Admission assessment
     b. Annual assessment
     c. Significant change in status assessment
     d. Significant correction of prior full assessment
     e. Significant correction of prior quarterly assessment
     f. Quarterly review
     g. A subset of items upon a resident transfer, re-entry, discharge and death
     h. Background (face sheet) information, for an initial transmission of MDS data on a resident who does not have been admission assessment.
  4. *Data Format*—The facility must transmit data in the format specified by HCFA or, for a state that has alternate RAI approved by HCFA, in the format specified by the state and approved by HCFA.
  5. *Resident-Identifiable Information*
     a. A facility may not release information that could identify residents to the public.
     b. The facility may release information that is resident-identifiable to an agent only in accordance with a contract under which the agent agrees not to use or disclose the information except to the extent the facility itself is permitted to do so.

- **Accuracy of Assessments**—The assessment must accurately reflect the resident's status.

- **Coordination**—A registered nurse must conduct or coordinate each assessment with the appropriate participation of health professionals.

- **Certification**
  1. A registered nurse must sign and certify that the assessment is completed.
  2. Each individual who completes a portion of the assessment must sign and certify the accuracy of that portion of the assessment.

- **Penalty for Falsification**
  1. Using Medicare and Medicaid, an individual who willfully and knowingly
     a. Certifies a material and false statement in a resident assessment is subject to a civil money penalty of not more than $1,000 for each assessment, or
     b. Causes another individual to certify a material and false statement in a resident assess-

ment is subject to a civil money penalty of not more than $5,000 for each assessment.
2. Clinical disagreement does not constitute a material and false statement.

### Comprehensive Care Plans

The facility must develop a comprehensive care plan for each resident that includes measurable objectives and timetables to meet a resident's medical, nursing and psychosocial needs that are identified in the comprehensive assessment. The care plan must deal with the relationship of items or services ordered to be provided (or withheld) to the facility's responsibility for fulfilling other requirements in these regulations.

A comprehensive care plan must be:

1. Developed within 7 days after completion of the comprehensive assessment.
2. Prepared by an interdisciplinary team that includes the attending physician, a registered nurse with the responsibility for the resident and other appropriate staff in disciplines as determined by the resident's needs. Also needed are the participation of a resident, the resident's family or legal representative to the extent practicable.
3. Periodically reviewed and revised by a team of qualified persons after each assessment.

The services provided or arranged by the facility must:

1. Meet professional standards of quality.
2. Be provided by qualified persons in accordance with each resident's written plan of care.

### Discharge Summary

When the facility anticipates discharge, a resident must have a discharge summary that includes:

1. A recapitulation of the resident's stay.
2. A final summary of the resident's status to include the items in the comprehensive assessment at the time of discharge. It is available for release to authorized persons and agencies with the consent of the resident or legal representative.
3. A post-discharge plan of care that is developed with the participation of the resident and his or her family that will assist the resident to adjust to his or her new living environment.

### Quality of Care
### 42 CFR, Sec. 483.25. Ch. IV (10-1-98)

Each resident must receive and the facility must provide the necessary care and services to attain or maintain the highest practicable physical, mental and psychosocial well-being in accordance with the comprehensive assessment and plan of care.

### Activities of Daily Living

Based on the comprehensive assessment of a resident, the facility must ensure that:

1. A resident's abilities in ADLs do not diminish unless circumstances of the individual's clinical condition demonstrates that diminution was unavoidable. This includes the resident's ability to:
   • Bathe, dress and groom.
   • Transfer and ambulate.
   • Toilet.
   • Eat.
   • Use speech, language or other functional communications systems.
2. A resident is given the appropriate treatment and services to maintain or improve his or her abilities.
3. A resident who is unable to carry out ADLs receives the necessary services to maintain good nutrition, grooming and personal and oral hygiene.

### Vision and Hearing

To ensure that residents receive proper treatment and assisted devices to maintain vision and hearing abilities, the facility must, if necessary, assist the resident:

1. In making appointments.
2. By arranging for transportation to and from the office of a medical practitioner specializing in the treatment of vision or hearing impairment or the office of a professional specializing in the provision of vision or hearing devices.

## Pressure Sores

Based on the comprehensive assessment of a resident, the facility must ensure that:

1. A resident who enters the facility without pressure sores does not develop pressure sores until the individual's clinical condition demonstrates that they were unavoidable.
2. A resident having pressure sores receives necessary treatment and services to promote healing, prevent infections and prevent new sores from developing.

## Urinary Incontinence

Based on the resident's comprehensive assessment, the facility must ensure that:

1. A resident who enters the facility without an indwelling catheter is not catheterized unless the resident's clinical condition demonstrates that catheterization was necessary.
2. A resident who is incontinent of the bladder receives appropriate treatment and services to prevent urinary tract infections and to restore as much normal bladder function as possible.

## Range of Motion

Based on the comprehensive assessment of a resident, the facility must ensure that:

1. A resident who enters the facility without a limited range of motion does not experience reduction in range of motion unless the resident's clinical condition demonstrates that a reduction in range of motion is unavoidable.
2. A resident with a limited range of motion receives appropriate treatment and services to increase range of motion to prevent further decrease in range of motion.

## Mental and Psychosocial Functioning

Based on the comprehensive assessment of a resident, the facility must ensure that:

1. A resident who displays mental or psychosocial adjustment difficulty receives appropriate treatment and services to correct the assessed problem.

2. A resident whose assessment did not reveal a mental or psychosocial adjustment difficulty does not display a pattern of decreased social interaction and/or increased withdrawn, angry or depressive behaviors unless the resident's clinical condition demonstrates that such a pattern was unavoidable.

## Nasogastric Tubes

Based on the comprehensive assessment of a resident, the facility must ensure that:

1. A resident who has been able to eat enough alone or with assistance is not fed by nasogastric tube unless the resident's clinical condition demonstrates that use of a nasogastric tube was unavoidable.
2. A resident who is fed by a nasogastric tube or gastrostomy tube receives the appropriate treatment and services to prevent aspiration pneumonia, diarrhea, vomiting, dehydration, metabolic abnormalities and nasopharyngeal ulcers and to restore, if possible, normal feeding skill.

## Accidents

The facility must ensure that:

1. The resident environment remains as free of accident hazards as is possible.
2. Each resident receives adequate supervision and assistive devices to prevent accidents.

## Nutrition

Based on a resident's comprehensive assessment, the facility must ensure that a resident:

1. Maintains acceptable parameters of nutritional status, such as body weight and protein levels, unless the resident's clinical condition demonstrates that this is not possible.
2. Is provided a therapeutic diet when there is a nutritional problem.

## Hydration

The facility must provide each resident with sufficient fluid intake to maintain proper hydration and health.

### Special Needs

The facility must ensure that residents receive proper treatment and care for the following special services:

1. Injections.
2. Parenteral and enteral fluids.
3. Colostomy, ureterostomy or ileostomy care.
4. Tracheostomy care.
5. Tracheal suctioning.
6. Respiratory care.
7. Foot care.
8. Prosthesis.

### Drug Therapy

- **Unnecessary drugs**—Each resident's drug regimen must be free from unnecessary drugs. An unnecessary drug is any drug when used:
  1. In an excessive dose (including drug therapy).
  2. For excessive duration.
  3. Without adequate monitoring.
  4. Without adequate indications for its use.
  5. In the presence of adverse consequences that indicate the dose should be reduced or discontinued.
  6. Any combination of the reasons above.
- **Antipsychotic drugs**—Based on a comprehensive assessment of a resident, the facility must ensure that:
  1. Residents who have not used antipsychotic drugs are not given these drugs unless therapy is necessary to treat a specific condition as diagnosed and documented in the clinical record.
  2. Residents who used antipsychotic drugs receive gradual dose reductions, drug holidays or behavioral interventions unless clinically contradicted in an effort to discontinue these drugs.

### Medication Errors

The facility must ensure that:

1. It is free of medication error of 5% or greater rates.
2. Resident or free of any significant medication errors.

### Medical Director
#### 42 CFR, Sec. 483.75(h2i), Ch. IV (10-1-98)

The facility must designate a physician to serve as medical director.

The medical director is responsible for:

1. Implementation of resident care policies.
2. The coordination of medical care in the facility.

### Physician Services
#### 42 CFR, Sec. 483.40, Ch. IV (10-1-98)

A physician must personally approve in writing a recommendation that an individual be admitted to a facility. Each resident must remain under the care of a physician.

### Physician Supervision

The facility must ensure that:

1. The medical care of each resident is supervised by a physician.
2. Another physician supervises the medical care of residents when their attending physician is unavailable.

### Physician Visits

The physician must:

1. Review the resident's total program of care including medications and treatments at each visit. (See the following text.)
2. Write, sign and date progress notes at each visit.
3. Sign and date all orders.

### Frequency of Physician Visits

1. The resident must be seen by a physician at least once every 30 days for the first 90 days after admission and at least once every 60 days thereafter.
2. A physician visit is considered timely if it occurs not later than 10 days after the date the visit was required.
3. All required physician visits must be made by the physician personally except as indicated in the following text.
4. At the option of the physician, required visits in skilled nursing facilities (SNFs) after the initial visit may alternate between personal visits by the

physician and visits by a physician assistant, nurse practitioner or clinical nurse specialist.

### Availability of Physicians for Emergency Care

The facility must provide or arrange for the provision of physician services 24 hours a day in case of an emergency.

### Physician Delegation of Tasks in SNFs

Except as indicated below, a physician may delegate tasks to a physician assistant, nurse practitioner or clinical nurse specialist who:

1. Meets the applicable definition:
   a. **Physician Assistant**—Meets state requirements regarding qualifications for assistance to primary care physicians.
   b. **Nurse Practitioner**—A licensed registered nurse meeting state requirements.
   c. **Clinical Nurse Specialist**—Licensed as such by the state.
2. Is acting within the scope of practice as defined by state law.
3. Is under the supervision of the physician.

A physician may not delegate a task when the regulations specify that the physician must perform it personally or when the delegation is prohibited under state law or by the facility's own policy.

### Performance of Physician's Tasks in NFs

At the option of the state, any required physician tasks in a nursing facility (NF) (including tasks that the regulations specify must be performed personally by the physician) also may be satisfied when performed by a nurse practitioner, clinical nurse specialist or physician assistant who is not an employee of the facility but who is working in collaboration with a physician.

## Dental Services
### 42 CFR, Sec. 483.55, Ch. IV (10-1-98)

The facility must assist residents in obtaining routine and 24-hour emergency dental care.

### Skilled Nursing Facilities

1. Must provide or obtain from an outside resource, routine and emergency dental services to meet the needs of each resident.
2. May charge a Medicare resident an additional amount for routine and emergency dental services.
3. Must, if necessary, assist the resident:
   a. In making appointments.
   b. By arranging for transportation to and from the dentist's office.
4. Must promptly refer residents with lost or damaged dentures to a dentist.

### Nursing Facilities

1. Must provide or obtain from an outside resource, the following dental services to meet the needs of each resident:
   a. Routine dental services to the extent covered under the state plan.
   b. Emergency dental services.
2. Must, if necessary, assist the resident:
   a. In making appointments.
   b. By arranging for transportation to and from the dentist's office.
3. Must promptly refer residents with lost or damaged dentures to a dentist.

## Laboratory Services
### 42 CFR, Sec. 483.75(j), Ch. IV (10-1-98)

The facility must provide or obtain clinical laboratory services to meet the needs of its residents. The facility is responsible for the quality and timeliness of the services.

1. If the facility provides its own laboratory services, the services must meet the applicable conditions for coverage of the services furnished by independent laboratories meeting state and local specifications.
2. If the facility provides blood bank and transfusion services, it must meet the applicable conditions for:
   a. Independent laboratories meeting state and local specifications, and

b. Hospitals with facilities for procurement, safe-keeping and transference of blood and blood products that are provided or readily available.

3. If the laboratory chooses to refer specimens for testing to another laboratory, the referral laboratory must be approved or licensed to test specimens in the appropriate specialties and/or subspecialties of service.

4. If the facility does not provide laboratory services on site, if must have an agreement to obtain the services only from a laboratory that is approved for participation in the Medicare program either as a hospital or as an independent laboratory, or from a physician's office.

The facility must:

1. Provide or obtain laboratory services only when ordered by the attending physicians.

2. Promptly notify the attending physician of the findings.

3. Assist the resident in making transportation arrangements to and from the source of service, if the resident needs assistance.

4. File in the resident's clinical record, laboratory reports that are dated and contain the name and address of the testing laboratory.

### Radiology and Other Diagnostic Services
### 42 CFR, Sec. 473.75(k), Ch. IV (10-1-98)

The facility must provide or obtain radiology and other diagnostic services to meet the needs of its residents. The facility is responsible for the quality and timeliness of the services.

1. If the facility provides its own diagnostic services, the services must meet the applicable conditions of participation for hospitals maintaining diagnostic radiological services.

2. If the facility does not provide diagnostic services, it must have an agreement to obtain the services from a provider or supplier that is approved to provide these services under Medicare.

The facility must:

1. Provide or obtain radiology and other diagnostic services only when ordered by the attending physician.

2. Promptly notify the attending physician of the findings.

3. Assist the resident in making transportation arrangements to and from the source of service, if the resident needs assistance.

4. File in the resident's clinical record, signed and dated reports of X-ray and other diagnostic services.

## QUALITY ASSESSMENT AND ASSURANCE

The CFR requires that resident care be audited for effectiveness. A monitoring or auditing program identifies issues, implements any needed changes and provides follow-up to determine effectiveness of such changes. To prevent problems and address others more efficiently before they become apparent, the facility must establish an audit system to continuously monitor the provision of services to the residents in accordance with its mission statement. Elements of such a system need to be outcome-oriented and include criteria for measuring department achievement in accordance with relative standards and policy, methods of ongoing review with triggers for immediate correction where safety is concerned, problem solving and corrective action, and communication of audit results to staff who can take steps to solve the problems and influence future results.

The mechanism for determining program success is the MDS, which provides a guideline for monitoring resident progress. Goals, criteria for measuring progress, treatment strategies by single disciplines of all staff, and changes related to normal aging and/or unavoidable disease process are all taken into account. A good way to determine if a resident is progressing is to observe changes in his or her functional levels as documented in the care plan. Items in the updated comprehensive assessment compared to objectives in the initial assessment indicate any changes in the resident's condition and functioning. Barbara Wisnom, in her paper "Quality Assurance: Is Your Practice Effective?" recommends the following when setting up and operating a system of examining activities:

1. Set up standards and criteria. Develop policies and procedures by which achievement can be monitored.

2. Monitoring and evaluation. Plan a system of on-going review and choose a method of selecting a representative sample of cases to be examined.
3. Problem identification. Set the system to make immediate correction of deficiencies affecting safety.
4. Corrective action. Take corrective action.
5. Follow-up. Assess results and share positive findings with the staff workers.

Measuring progress by use of the comprehensive assessment is accomplished by an interdisciplinary team composed of the following people:

1. Physician—a medical doctor or a psychiatrist. He or she is able to prescribe.
2. Physical therapist—deals with disorders of motion as a result of a disabling disease such as stroke.
3. Occupational therapist—aids in the recovery of skills. (The difference between the physical therapist and the occupational therapist is that the occupational therapist deals more with retraining in the activities of daily living and the physical therapist deals with ambulation.)
4. Social worker—evaluates the socio-behavioral response of the resident to disability, how the residents adapt and motivational factors.
5. Speech pathologist—evaluates and tests communication disorders. He or she may provide therapy for speech or swallowing disorders.
6. Audiologist—tests hearing, prescribes hearing aids and teaches the resident how to use them.
7. Dietitian/nutritionist—sees that nutritional needs are met according to the physician's orders.

The facility must have a comprehensive permanent quality assessment and assurance committee as a part of operations. This committee is familiar with available resources (i.e., outpatient or other independent specialized services) in the community and monitors the quality of facility service in areas such as utilization review, infections control, and safety and pharmacy. Additionally, there should be an audit committee looking at falls, pressure sores and other incidents occurring in the facility. The CFR states that the quality assessment and assurance committee must meet at least quarterly to determine what quality assurance activities are needed and to prepare a plan of corrections for deficiencies. The committee must consist of the director of nursing

services, a physician designated by the facility and three other staff workers.

When a surveyor inspects a nursing facility, he or she may talk directly to the residents and their families, along with checking for proper compliance. The findings of the quality assessment and assurance committee are not subject to the review of state inspection survey team scrutiny. The survey team may review these records only as necessary to prove compliance with the requirements that a quality assessment program and committee exist.

The administrator must be aware of the findings and actions of the quality assessment and assurance committee and of any consultant reports. The department heads and administrator work together to pinpoint related problems and work out solutions. Rounds by personnel who are familiar with state and federal requirements (including nursing, maintenance or administrative) will help spot problems in areas of resident care, physical environment and resident rights. Hiring of an independent presurvey team can provide the governing body and administrator with an overview of each department pointing out any problems and with recommendations for corrections, relevant policy and procedure, and staffing.

**Quality Assessment and Assurance**
**42 CFR, Sec. 483.75(o), Ch. IV (10-1-98)**

For the facility to participate in Medicare and/or Medicaid, the following conditions relating to the quality assessment and assurance committee must be met.

A facility must maintain a quality assessment and assurance committee consisting of:

1. The director of nursing services.
2. A physician designated by the facility.
3. At least three other members of the facility's staff.

The quality assessment and assurance committee:

1. Meets at least quarterly to identify issues with respect to which quality assessment and assurance activities are necessary.
2. Develops and implements appropriate plans of action to correct identified quality deficiencies.

A state or the Department of Health and Human Services (HHS) secretary may not require disclosure of the records of such committee, except when such disclosure is related to the compliance of such committee with these requirements. Good faith attempts by the committee to identify and correct quality deficiencies will not be used as a basis for sanctions.

## Terms and Concepts

**Excess Disability**—An avoidable dysfunction. Examples are extra confusion of residents because they need hearing aids or proper glasses or they incur clinical depression. Excess disability may be associated with:

- **Learned Helplessness**—The behavior of individuals who believe that nothing they do will affect what happens to them. This often occurs in an institutional setting where there are few choices and little control.

- **Institutional Totality**—Standardization and "bulking together" residents for the purpose of watching and controlling them by a relatively small staff. This often entails loss of privacy, autonomy and individuality which can lead to passivity, dependence and regression.

**Medication Error**—The difference between what the physician prescribes and what is given to a resident.

**Minimum Data Set**—A form (RAI) used by the team for the comprehensive assessment. It serves as the basis for the comprehensive care plan. A registered nurse certifies the MDS and each of the other health professionals signs his or her part of the document. Triggers indicate that further investigation is needed and Resident Assessment Protocols (RAPs) are guidelines for studying and treating the problem; these forms are used in conjunction with the MDS.

**Nursing Facility**—Replaces the terms skilled nursing facility and intermediate care facility (ICF) to indicate that both are held to the same standards of care under Medicaid.

**Ombudsman**—Investigates and attempts to resolve complaints made by residents and their families. Each state must set up an office of ombudsman under the Older Americans Act of 1965.

**Physician Extenders**—Nurse practitioners, clinical nurse specialists and physician assistants.

**Preadmission Screening and Annual Resident Review** (PASARR)—Designed to ensure appropriate placement of persons with mental retardation or serious mental illness. To be admitted, these persons must require the kind of care offered by the nursing facility.

**Perspective Payment System** (PPS)—A payment using diagnosis-related groups, based on the kind of illness regardless of the cost or the length of time required to care for a particular resident.

**Resident Care System** (RCS)—Includes MDS, assessment and care plans, resident flowcharts and psychotropic and physical restraint information.

**Significant Medication Error**—An error that causes a resident extreme discomfort or jeopardizes his or her health or safety. A facility may incur a sanction for any significant medication error or for more than 5% medication errors overall.

## BIBIOGRAPHY

Code of Federal Regulations, Title 42, Parts 430 to end, 10-1-98.

Davis, W. 1994. *Introduction to health care administration*. Bossier City, LA: Professional Printing & Publishing.

Department of Health and Human Services, Health Care Financing Administration. 1995. *Interpretive Guidelines: State Operations Manual #250*. Baltimore, MD.

Haffenreffer, D.P., and M.F. Gold. 1991. Introduction to health care administration. *Provider*.

National Association of Boards of Examiners for Nursing Home Administrators. 1997. *NAB study guide*, 3rd ed. Washington, DC.

Peppen, H. 1982. *Fundamentals of care of the aging, disabled and handicapped*. New York: Charles C Thomas Publisher.

*Taber's cyclopedic medical dictionary*. 1993. 17th ed. A.F. Davis Co.

Wisnom, B. 1989. Quality assurance: is your practice effective? In: *Rehabilitation Nursing: Process and Application*, ed. S. Dittmar. St. Louis, MO: C.V. Mosby.

# Appendix 7–A

## Glossary of General Medical Terminology

**Activities of Daily Living (ADLs)**—Dressing, washing and eating.

**AIDS**—Acquired immune deficiency syndrome.

**Abrasion**—Injury that rubs off the surface skin.

**Acute**—Sharp, severe, having a rapid onset.

**Airborne Infection**—Transfer of infection by droplets of moisture containing the causative agent without direct contact between individuals.

**Alcoholism**—Morbid results of excessive or prolonged use of alcohol.

**Alopecia**—Loss of hair from skin.

**Ambulatory**—Walking or able to walk, not confined to bed.

**Amputation**—Removal of a limb generally by surgery.

**Angina Pectoris**—Pain in the chest.

**Anorexia**—Absence of appetite.

**Anuria**—Suppression of urine.

**Aphagia**—Inability to swallow.

**Aphasia**—Loss or impairment of capacity to use words as symbols of ideas.

**Aponea**—Temporary suspension of respiration or breathing.

**Arteriosclerosis**—Thickening and hardening of the arteries.

**Arthritis**—Acute joint inflammation.

**Asepsis**—Exclusion of micro-organisms producing decay.

**Aseptic Technique**—Protection against infection by the use of sterile technique.

**Aspirate**—To remove material from a body cavity.

**Ataxia**—Failure or irregularity of muscle coordination.

**Atherosclerosis**—A type of arterosclerosis that causes deposits of fat or plaque to form on the inner walls of the arteries.

**Atrophy**—Reduction in size of an organ or cell. Degeneration.

**Autopsy**—Postmortem examination of the body.

**Bedridden**—Permanently confined to bed.

**Benign**—Not endangering health or life, not malignant.

**Blood Pressure**—The pressure exerted by blood within the arteries.

**Botulism**—Food poisoning due to toxins.

**Bypass**—Surgical procedure to divert the flow of blood from normal anatomic courses.

**Carcinoma**—A malignant neoplasm.

**Cardiology**—Study of function, structure and diseases of the heart and blood vessels.

**Cataract**—Partial or complete opacity of the lens of the eye or its capsule.

**Cephalalgia**—Headache.

**Cerebrovascular Accident (CVA)**—Stroke.

**Chemotherapy**—Prevention or treatment of infective disease by chemicals.

**Chronic**—Long continued, of long duration, recurring frequently.

**Circulatory System**—Includes the heart, blood vessels and circulation of the blood throughout the body.

**Colostomy**—Formation of an artificial anus in the anterior abdominal wall.

**Coma**—State of unconsciousness caused by disease, injury or poison.

**Comatose**—In a condition of coma.

**Communicable**—Transmissable from one person to another.

**Congenital**—Existing at birth.

**Congestive Heart Failure (CHF)**—Condition where the heart is unable to maintain adequate circulation of blood.

**Constipation**—A decrease in the frequency of bowel movements.

**Contagious**—Transmission from one person to another.

**Contracture**—Progressive stiffening in the muscles, tendons and ligaments surrounding the joints.

**Contusion**—A bruise, an injury.

**Convalescent**—The time spent in recovery.

**Coronary Thrombosis**—Clot in a blood vessel.

**Cyanosis**—A bluish tinge in the color of mucous membranes and skin due to oxygen reduction.

**Cystitis**—Inflammation of the urinary bladder.

**Debilitated**—A person who is infirm and weak.

**Debridement**—Removal of foreign material or dead/damaged tissue from a wound.

**Decubation**—Period of recovery from an infectious disease.

**Decubitus Ulcer**—Bedsore.

**Degenerative**—Cells undergoing deterioration.

**Dehydrated**—Removal of water from body.

**Diabetes**—Metabolic disturbance.

**Diagnosis**—The act/art of determining the nature of a disease.

**Dialysis**—Separation of substances from one another in solution.

**Diarrhea**—Loose or watery stools and increase in bowel movements to usually more than two a day.

**Diverticulitis**—Inflammation of the diverticulum (pouch springing from a hollow organ such as intestine or bladder).

**Drug Interaction**—Two or more drugs taken at the same time which may produce an unwanted effect.

**Edema**—Excessive accumulation of fluid in the tissue spaces.

**Elderly**—Generally referring to individuals over age 65.

**Embolism**—Occlusion (shutting) of a artery by a blood clot.

**Emesis**—Vomiting

**End-Stage Renal Disease (ESRD)**—Failure of kidneys to perform essential functions.

**Endemic**—Disease confined to a certain region.

**Epidemiology**—Study of the prevalence of disease.

**Epilepsy**—Disorder of the central nervous system

**Etiology**—Science or study of the cause of diseases.

**Equilibrium**—State of balance.

**Forensic Medicine**—Application of medical knowledge to questions of law.

**Functionally Dependent Elderly**—Individuals in whom illnesses, disabilities or social problems have reduced their ability to perform self-care and household tasks.

**Gangrene**—Death of part of the body due to a failure of the blood supply.

**Geriatrics**—Branch of medical science that is concerned with the diseases and problems of old age and aging people.

**Germicide**—An agent that destroys germs.

**Geroderma**—Appearance of senility brought about by premature loss of hair, wrinkling of the skin, and general atrophy.

**Gerodontics**—Branch of dentistry dealing with dental problems of the aged.

**Gerontology**—Study of the aging process, including clinical, biological, psychosocial and historical aspects of aging.

**Glaucoma**—Eye disease marked by heightened intraocular tension.

**Gout**—An inherited condition which usually develops in men between the ages of 40 and 60. It results from an excess of uric acid in the blood causing severe inflammation.

**Heart Attack**—Damage to the heart muscle due to insufficient blood supply.

**Hematoma**—Blood that clots to form a solid mass, tumorlike swelling.

**Hemiparesis**—Loss of muscular pain on one side of the body.

**Hemiplegia**—Paralysis of one side of the body.

**Hemophilia**—Prolonged coagulation time and abnormal bleeding.

**Hemorrhage**—An escape of blood from the vessels by flow through ruptured walls.

**Hepatitis**—Inflammation of the liver.

**Hereditary**—Congenital.

**Herpes**—Acute inflammation of the skin or mucous membrane.

**High Blood Pressure (HBP)**—Hypertension usually of unknown etiology

**Hydrotherapy**—Treatment involving various forms of water.

**Hypertension**—High blood pressure.

**Hypertrophy**—Increase in the size of an organ independent of natural growth.

**Immunity**—The state of being resistant or not susceptible to a disease.

**Incipient**—Just beginning to exist or appear.

**Incontinent**—Inability to control natural evacuations (feces, urine).

**Infection**—An illness caused by an organism such as virus, bacteria or fungus.

**Inflammation**—Reaction of tissues to injury.

**Intravenous Injection**—Administered within the vein.

**Jaundice**—Yellowness of the skin, mucous membranes and secretions.

**Laceration**—A tear, the act of tearing.

**Laryngology**—Field of medicine for treatment of diseases of the larynx.

**Long-Term Care**—Medical and social care given to those with severe chronic impairments.

**Lymphosarcoma**—A malignant tumor of lymphatic tissue.

**Malaise**—General feeling of illness sometimes accompanied by restlessness and discomfort.

**Malignant**—Virulent, threatening life (i.e., malignant tumors).

**Malnutrition**—Imperfect nutrition.

**Metastasis**—The transfer of disease from a primary focus to a secondary site by conveyance of causal agents or cells.

**Modality**—A method of therapy.

**Monoplegic**—Paralysis of one limb.

**Morbidity**—The quality of disease or being diseased. The ratio of the number of sick individuals to the total population.

**Mortality**—The death rate.

**Multiple Sclerosis**—Progressive disease characterized by disorder of nerve fibers of heart and spinal cord.

**Nausea**—Feeling of discomfort in the region of the stomach.

**Nephritis**—Inflammation of the kidney.

**Nonambulatory**—Bedridden.

**Nutrition**—Pertaining to the body's need for food.

**Obese**—Extremely fat, corpulent.

**Occupational Therapy**—The use of purposeful activity to those who are limited by physical injury or illness.

**Osteoporosis**—A condition resulting in decreased bone mass.

**Palliative**—Relieving or alleviating suffering.

**Paraplegia**—Paralysis of the lower limbs.

**Pathogenic**—Pertaining to the capacity to produce disease.

**Pathological**—Changes in the cells, the basis of disease.

**pH**—Scale representing the relative acidity of a solution. Alkaline is pH7 or above; under pH7 is acidic.

**Phlebitis**—Inflammation of a vein.

**Physical Therapy**—The treatment of disorders with physical agents and methods such as massage and therapeutic exercise.

**Physician's Desk Reference (PDR)**—Reference for medications and their effects.

**Physiology**—Science of active body functions.

**Pituitary**—Master gland influencing other glands.

**Placebo**—Substance substituted for a medication.

**Pneumonia**—An acute inflammation of the lungs usually created by inhaled pneumococci or other bacteria, virus or fungi.

**Prognosis**—Prediction of the duration, course and termination of a disease.

**Prone**—Lying with face downward.

**Ptomaine**—An amino compound resulting from the decomposition of proteins or dead animal matter by microorganisms.

**Quadriplegia**—Paralysis affecting the four extremities.

**Rehabilitation Therapy**—The restoration of an individual or a part of the body to normal or near normal function after a disabling disease or injury.

**Rheumatism**—Refers to a disease of the joints, muscles, bones and includes most forms of arthritis.

**Rheumatoid Arthritis**—A chronic, destructive, collagen disease characterized by inflammation of the synovium.

**Salmonella**—Pathogenic species of bacteria causing gastrointestinal symptoms.

**Sarcoma**—A malignant neoplasm derived from connective tissue, muscle or bone. Usually named after the tissue of origin, i.e., fibrosarcoma (connective tissue) or osteosarcoma (bone).

**Shingles**—Form of herpes.

**Spasm**—Sudden muscular contraction.

**Spasmodic**—Pertaining to or characterized by a spasm.

**Subcutaneous**—Beneath the skin, hypodermic.

**Supine**—Lying on the back, face upward.

**Syndrome**—A group of signs and symptoms that collectively characterize or indicate a particular disease or abnormal condition.

**Symptoms**—Phenomena of disease leading to complaints on the part of the patient.

**Thorax**—The chest.

**Toxin**—Poison.

**Trauma**—A wound or injury.

**Triplegic**—Paralysis of three extremities.

**Tumor**—A swelling, new growth of cells or tissue.

**Ulcers**—An open sore or lesion of the skin or mucous membrane accompanied by casting off of the inflamed necrotic tissue.

**Vasodilator**—Agent producing dilation of blood vessels.

**Vertigo**—The sensation that the outerworld is revolving about the patient.

**Virus**—A small parasitic microorganism.

**Vital Signs**—Signs pertaining to life.

# Appendix 7–B

## Glossary of Prefixes

A prefix is one or more syllables placed in front of a word to describe a particular relationship.

**a, an-** —Without (i.e., asepsis, without infection).

**ab-** —From, off, away from (i.e., abacterial, non-bacterial).

**acr- or acro-** —Relating to an extremity, top or summit (i.e., acro-arthritis, arthritis effecting the extremities).

**adeno-** —Gland or glands (i.e., adenocellulitis, inflammation of the gland).

**ambi-** —Both (i.e., ambilateral, relating to or affecting both sides).

**ana-** —Back, up, again, through (i.e., anabolism, the building up of constructive metabolism).

**angio-** —To a vessel (i.e., angioma, a tumor composed of blood or lymphatic vessels).

**ante-** —Before, preceding, in front of, prior to (i.e., anteaural, before or in front of the ear).

**antero-** —Front or before (i.e., anteromedian, in front and toward the middle).

**anti-** —Signifying against or opposed to (i.e., anti-allergic, a therapeutic agent that inhibits, arrests or prevents an allergic reaction).

**apo-** —Away from (i.e., apoclesis, aversion to eating).

**arterio-** —Pertaining to the arteries (i.e., arteriogram, X-ray of an artery).

**arthro-** —Relating to the joints (i.e., arthrocele, any swollen joint).

**atel-** —Imperfect or incomplete development (i.e., atelectasis, imperfect expansion of the lungs at birth).

**auto-** —Pertaining to oneself (i.e., autoanalysis, analysis by a patient of his or her own mental disorder).

**bi-** —Two (i.e., bilateral, relating to two sides).

**bio-** —Relation to or connection with life and living organisms (i.e., biochemistry, the chemistry of living tissues or of life).

**blast-** —Denoting a sprout, shoot, germ, or formative cell (i.e., blastoma, a term employed to indicate that a tumor originated from embryonal cells).

**blepharo-** —Relating to the eyelid (i.e., blepharoatheroma, a sebaceous cyst of the eyelid).

**brady-** —Slow (i.e., bradycardia, a slow heart beat.)

**broncho-** —Relating to the bronchi (windpipe; i.e., bronchocele, a swelling or dilation of a windpipe).

**bucco-** —Pertaining to the cheeks (i.e., buccolabial, pertaining to the cheek and the lip).

**carcin, carcino-** —Pertaining to cancer (i.e., carcinoma, a malignant neoplasm or growth).

**cardio-** —Pertaining to the heart (i.e., cardiogram, a record of the heart's pulse taken through the chest wall).

**cata-** —In accordance with, downward or against (i.e., catatropia, turning of both eyes downward).

**celio-** —Pertaining to the abdomen (i.e., celioscopy, an examination of the abdominal wall by cystoscope).

**cephalo-** —The head (i.e., cephalic, pertaining to the head).

**cervico-** —Relation to the neck (i.e., cervicovesical, pertaining to the urinary bladder and the cervi uteri).

**chiro-** —Pertaining to the hand (i.e., chiroplasty, plastic operations on the hand).

**chole-** —Pertaining to bile (i.e., cholecystitis, inflammation of the gall bladder).

**chondro-** —Composed of cartilage or connection with cartilage (i.e., chondrocostal, relating to the ribs and their cartilages).

**circum-** —On all sides or around (i.e., circumcorneal, around or about the cornea).

**co, com-** —Together (i.e., complication, a disease associated with another disease).

**contra-** —Against, contrary or in opposition (i.e., contraception, prevention of conception).

**counter-** —Against (i.e., counteraction, action of a drug or agent opposed to that of some other drug or agent).

**cranio-** —Pertaining to the head (i.e., craniotomy, excision of a part of the skull).

**crypto-** —Hidden, secret or covered (i.e., cryptogenic, of unknown or obscure cause).

**cysto-** —Pertaining to the bladder or cyst (i.e., cystocele, meaning prolapse of the bladder into the vagina).

**cyto-** —Connection with, relation to, a cell (i.e., cytolysis, the disintegration or dissolution of cells).

**de-** —Down or away from (i.e., deactivation, process of becoming inactive).

**deca-** —Ten (ie., decameter, a metric measure of length equal to ten meters).

**demi-** —Half (i.e., demibain, one-half bath).

**derm-** —Pertaining to the skin (i.e., dermatitis, inflammation of the skin).

**dextro-** —Right (i.e., dextrocerebral, located in the right cerebral hemisphere).

**di-** —Double or twice (i.e., diarthric, relating to two joints).

**dia-** —Through, between, apart (i.e., diaderm, through the skin).

**dys-** —Difficult or painful (i.e., dysbasia, difficulty in walking).

**e, ecto, ex-** —Out or away from (i.e., ectoderm, outermost layer of the skin).

**em, en-** —In (i.e., embolic, pushing or growing in).

**enceph, alo-** —A condition in the brain or head (i.e., encephalomyelitis, inflammation of the brain and spinal cord).

**endo-**—Within (i.e., endometrium, the mucous membrane lining the uterus).

**entero-** —Some relationship to the intestine (i.e., enterocenthesis, a surgical puncture of the intestine).

**epi-** —Above or over (i.e., epicardium, the top layer of the paracardium).

**extra-** —Outside of or in addition (i.e., extracranial, outside of the cranial cavity).

**fibro-** —Pertaining to fiber (i.e., fibrocarcinoma, a carcinoma with fibrous elements).

**galacto-** —Pertaining to milk (i.e., galactosis, secretion of milk by the mammary glands).

**gastro-** —Stomach or belly (i.e., gastroenteritis, inflammation of the stomach and intestines).

**glosso-** —Tongue or pertaining to the tongue (i.e., glossodynia, pain in the tongue).

**glyco-** —Relationship to sweetness (i.e., glycolysis, the hydrolysis of sugar in the body).

**gyn, gyne, gyneco-** —Pertaining to a woman (i.e., gynecology, the science of the diseases of women, especially those pertaining to the sexual organs).

**helio-** —Pertaining to the sun (i.e., heliophobe, one who is morbidly sensitive to the effects of the sun's rays).

**hem, hemo, haemo-** —Pertaining to the blood (i.e., hematolysis, destruction of the red cells).

**hemi-** —Half (i.e., hemicrania, pain or headache on one side of the head only).

**hepato-** —Liver (i.e., hepatosis, enlargement of the liver due to an obstructive dilation or inflammation).

**hetero-** —Different from or other (i.e., heteroerotism, the direction of the sexual desire toward another person or toward any object other than oneself).

**histo-** —Relationship to the tissues (i.e., histolysis, disintegration of organic tissue).

**homeo-** —A similarity (i.e., homeomorphous, like or similar in form).

**hydro-** —Pertaining to water (i.e., hydrocele, an accumulation of fluid in the sac of the testis).

**hyper-** —Excessive, over or above (i.e., hypertension, high blood pressure).

**hypno-** —Pertaining to sleep (ie., hypnosis, a state of sleep or trance).

**hypo-** —Deficiency or lack of (i.e., hypotension, diminished or low blood pressure).

**hystero-** —Some relationship to the uterus (i.e., hysterectomy, removal of the uterus).

**ileo-** —Relationship to the ileum (i.e., ileum, lower portion of the small intestine).

**im, in-** —In (i.e., implanation, the act of setting in an organ).

**infra-** —Below or beneath (i.e., infracardiac, situated below or beneath the heart).

**inter-** —Between (i.e., intercostal, between the ribs).

**intra-** —Within (i.e., intraoral, within the mouth).

**intro-** —Within (i.e., introversion, a turning within).

**juxta-** —Near or by (i.e., juxta-articular, near a joint).

**kerato-** —Relating to the cornea or relating to a condition of horny tissue (i.e., keratoderma, a horny condition of the skin).

**labio-** —Relationship to the lip (i.e., labicervical, pertaining to the lip and the neck).

**lacto-** —Relationship to milk (i.e., lactiferous, secreting milk).

**leuko-** —Pertaining to anything white (i.e., leukotrichia, whiteness of hair).

**macro-** —Relating to anything large (i.e., macrocyte, a giant red cell).

**mast, masto-** —Relating to the breast (i.e., mastectomy, amputation of a breast).

**mega-** —Anything that is large or great (i.e., megalomelia, gigantism of one limb).

**meso-** —Relating to the middle or something that is situated in the middle (i.e., mesoderm, in the middle of the skin).

**meta-**—Between, after, beyond or transformation (i.e., metabolic failure, advanced progressive debility characterized by failure of mental and physical functions).

**metro-**—Relationship to the uterus (i.e., metrodynia, pain in the uterus).

**micro-**—Anything small (i.e., microglossia, abnormal smallness of the tongue).

**multi-**—Many (i.e., multiglandular, pertaining to several glands).

**myce, myco-**—Pertaining to fungus (i.e., mycology, the science of fungus).

**myel, myelo-**—Pertaining to the spinal cord or to bone marrow (i.e., myeloencephalitis, inflammation of both spinal cord and brain).

**myo-**—Relating to the muscle (i.e., myocarditis, inflammation of the heart muscle [myocardium]).

**necro-**—Relating to death (i.e., necrocytosis, death of cells).

**nephro-**—Pertaining to the kidney (i.e., nephritis, inflammation of the kidney).

**ob-**—Against, in front of or toward (i.e., obstruent, obstructive or tending to obstruct).

**odonto-**—Relating to the teeth (i.e., odontology, the branch of science dealing with diseases of the teeth).

**oligo-**—Little or a deficiency (i.e., oligemia, a diminishing of the blood quantity).

**omo-**—Pertaining to the shoulder (i.e., omohyoid, pertaining jointly to the scapula and the hyoid bone).

**oo-**—Egg (i.e., oocyte, an egg cell before the completion of its maturity).

**oophor, oophoro**—Pertaining to an ovary (i.e., oophoroma, malignant ovarian tumor).

**ophthalm-**—Relating to the eye (i.e., opthalmia, severe inflammation of the eye).

**opto-**—Relating to vision (i.e., optometrist, one who measures the degree of visual powers using a refractor).

**orchi-**—Pertaining to the testicles (i.e., orchiectomy, surgical removal of the testicles).

**ortho-**—Straight or normal (i.e., orthograde, walking or standing in a straight or upright position).

**osseo-**—Relating to the bones (i.e., ossicle, a small bone).

**osteo-**—Pertaining to the bones (i.e., osteocyte, a bone cell).

**oto-**—Relating to the ear (i.e., otologist, a physician specializing in the diseases of the ear).

**ovario-**—Relating to the ovary (i.e., ovariocele, a tumor or hernia of the ovary).

**oxy-**—Sharp or acute (i.e., oxyesthesia, a condition of increased acuity of sensation).

**pachy-**—Thick (i.e., pachydermia, abnormally thick skin).

**pan-**—Relating to all (i.e., panacea, a cure-all).

**para-**—Beyond or beside (i.e., paradental, near or beside a tooth).

**patho-**—Disease (i.e., pathogenic, pertaining to the capacity to produce disease; a pathogenic microorganism).

**per-**—Through or excessively (i.e., performation, a hole made through a part or wall of a cavity).

**peri-**—Around (i.e., peribronchitis, inflammation of the tissue around the bronchi).

**phlebo-**—Relating to a vein (i.e., phleborrhexis, rupture of a vein).

**photo-**—Light (i.e., photodynia, a pain arising from too much light).

**platy-**—Broad or flat (i.e., platycephalic, a person having a skull with a flat vertex).

**pluri-**—Many (i.e., pluripara, a woman who has given birth to several children).

**pneumo-**—Ear or lung (i.e., pneumocephalus, the presence of air or gas within the cranial cavity).

**polio-**—Gray (i.e., poliomyelitis, inflammation of the gray matter of the spinal cord).

**poly-**—Many (i.e., polycystic, containing many cysts).

**post-**—After (i.e., postconvulsive, coming on after a convulsion).

**pre-**—Before or in front of (i.e., precardiac, in front of the heart).

**pro-**—Before or in front of (i.e., process, a course of action).

**proct, procto-**—Relating to the anus (i.e., proctology, the science of the anatomy of diseases of the rectum and anus).

**pseudo-**—False (i.e., pseudomalady, an imaginary illness).

**psycho-**—Pertaining to the soul or mind (i.e., psychotropic, capable of altering brain function through stimulation or sedation).

**pyelo-**—The pelvis (i.e., pyeloplasty, plastic repair of the renal pelvis).

**pyo-**—Signifying pus (i.e., pycephalus, pus within the brain or cranium).

**rachi-** —Spine (i.e., rachiocampsis, curvature of the spine).

**re-** —Back (i.e., reacquired, acquired a second time).

**retro-** —Backward or behind (i.e., retroaction, reverse action).

**rhino-** —Nose (i.e., rhinoplasty, plastic surgery of the nose).

**salpingo-** —Relating to the fallopian tube (i.e., salpingoperitonitis, an inflammation of the uterine tube).

**sarco-** —Flesh (i.e., sarcobiont, living on flesh).

**semi-** —Half (i.e., semicoma, condition of partial coma).

**septi-** —Poison (i.e., septicemia, disease produced by poisonous products in the blood stream).

**staphyl-** —Pellet or uvula (i.e., staphylectomy, operation for the removal of the uvula).

**stereo-** —Solid (i.e., stereoblastula, a solid blastula).

**sub-** —Under (i.e., subclavian, lying under the clavicle).

**super-** —Above (i.e., supernormal, superior to the average).

**supra-** —Above or over (i.e., subrapubic, above the pubis).

**sym, syn-** —Together with (i.e., symactosis, malformations caused by the abnormal growing together of parts).

**teno-** —Relating to a tendon (i.e., tendonitis, inflammation of a tendon).

**thermo-** —Relating to heat (i.e., thermogenics, the science of production of heat).

**trache, tracheo-** —Relating to the trachea (i.e., tracheoplasty, plastic surgery of the trachea).

**trans-** —Across or through (i.e., transfuse, to perform a transfusion).

**tricho-** —Hair (i.e., trichoesthesia, the sensation received when hair is touched).

**ultra-** —Beyond or excess (i.e., ultrasonic, pertaining to sounds with frequencies above those normally heard).

**uni-** —One (i.e., unicellular, composed of but one cell).

**vaso-** —Vessel (i.e., vasoconstriction, constriction of the blood).

**zoo-** —Pertaining to an animal (i.e., zoopsia, the seeing of animals).

# Appendix 7–C

# Glossary of Suffixes

A suffix is one or more syllables added to the base of a word to indicate or describe a relationship.

**-ac**—Pertaining to (i.e., cardiac, pertaining to the heart).

**-ad**—Toward, to, at (i.e., cephalad, toward the head).

**-aemia**—Denotes a condition of the blood (i.e., glycemia, sugar in the blood).

**-al**—Pertaining to or characteristic of (i.e., hematal, pertaining to blood or blood vessels).

**-algia**—A painful condition (i.e., dermatalgia, pain, burning or other sensations of the skin).

**-asis, -iasis**—State or condition resulting from (i.e., cholelithiasis, the presence or formation of billiary concretions).

**-blast**—Denotes an immature cell (i.e., hematoblast, a cell from which red blood corpuscles are developed).

**-cele**—A hernia (i.e., meningocele, hernial protrusion of the meninges).

**-centesis**—Puncture (i.e., paracentesis, a puncture of the body cavity).

**-clasis**—Breaking (i.e., thromboclasis, the breaking up of a blood clot).

**-cleisis**—Closure (i.e., colpocleisis, a closure of the vagina).

**-coccus**—Round bacterium (i.e., dermococcus, round bacteria found in the skin).

**-culum**—Diminion (i.e., tuberculum, a tubercle or small prominence).

**-cyst**—Sac or bladder containing fluid (i.e., microcyst, a small cyst).

**-cyte**—A hollow vessel (i.e., hematocyte, any mature blood vessel).

**-cytosis**—A condition having to do with a cell or cells (i.e., lymphocytosis, having more than the normal lympocytes in the blood).

**-dynia**—A painful condition (i.e., cardiodynia, pain in the heart).

**-ectasia, -ectasis**—Dilation, expansion, stretching (i.e., venectasia, dilation of the veins).

**-ectomy**—Excision of (i.e., gastrectomy, removal of the stomach).

**-ethesia**—Denoting sensation (i.e., anesthesia, lack of sensation).

**-graph, -graphy**—Pertaining to that which is written or a process of recording (i.e., encephalograph, an instrument that records the brain waves).

**-ia**—Denoting a diseased condition (i.e., trachealgia, pain when hair is touched).

**-ible**—Capacity or ability (i.e., visible, the ability of being seen).

**-ician**—One skilled in (i.e., optician, one skilled in making lenses).

**-ist**—One who practices a given art (i.e., dermatologist, a doctor who specializes in skin diseases).

**-itis**—Inflammation (i.e., dermatitis, inflammation of the skin).

**-ity**—Quality (i.e., density, the quality of being dense).

**-lith**—Stone (i.e., nephrolith, a calculus, renal stone in the kidney).

**-logy, -ology**—The science of (i.e., dermatology, the science of skin).

**-mania**—Pertaining to an insane desire (i.e., kleptomania, one who has a desire to steal).

**-oid**—Like or similar in shape (i.e., thromboid, like or resembling a thrombis).

**-oma**—Indicating a morbid condition (i.e., carcinoma, a malignant cancer).

**-opia**—Denoting sight or vision (i.e., corectopia, malposition of the pupil).

**-orexia**—Appetite, desire (i.e., anorexia, lack of appetite).

**-ory**—Pertaining to (i.e., circulatory, pertaining to the circulation).

**-oscopy, -scopy**—An inspection, viewing of (i.e., sigmoidoscopy, an inspection of the sigmoid).

**-otomy, -tomy**—A cutting or an incision (i.e., nephrotomy, an incision of a kidney).

**-ous**—Full of, having, possessing (i.e., fibrous, composed of fibers).

**-pathy**—Suffering disease (i.e., neuropathy, any nerve disease).

**-pexy**—Fixation of (i.e., hysteropexy, fixation of a displaced uterus).

**-phasia**—Speech (i.e., aphasia, loss of the power of speech).

**-phobia**—Fear (i.e., hydrophobia, abnormal fear of water).

**-plasty**—Repair of (i.e., dermaplasty, repair of the skin).

**-pnea**—Breath (i.e., dyspnea, labored or difficulty breathing).

**-ptosis**—A falling of (i.e., hysteroptosis, falling or prolapse of the uterus).

**-rhythmio**—Rhythmical action (i.e., arrhythmia, any variation from normal rhythm of the heart).

**-rhagia**—A flowing (i.e., menorrhagia, an excessive menstruation).

**-rhaphy**—Sewing of (i.e., colporhaphy, suturing the vaginal wall).

**-rhea**—Discharge (i.e., diarrhea, watery unformed discharge from the bowel).

**-spasm**—A spasm of (i.e., idiospasm, a spasm of a limited area).

**-stasis**—Standing still, position (i.e., hemostasis, the checking of the flow of blood).

**-taxis**—Order, arrangement (i.e., thermotaxis, a normal adjustment).

**-tion**—A condition, action (i.e., preparation, the act or process of making ready).

**-tripsy**—A crushing (i.e., lithotripsy, crushing of stones in the bladder).

**-trophia**—Nutrition (i.e., hypertrophia, enlargement).

**-ure**—An act (i.e., culture, state of being cultured).

**-uria**—Urine (i.e., albuminuria, presence of albumin in the urine).

# Appendix 7–D

## Medical Abbreviations

aa—of each.

ad lib—at pleasure, as much as needed.

ac—before meals.

ad—to, up to.

adv—against.

alt dieb—every other day.

alt hor—every other hour.

alt noct—every other night.

ante—before.

aq—water.

aq dist—distilled water.

bib—drink.

bid—twice daily.

BMR—basal metabolic rate.

BP—blood pressure.

C—celsius or centrigrade.

c̄—with.

CA—cancer, carcinoma.

cap—capsule.

cc—cubic centimeter.

cf—compare.

cn—tomorrow night.

CNS—central nervous system.

CSF—cerebral spinal fluid.

CV—cardiovascular.

D & C—dilation and curettage.

decub—dying down.

def—defecation.

DNI—do not intubate.

DNR—do not resuscitate in case of medical emergency.

e.g.—for example.

EKG—electrocardiogram.

ENT—ear, nose and throat.

F—Fahrenheit.

GB—gall bladder.

G, gm—gram.

Gr, gr—grain.

GT or gt—drop.

Hypo—hyperdermic.

H—hour.

hs—at bedtime.

IM—intramuscular.

In d.—daily.

IV—intravenous.

liq—liquid solution.

mm—millimeter.

no—number.

noct—at night.

O—pint.

Omn hor—every hour.

Omn noct—every night.

OD, od—right eye.

OS, os—left eye.

PC—after meal.

prn—whenever necessary.

prog—prognosis.

PT—physical therapy.

Px—physical exam.

q—every.

q d—every day.

q h—every hour.

q 2h—every 2 hours.

qid—4 times a day.

qs—sufficient quantity.

quotid—daily.

sol—solution.

SOS—as necessary.

stat—at once.

syr—syrup.

tid—three times daily.

TPR—temperature, pulse, respiration.

USP—U.S. Pharmacopeia.

ung—ointment.

vin—wine.

WBC—white blood cells.

%—male.

&—female.

# Appendix 7–E

# Drugs and Their Effect

**Anesthetic**—A drug that causes insensitivity to pain by depressing the central nervous system.

**Antiseptic**—Slows down growth of bacteria. Does not kill all bacteria (i.e., hydrogen peroxide).

**Antacids**—Neutralizes the acid in the stomach (i.e., Amphojel).

**Antitoxin**—Neutralizes bacterial toxins in infections (i.e., tetanus antitoxin).

**Antibiotics**—Destroys microorganisms in the body (i.e., penicillin).

**Analgesic**—A drug that relieves pain; may be narcotic or non-narcotic (i.e., aspirin, Tylenol).

**Anticoagulants**—Depresses the coagulation of blood.

**Antihypertensive**—Medicine used to lower blood pressure.

**Antianemics**—Used in treatment of anemia (i.e., liver extract).

**Anthelmintus**—Kills worms in the gastrointestinal tract (i.e., chiniofon).

**Anticonvulsant**—Prevents or controls convulsions (i.e., Dilantin, IV Valium, phenobarbitol).

**Antidote**—Used to counteract poisons.

**Antispasmodics**—Relieves smooth muscle spasm (i.e., atropine sulfate).

**Astringents**—Used to constrict skin and mucous membranes by withdrawing water (i.e., alum).

**Antitussive**—Controls coughing (i.e., Robitussin).

**Cathartics, laxatives, purgatives**—Induces bowel movements (i.e., cascara sagrada).

**Carminatives**—Reduces flatulence (bloating).

**Caustics**—Destroys tissue by local application (i.e., silver nitrate).

**Chemotherapeutics**—Used to cure disease.

**Coagulants**—Stimulate coagulation of blood.

**Diaphoretics**—Used to induce perspiration.

**Disinfectants**—Destroys pathogenic organisms (i.e., Zephiran Chloride).

**Diuretics**—Stimulates elimination of urine (i.e., Thiomirin).

**Emetics**—Induces vomiting (i.e., warm salt water).

**Emollients**—Used to soften and soothe tissue (i.e., cold cream).

**Expectorant**—Used to induce coughing.

**Generic Substitution**—Different brand or unbranded drug substituted for a legend drug.

**General Anesthetic**—Administered to the whole body and produces unconsciousness.

**Hypnotics**—Assists patient to fall asleep (i.e., Nembutal).

**Hypotensive**—Helps lower blood pressure.

**Hypertensive**—Helps raise blood pressure.

**Local Anesthetic**—Used to anesthetize only one specific region of the body.

**Miotics**—Constricts pupil of eyes.

**Mydriatic**—Dilates pupil of eyes.

**Palliative**—Relieves symptoms but does not cure (i.e., aspirin, antibiotics).

**Parenteral Drugs**—Administered by injection (i.e., intravenous-intramuscular substances).

**Placebo**—Substance that has no medicinal value.

**Sedatives**—Relieves anxiety and emotional tensions (i.e., Phenobarbitol).

**Tonics, stimulants**—Used to stimulate body activity (i.e., quinine).

**Topical**—Applied to a specific area of the body (i.e., ointments, lotions).

**Tranquilizer**—Reduces mental tension and anxiety (i.e., Librium, Thorazene).

**Vasoconstrictors**—Constricts blood vessels.

**Vasodilators**—Dilates blood vessels.

# Appendix 7–F

# Equipment Used in Long-Term Care Facilities

**Aspirator**—Used to draw fluids from the body by suction.

**Audiometer**—Instrument to test hearing acuity.

**Autoclave**—Machine used to sterilize equipment.

**Catheter**—Hollow metal, glass or soft/hard rubber tube for introduction into a cavity to discharge the fluid contents.

**Disposables**—Underpads and other medical supplies used only once.

**Electrocardiograph (ECG or EKG)**—An instrument that measures electrical impulses generated by the heart.

**Foley Catheter**—Used in urinary tract infections.

**Gastroscope**—Instrument inserted in the mouth and down the esophagus to the stomach to view the stomach.

**Indwelling Catheter**—Catheter allowed to remain in the bladder.

**Levine Tube**—Tube inserted through the nose into throat and stomach.

**Life Support System**—Electric equipment used to maintain patient's life, such as catheters, dialysis machines or respirators.

**Medical Supplies**—Basic medical supplies, such as crutches or dressing.

**Nasogastric Tubes**—Feeding tubes.

**Oxygen Apparatus**—Oxygen tubes, tanks or carriers.

**Sphygmomanometer (Cuff)**—Instrument to take blood pressure.

**Sphygmotonometer**—Instrument used to measure blood pressure.

# Appendix 7–G

# Medical Specialists

**Allergist**—A physician who treats and diagnoses reactions and sensitivities to various substances such as foods, pollens and dust.

**Anesthesiologist**—A physician who supervises and administers anesthesia during operations and other medical procedures.

**Anesthetist**—A technician who renders anesthetic.

**Cardiologist**—A physician who specializes in the diagnosis and treatment of heart disease.

**Chiropodist**—A trained professional but not a medical doctor, who treats ailments (such as corns or bunions) affecting the feet.

**Chiropractor**—A trained professional but not a medical doctor, who restores normal function by manipulation of structures of the body.

**Dermatologist**—A physician who diagnoses and treats disease of the skin.

**Endocrinologist**—A physician who specializes in disorders affecting the endocrine system. The endocrine system includes such glands as the pituitary, thyroid, pancreas and adrenals, which secrete certain hormones into the blood stream.

**Exondonist**—A dentist who specializes in the extraction of teeth.

**Gastroenterologist**—A physician who treats and diagnoses disease of the digestive tract.

**General Surgeon**—A physician who specializes in operative procedures to treat illnesses or various injuries.

**Geriatrician**—A physician who concentrates on the treatment of elderly persons.

**Gerontologist**—One who studies aging and deals with problems or diseases of the aged.

**Gynecologist**—A physician who specializes in diseases of the female reproductive organs.

**Hematologist**—A physician who specializes in diseases of the circulatory system.

**Internist**—A physician who specializes in the diagnosis and the treatment of diseases usually for adults.

**Nephrologist**—A physician specializing in diseases of the kidney.

**Neurologist**—A physician who diagnoses and treats diseases of the brain, nerves and spinal cord.

**Obstetrician**—A physician who specializes in the care and treatment of women before, during and after childbirth.

**Oncologist**—A physician who specializes in the study and treatment of cancer.

**Ophthalmologist**—A physician who diagnoses and treats eye diseases and disorders, and prescribes corrective eye glasses.

**Optician**—A technician (not a physician) trained to grind lenses and to fit eye glasses.

**Optometrist**—A trained professional (not a physician) who gives limited eye care (testing vision, correcting focusing errors and prescribing glasses).

**Oral Surgeon**—A dentist specializing in surgical techniques for correcting deformities, injuries and treating diseases in or adjacent to the mouth.

**Orthodontist**—A dentist who specializes in treating and correcting malformations of the jaw and teeth.

**Orthopedist**—A physician who specializes in diseases and injuries to bones, muscles, joints and tendons.

**Osteopath**—A doctor of osteopathy. A physician who uses methods of diagnosis and treatment, placing special emphasis on the interrelationship of the musculoskeletal system to the other body systems.

**Otologist**—A physician who specializes in diseases of the ear.

**Pathologist**—A professionally trained person or physician who specializes in examination of body tissues under laboratory conditions.

**Pediatrician**—A physician who specializes in diagnosis and treatment of diseases of children and adolescents.

**Pedodontist**—A dentist specializing in dental care of children.

**Periodontist**—A dentist specializing in treating diseases of the gums.

**Plastic Surgeon**—A physician who practices restorative surgery.

**Podiatrist**—A specialist in treating diseases of the feet.

**Proctologist**—A physician who specializes in the diagnosis and treatment of the large intestine, particularly the anus and rectum.

**Radiologist**—A physician who specializes in the use of X-rays in treatment and diagnosis of injury or disease.

**Rheumatologist**—A physician specializing in arthritis.

**Urologist**—A physician who specializes in the diagnosis and treatment of diseases of the kidney, bladder and reproductive organs.

# CHAPTER 8

# Resident Care Management: Psychology of Resident Care

## PSYCHOLOGICAL ASPECTS OF AGING

Psychology has been defined as the science that studies the function of the mind by taking into consideration the behavior of the individual and such attitudes as sensation, perception, hearing, response behavior, learning and intelligence. This section will discuss psychology as it applies to the aging person.

### Social Aspects of Aging

One immediate problem confronting a study of psychology of the aging is the definition of the aging. The National Institute of Child Health and Human Development somewhat arbitrarily has designated the beginning of the process of aging at 21. Although degenerative processes are occurring in the human body before birth, physiological aging is considered to begin from the moment of birth. Generally speaking, psychologists have determined that both progressive and regressive processes occur at all stages of life, taking on certain characteristics of development: early childhood, a plateau, the period of concern about retirement and a gradual decline. Generally, in our society, people over the age of 65 are termed elderly. Frail elderly are those persons who cannot maintain social contact or households without ongoing assistance from others. Functionally disabled elderly are those who cannot perform self-care or household tasks independently due to illness, disability or social problems.

It is estimated that there were 34 million people 65 years of age or older in the United States as of July 1996. Some of the social considerations involved in aging include the areas of retirement, the relationship of the elderly to their children, and the degree of satisfaction the elderly have with life.

### Retirement

Retirement affects both men and women to varying degrees. The man is the one usually employed at a full-time job and much of his social interaction in preretirement years has been through his occupational status. With many women working today, some of the problems attendant with the male retiree applied to the female retiree. Adjustability to the retirement stage of life depends upon several factors including the nature of work done during occupational years and the mental attitude of the retiree. Although individuals who were unhappy while working often are unhappy as retirees, retirement crises among the elderly vary with individual lifestyles and attitudes. Generally, many older people become less involved with the world; their scope of interest becomes narrower as the environment becomes younger and less meaningful. Toward the final years, a tendency develops to withdraw from reality and live on memories.

### Relationship to Children

Whether elderly parents have children living near them or are geographically separated, some sort of frequent contact occurs. It is assumed that most older parents desire a great deal of contact with their children. However, studies have indicated that both the children and the parents want a certain degree of independence. Both prefer to have separate living arrangements. The middle generation (45 to 65) often provides financial and emotional support to both younger and older generations, generally with the women shouldering most of the responsibility for the care of elderly relatives.

### Satisfaction with Life

Along with the realization of becoming older, a person is faced with many losses at a time when emotional and physical well-being and energies are decreasing. This social aspect of retirement involves many aspects and has no single solution. An older person is an individual and cannot be stereotyped or categorized as to behavior. Each individual will find new ways to adapt, accepting perhaps a situation which he or she previously would have tried to master.

Some psychologists view old age as a period of harvest where the fruits of one's previous efforts are gathered and feel that society must have available some sort of "rewards" to help the elderly feel accepted and enjoy this phase of life. Social programs must be based on the general and specific needs of each older person. Problem areas must be identified, realizing that future generations of older people will not necessarily have the same social problems as our older people today. Some consideration might be given to the following to help the elderly cope:

- **Planning for Old Age**—Training for leisure activities, retirement counseling during middle age and participation in community mental health activities are items to be considered here.
- **Psychological Support**—Establish effective methods to handle the increasing leisure time resulting from the shortened period of work and increased life expectancy. Removal of severe stressful situations, creation of a beneficial physical environment and proper stimulation of mental functions are important factors.
- **Interpersonal Support**—Help the aged person to maintain independence, community/social involvement and the sense of dignity and self-esteem with assistance programs and good long-term care facilities.

- **Economic Support**—Assist the elderly to maintain financial independence and provide the basic needs of food, shelter, clothing and protective legal support.
- **Medical Support**—Medical services must be delivered to the elderly at a reasonable cost, including drugs, prosthetic devices and health care facility stays.

### Senescence

Writers have indicated that old age is a time of backing away from society and from usual occupational activities. This is manifested by a decrease in physical and psychological energy. The elderly person goes through a period where he or she reviews life as it has been lived in an attempt to make the remaining years more meaningful. Some look back with nostalgia, whereas others become depressed, anxious or suicidal.

This period is termed senescence, which is defined as the process of becoming aged. Senescence involves psychological, biological and sociological aspects and the changes, responses, realizations and related adjustments. Essentially, this is a time of many losses and adaption to them. Losses of loved ones, friends, independence, responsibility and being needed represent a bit-by-bit loss of one's self that will terminate in death. Self-image and motivation may be threatened as aging isolates the individual from many of the roles previously filling his or her life.

Senescence has very little to do with senility. Senility is defined as pathological (disease-related) changes affecting mental ability. Senility regression is a gradual withdrawal and tendency to live in one's memories and sometimes occurs in late senescence. Complete senile regression involves a total break with reality and total involvement in the past.

### Stress and Grief

Stress and grief are among the several psychological changes and reactions to be taken into account in relation to senescence. It has been pointed out that health is not merely an absence of disease but the ability to cope with stress as well. The ability to cope with stress is in the ego or concept of self: the strength and maturity of the ego affect the degree of adjustments to the environment. If an individual is confronted with a conflict and successfully handles the problem, he or she will gain a certain amount of self-confidence. Conversely, if unable to cope with stress, crisis will be experienced and depression may occur.

Stress arises when one becomes anxious. Fear is an aspect of stress and is a normal reaction to danger or injury. Dangers can be real or imaginary. A person reacting mildly to imagined dangers is said to have a neurotic behavior pattern. Reaction that severs the relationship with reality is said to be psychotic. Fear can be intensified in conditions of powerlessness. Loss of mastery over bodily functions can be perceived as menaces in an institutional environment.

Grief that occurs when damage actually takes place is considered a part of senescence inasmuch as the person attaining old age has experienced the loss of loved ones, friends and colleagues. Traits of depression and grief are understandably quite common in the aging. A difference arises between grief and depression. A grief reaction is an emotional response, whereas depression is a pathological emotional reaction involving prolonged sadness, inactivity and self-depreciation. Grief reaction involves a clear and conscious recognition of an actual loss. Following the initial emotional shock, a realization emerges of the significance and the ramifications of the loss. Episodes of specific physiological sensations of distress and waves of sadness recur. The feelings of grief and sadness are expressed verbally and nonverbally. Toward the end of the grief reaction, a resolution appears that involves a redirecting of energy and interest toward new people, goals and activities.

### Personality

Generally, an older person who is in good health shows very little personality change. Psychological testing, however, has found that middle-aged persons respond differently than those who are aged: the middle-aged person seeing himself or herself as energetic and the older person seeing himself or herself as more withdrawn and conforming. Different personality types characterized by the ability to adjust to aging include the:

1. Mature person who is well-adjusted and continues to look at the world with a positive attitude.
2. Rocking chair person who relies on others and does not overly exert himself or herself.

3. Armored person who has developed a pattern of defense toward anxiety.
4. Angry person who blames everyone for his or her problems.
5. Self-hater who blames himself or herself for any problems and frustrations.

### Problems of Aging

In order to support and cope with individual residents, some of the areas affecting the behavior of aging persons to be considered and understood by those working with the elderly are discussed below.

### Intelligence

Intelligence has been defined as the ability to perceive qualities and attributes of the objective world and to employ purposefully a means toward the attainment of an end. It involves abstract thinking and problem solving.

Intelligence is measured in part by intelligence quotient (IQ), a figure determining intelligence in relationship to chronological age. Most of these intelligence tests are geared to measure specific qualities, such as vocabulary, spatial relationships, reading ability, comprehension ability and mathematical ability.

The process of becoming older in itself does not seem to adversely affect performance on IQ tests because so many variables come into the picture. Persons from varied social, economic and cultural backgrounds often score differently on these tests. Some psychologists have concluded that IQ scores decline with age, whereas some are quick to point out that studies have shown there is little change with advanced aging. Motivation to do well on these intelligence tests is an important aspect of performance. This is generally lacking in older persons who do not find such tests meaningful to the interests in their lifestyle. Serious psychological illness also can adversely affect IQ scores.

General intelligence is a trait that maintains itself into old age, providing the individual uses his or her mind and there has not been undue physical deterioration.

### Response Reactions

Although some reactions (i.e., spontaneous speech) seem to be unaffected with age, generally speaking a person's response to stimuli is lower with age. Young people's reactions appear to be quicker to changing situations whereas the older person will approach new environments and situations at a slower rate. The older person will approach unfamiliar problems or materials at his or her own rate and will not usually be influenced to move at a faster pace. Indications are that the older person needs more time to respond to a given situation.

### Learning Ability

Although the physiological aging process and slowing down of responses affect learning skills in older persons, there are other factors to consider. The older person has a vast area of experience and knowledge to meet various situations, but the rate of retrieval of such information may be slowed. Lack of motivation and interest in particular subjects have definite adverse effect on the ability or willingness to learn.

### Ability to Move About

A definite relationship exists between aging and the ability to move around. The slowing of reaction to stimuli, decreased motor function, worsening coordination, disease and the development of behavior patterns over the years affect the older person in mobility. After age 65, many are involved in falls. It has been asserted that, compared to younger drivers, older people are generally involved in more accidents, not because of speeding, but because of slower reactions to external stimuli affecting visual acuity and the necessary coordination of responses in driving.

### Sensory Perception

Generally with the process of aging, a loss of acuity relating the sensory perceptions of hearing, seeing and smelling occurs. Although severe losses may reach the stage where medical devices may not help impairment, the effect of such loss can vary and often may be compensated by the use of artificial devices (such as hearing aids or glasses). Some accept these losses better than others. The ability to compensate is tied in with the individual's attitude and behavior pattern that have developed over the years. Adjustments in personal lifestyle and behavior are often involved.

### Memory

Older people tend to have a problem with short-term memory, especially if the experience to be remembered is of a personal nature. Psychologists maintain that retention of recent experience is impaired more than long-term memory for past events. There may be some difficulty ascertaining the time sequence of recent events. This difficulty contributes to disorientation. In a familiar environment, memory problems tend to be at a minimum; when a resident first enters the new environment of the nursing facility, memory problems may be evident but should lessen after the adjustment period.

### Security

For a long time, mental health professionals have continued to support the theory that conquering an environment and feeling competent in a particular area is extremely essential in humans and does not diminish with the aging process. An older person tends to view new environments and situations as threats to security rather than challenges as do younger persons.

## PERSONAL AND SOCIAL CARE

### Admission to the Nursing Facility

Admission to a nursing facility is viewed as the final realization of loss of many former activities and relationships. It represents a large change in lifestyle, coupled with a variety of physical and emotional responses (separation reaction). The resident experiences an emotional shock that leaves a deep psychological impression (trauma) when entering the nursing facility. During what is called the "first month syndrome," a newly admitted resident will deteriorate emotionally before gradually adapting to the new surroundings—usually at the end of a 30-day period. After that period, the resident will take more interest in the facility and its activities.

Some maintain that the more the facility is like the personal home of the resident, the easier it will be to adapt. More realistically the primary factor in the ability to adjust is connected with the personality and habits the resident has acquired during younger years. Recognition, acknowledgement and acceptance of the resident's feelings are essential in the admission process. The staff's sincere understanding and concern will ease this adjustment to new surroundings.

The first dominant emotion an individual experiences upon admittance is that of helplessness. Helplessness is defined as a loss of control over the outcome of one's life in connection with daily living activities and experiences. A new resident entering the home may feel the loss of control over immediate routine and everyday activities to physical illness, loss of privacy and a regimented environment. In younger years or before affliction with disease, many were looked up to for guidance by their families and had a complete sense of independence. The need to turn to others outside of family and friends for help, particularly assistance in the performance of simple tasks, creates a feeling that this time is the beginning of the end. The resident usually will have mixed feelings of guilt, shame, failure and embarrassment that he or she must turn to strangers for assistance. Such anxiety about the future, self-worth, security and companionship can manifest itself in the resident's blame of others for his or her problems. Because of dependence on the staff for care, and fear of retribution, the resident may use family to speak on his or her behalf concerning his or her complaints, needs or desires. Thus, it is important that the resident be given an opportunity to solve problems, to perform tasks if desired and to become involved in activities to restore a feeling of competency and importance.

The second dominant emotion experienced is hopelessness—a feeling that no meaningful future, no expectations of good success or of contributions to others and the community will occur. When a person has despair, life holds little meaning. Many residents have had traumatic experiences in recent years. This coupled with the idea that going to a nursing facility is going to a place to die quite naturally causes depression and despair. The staff needs to recognize the characteristics of such feelings and help each resident understand that they are sincerely interested and concerned and that the nursing facility is a type of physical and emotional support by the younger generation.

When the resident first comes to the nursing facility, he or she is usually unfamiliar with the established routine. Because new situations often appear as threats, a resident may experience some disorientation initially. This is a new environment usually with few or no acquaintances and friends and little with which to identify. Memory difficulty seems to contribute to the problem of disorientation in the older person; this tends to be at a minimum level in a familiar environment. The resident may exhibit fear that if he or she does not adjust or follow the rules, basic needs (food, shelter, care) may not be met. Other fears include those of losing former relationships, being put somewhere to die and being in a place among those who are ill and/or mentally disabled.

Thus, the newly admitted resident may be feeling rejected by his or her loved ones because of their consent to his or her staying in the nursing facility. He or she may feel hostile and angry toward members of the family who participated in this decision or angry at the position in which their aging and health has put them. Although the generation gap of today seems to preclude the pattern of the elderly being with the younger people in the same home, some cultures in America continued to place a great emphasis on the belief that the younger generation should care for members of the family in their homes during their aging years. Only in recent times have social and economic trends caused families to rely on institutions to provide care customarily provided at home. Tied up with the feelings of rejection and hostility are those of grief in relation to previous losses and the present ones of home, independence, family, friends and abilities to function.

## Interpersonal Relationships with the Elderly

Following are some guidelines, thoughts and tips for those who care for and work with the elderly.

### Sensitivity

Older persons are easily hurt and may be especially sensitive in situations where individual limitations are apparent. All who help the elderly walk a thin line between being overly protective and safely guarding the older person's best interests. Kind and firm persuasion to assist the older person to accept handicaps and use the assets and abilities retained allows the individual to make decisions and retain autonomy.

### Troubles

When an older person is upset or troubled, the tendency is to try to divert attention to what a wonderful day it is, how much there is for which to be thankful, or options to remedy the upsetting condition. However, asking why the person seems troubled, encouraging a sharing of feelings and just listening is considered a more constructive approach and will help even if it may or may not solve the problem.

## Complaints

Usually, the individual who constantly complains about anything and everything actually may be saying, "I feel neglected. Nobody around here likes me or gives me any attention." This person may be too proud to admit such feelings outright or may not know the real reason he or she acts this way. Obviously, this individual needs more attention than is being received; attitude (such as a brief pleasant remark, a pat or hug) rather than words will convey a message that he or she is recognized and will help lessen constant complaints.

## Personal Complaints

Some people have a tendency to exaggerate the aches and pains they are experiencing. Such an individual often is seeking attention. Scolding, challenging honesty in this area, or pointing out that others are suffering more are not helpful, comforting or constructive ways to get at the problem. A little kindness, attention, sympathy and an attempt to change the subject will go further toward alleviating the situation.

## Hostility

Often one of the most difficult things to learn and accept is not to be offended personally by unkind or insulting remarks sometimes made by older persons. Many times such hostility is directed at a frustrating situation, not personally at the receiver who happened to be the first contact. Realizing that this may be the case can encourage a more assured positive reply such as: "I'm sorry you feel that way." Suppress a hostile response that tends only to increase the tension.

## Memory Loss

Individuals with severe memory loss usually have lost the ability to reason or think logically. Prompt and correct information is the best response to questions asked by persons with such memory loss. Counterquestioning may foster undue stress and frustration rather than stimulate thinking.

## Grief

What should be done when an older person cries? Although the first reaction is to offer assurances that everything will be all right, the greatest help to this person is to allow him or her to cry. Ask about the problem and listen carefully to the answer. Let the unhappy person know that caring support and help are available.

## Administrator's Relationships within the Facility

### To Residents

The administrator has two major concerns in operating the nursing facility and is more involved with the residents than the hospital administrator who is concerned essentially with the management of the hospital where patient involvement is minimal. The nursing facility administrator must practice management principles and become directly involved in the lives of the residents. A nursing facility resident may spend the rest of his or her life there. The administrator becomes very important as she or he will have a significant role to play in the resident's quality of life. Thus, he or she must be aware of the interpersonal relationships with each resident. The administrator should assist the governing body to establish policy consistent with an environment that will assist the resident therapeutically and see that the required care is given according to primary objectives and mission of the facility.

As the authority figure in the facility, the administrator needs to understand the emotional problems of residents. Ideally, he or she should meet with each resident before admission and explain the goals and objectives of the facility. The prospective resident should be given an opportunity to express any doubts or feelings regarding admission. The administrator may visit also with the resident and family in the office, or any other place with sufficient privacy soon after admittance to welcome him or her as a new resident. Residents should be encouraged to visit with the administrator whenever they feel the need to do so. It is important to let each resident know that it may take a little time to become accustomed to the new environment and that this is quite normal.

Mental health professionals suggest that the administrator can help make the resident's stay a more pleasant experience by helping him or her cope with emotional problems. With the assistance of the staff, the administrator can enhance the self-image of the resident; the example set will permeate through the entire staff. Recommendations include:

1. Call the resident by his or her name using Mr., Mrs. or Miss; do not use terms such as grandma or grandpa. Recognition as an individual will help the resident to retain identity, respect and dignity. He or she will feel more like a person than a number or disease entity.

2. Take preventive measures relative to the emotional problems by adequately preparing the resident for admission to the facility. Information should be obtained on the sociological background and former environment, history of past occupations, interest, dietary habits and likes and dislikes of each resident. Such a visit indicates interest in the potential resident and will provide opportunity for questions, input into roommate selection and meeting some of the staff members.

3. After being admitted to the facility, the resident usually gives up the right to make certain decisions including some daily living activities. Decisions pertaining to clothing, room arrangements, colors, menus, programs and entertainment should be encouraged. Some facilities have established resident committees to encourage and assist with such choices.

4. Set goals and objectives with input from residents and families as feasible, so they are resident-oriented. This means programs should evolve around the problems of the resident and planned so that most who are able can participate. When feasible, jobs such as carrying messages, folding napkins or distributing supplies can be given to residents so they may feel wanted and useful.

5. Encourage the resident to establish friendly relationships with the other residents of like temperament and personality.

6. For those residents not properly motivated, use remotivational techniques.

7. Some studies indicate that 49% of nursing facility residents would qualify for institutionalization in mental facilities. Residents with severe or acute emotional problems should be always under the guidance and supervision of a qualified physician.

### To the Family

The administrator, in addition to developing satisfactory interpersonal relationships with the residents, must understand and develop good relationships with the family of each resident. Both the nursing facility and the family have an essential role to play in providing care and need to assist one another in fulfilling this role. Families may be highly critical of facility conditions and procedures for a variety of complicated and interrelated reasons. The placing of a family member in the facility is traumatic for the family as well as the resident. To work effectively with families, the administrator should be aware of the reactions of close relatives to the admission of the family member. The varying degrees of behavior depend upon the interrelationships of the resident and the family. Emotional problems previously repressed in the family environment may come forth.

In some cases, the family will abandon the total responsibility for the resident's care. This kind of reaction displays itself by infrequent visitation and hostility toward any mention of the resident. The family may reject completely the further existence of the loved one because of their own feelings of guilt in the decision not to care for him or her at home. Any relief felt at the time of admission will add to these guilt feelings.

Other relatives react by attempting to dominate the life of the resident and criticizing the nursing facility. The discomfort, stress, guilt and/or anger accompanying the decision to admit a family member may be displaced onto the facility staff and administrator. The relative admitting the resident will emphasize the apparent inadequacies of the facility as a substitution for his or her inability to provide the needed care at home and to display his or her love and concern. This family member may be extremely sensitive to the criticism of other family members and is trying to make sure the best care is given.

Unusual visitation privileges often are requested by a spouse remaining at home. When two people have lived together for a long period of time, to see the other undergo physical and psychological deterioration has a traumatic effect. The disruption of a happy family life causes much grief when one of the parties is admitted to a nursing facility.

Generally, families expect care, treatment and activities on an ongoing well-organized basis. The premises are to be attractive, comfortable, well-maintained and well-ventilated. The residents are clean and well-groomed, and the staff is responsive and kind. Some residents may lose control of body functions, lack concern about dressing habits and personal appearance and/or seem depressed. Relatives often will not accept these facts as reasons when they come to the facility and see their relative or other residents dirty or untidy. In the eyes of the relative, the nursing facility is not doing its job. Procedures must be put in place to keep the residents well-groomed and dressed, accidents handled promptly and the facility neat, orderly and well-ventilated at all times. The administrator should reassure the family that everything is being provided as discussed prior to admission.

A lack of objectivity often is found among relatives concerning the condition or further deterioration of their family member. A loved one may not appear as deteriorated or sick as he or she does to the staff; families know the personality and unique behavior patterns of their member and have learned to accept them over a period of many years. To them the other residents are the ones who appear sick. One of the most difficult things for a relative to do is to accept the fact that the loved one is really sick and that his or her condition may become worse. Many individuals will not accept the fact of illness, particularly if their family member has been free from disease for many years. Nor will they accept the fact that a person's behavior may change in a new environment. They may not visit frequently enough to see subtle changes. If their loved ones act strangely or appear deteriorated, families may blame it on the staff.

It is a challenge to the institution and the family to assist each other in providing the best institutional care. Families can have unreasonable grievances and/or expectations that need to be met with openness and empathy to resolve role conflicts and focus on the real issues concerning the resident. The administrator is sometimes a buffer and tries to bring objectiveness among the family, residents, physicians and staff. He or she must be responsive to the family but not to the point where resident care is adversely affected. Good communication is essential to conflict resolution and creation of support for those dealing with the various situations, reactions and emotions in the nursing facility environment.

Guidelines for building the comfort and security of the family and generally improving facility relationships with the family include:

1. Indicate willingness to listen and cooperate by checking the facts of complaints thoroughly and with an open mind. Get back to the family. Show sincere concern by listening, asking questions and clarifying facility policies.
2. Maintain an effective flow of information by anticipating and providing all necessary information concerning the operation of the facility, external and internal rules, and regulatory procedures to family members.
3. Maintain ongoing and clear communications concerning the nontechnical aspects of the facility's job and family responsibilities. Regularly scheduled conferences can keep the family informed and clarify policies and roles in the resident's care.
4. Be as factual as possible concerning the family member's medical conditions and expectations. The family needs to know the care the resident is receiving and be involved in related decisions as much as they want to be. Help the family understand the special problems associated with aging.
5. Train the staff to understand that troublesome behavior on the part of the family or resident may be indicative of a family or facility problem. Explain family and nursing facility relationships. The family must become comfortable and secure with the key personnel providing most of the care to their relative.
6. Enlist the assistance of family-member volunteers and residents to help orient families of newly admitted residents to the facility and staff. Support groups where families get together and talk can help to involve the family in the resident's care on an ongoing basis.

### Resident Councils and Family Groups

The Code of Federal Regulations (CFR) supports the formation of independent resident councils and family groups. (See Chapter 6 on resident's rights and freedom of association and communication in privacy.) Residents or families are not required to organize. Should either one or both desire to do so, the facility is required to provide private space for group meetings, designate a staff member (if the group so desires) to assist with written requests, and to listen and respond to grievances and recommendations concerning proposed operational and policy decisions. The groups plan resident/family activities and participate in educational and other programs involved with the facility community.

## Staff Relationships within the Facility

### To Residents

The nursing facility staff who come into frequent contact with the residents have a significant role in their physical and mental well-being. An attitude of sincere care, interest and respect is as important as technical skills in care of residents. During the adaptation period, the resident is likely to choose a member of the staff with whom he or she wishes to interact, with the personality of the staff member reminding him or her of loved ones with whom relationships were pleasant. Conversely, he or she may reject staff members reminiscent of those in the family disliked or not gotten along with.

### To the Family

The staff needs to be sensitive to the needs of the family members as well as those of the resident. Families and institutional staff have mutual interest in providing care. Good communication and an understanding of the process of handling varying emotions and situations from preadmission throughout the resident's stay can alleviate stress and provide support for all involved. Staff members should learn the needs and interests of the residents under their care and the others in the facility. The primary nurse plays an important role in helping the family through grief at times of crisis or death by providing sensitive notification, ensuring family privacy and comfort, and simply talking with the family members if they desire.

### Orientation and Training

Several points an administrator can include in the training of his or her staff to help meet the mental and emotional problems of the aging are:

1. Orient staff members to understand the trauma of entering a nursing facility, the important therapeutic role played by the facility in the life of each resident and the relationships of family, resident and staff members.
2. Educate the staff to appreciate the fact that the older person is also a complex being with a combination of biological, psychological and sociological needs—some of which are unique to the elderly and which must be satisfied. Nursing personnel need to demonstrate sincere care, but must control involvement and handle the occasional disagreeable outbursts of the elderly.
3. Impress upon the minds of the staff that the modern nursing facility—while providing room, board, and medical and personal assistance—is also a key factor in the quality of the resident's life. Stress the fact that the facility places emphasis on the individual resident and his or her physical, spiritual and emotional needs. Programs are designed to meet each person's needs. The facility is a place to have, participate and find some peace and fulfillment.
4. Emphasize that the purpose of the facility is to care for residents—not to keep them. Staff members should know each resident as a person and be interested, kind and considerate.
5. Train staff members in the death and dying process, including self-awareness and the handling of grief.

## Death and Dying

Elisabeth Kubler-Ross has identified and described five stages through which most people will pass when moving toward an acceptance of death. Throughout this process, there is usually hope for continued existence—a cure, a medicine or a breakthrough in research. The length of time spent in each stage varies with each individual from several seconds to many months; the nature of illness has some bearing on this. Although each person will react differently to impending death depending on personality and past lifestyles, all are terminally ill.

- **Denial (Stage 1)**—Most people initially will reject a diagnosis of terminal illness. Some will seek alternative options. This disbelief will allow time to mobilize other defenses while discussing and arranging personal affairs in face of the new situation.

- **Anger (Stage 2)**—Next, individuals will become angry, feeling helpless to control their own fate. They may ask that if many things are left to accomplish, why are they chosen to die? This anger can become displaced and projected to those in the immediate environment; however, ventilation of personal rage without judgment helps to alleviate that rage.

- **Bargaining (Stage 3)**—This relatively short but difficult phase is the beginning of a person's acceptance of his or her own fate. It often involves an evaluation of the past and can bring on guilt feelings for acts accomplished or not accomplished in the past. Often the resident will try to bargain for "a few good days or more days" in return for good behavior or a life dedicated to God or church.

- **Depression (Stage 4)**—Depression will set in as one realizes that he or she will die and that nothing can be done about it. At first, a reactive depression appears in which the individual is vocal and concentrates on what is lost (such as opportunity, relationships, occupations or home). Next comes preparatory depression—the transition between the struggle for life and the acceptance of death. This is a more silent, contemplative time.

- **Acceptance (Stage 5)**—Most people die in the stage, which is almost void of feelings; there is no fear or despair. The elderly feel that they have lived a full life, and tend to reach the stage more quickly. Although the individual gradually withdraws from the world, the need to live to the end with dignity is always there. Communication is more nonverbal than verbal at this time.

The caring and support of the nursing staff are important throughout these stages. Patience, empathy and tact are vital to help both the resident and the family through their denial to acceptance of pending loss. Many retain hope until the final moment of their lives but will want to share thoughts, fears and loneliness concerning death and dying. Sometimes practical concerns (such as property, wills, letters or services of the clergy) need action. Some of the ways to offer support and assist in coping with terminal illness and death are through offering assistance, sympathetically listening, communicating and sharing feelings, reassurance, pro-

viding a silent presence, touching and helping the dying person to share, ventilate feelings and resolve differences with family members.

### Depression

Although depression is a significant and common psychiatric disorder among the elderly in the community—and more so in nursing facilities—it is treatable. Severe losses, psychosocial changes (such as retirement, loss of role, deaths of family members and friends or increased dependency), physical illness and genetic factors can lead to deep disturbances in mood, most commonly resulting in depression. Undiagnosed and untreated depression can lead to significant interference with quality of life, distressed to staff and, at worst, suicide. The staff needs to be aware of signs of depression, including feelings of sadness, worthlessness and guilt; loss of appetite and weight; diminished interest in people and activities; and inability to enjoy life. A social worker should visit with residents who are withdrawn and isolated to determine the depth of depression. Positive reactions and discussion of previous enjoyments indicate a milder depression where residents will respond, join in some activity and move toward better self-concept. Reaction indicating that nothing is enjoyed, things only get worse and there is no purpose to life may require specialized psychiatric treatment as determined by the interdisciplinary care team.

### Resident Relationships within the Facility

#### To Other Residents

A nursing facility must be efficient in giving resident care while providing an environment conducive to quality community life. This concerns the resident's relationship to others, right of privacy, respect as an individual, room assignment and handling severe mental problems. How these resident relationships are dealt with conveys the attitude of the facility and staff.

Many residents experience a long stay in the facility, and each has a right to his or her own living space, a place for belongings, some time to himself or herself, and privacy for treatments, visiting, relaxing and other activities. The resident often interprets a nursing facility as a roadblock to independence and becomes very sensitive to invasion of privacy. In an institutional environment, this right to privacy can be often overlooked, resulting in indignation and other emotional consequences. Some considerations in this area include knocking at the door to give some control over who enters; using proper draping and adequate screens or curtains when giving treatment; closing the door while the resident is bathing to keep others from seeing his or her body; not listening in on family conversations; and not discussing the resident's condition in front of others. (It is hard to establish relationships with peers under these circumstances.)

Each resident has a right to be treated with dignity and respect. Respect of space and personal belongings adds to self-worth and personal dignity. Each resident should be addressed in an acceptable manner to identify him or her as an individual in the desired way. An attitude of respect will filter from the administration and staff to the residents and toward each other.

The room assignment of the resident will affect his or her behavior pattern toward others. The resident should be assigned a cheerful comfortable room, providing space for clothing and other personal belongings. If the resident is to share a room, compatibility of the personalities is important; persons with mental problems should not be put with those who are alert. Confused residents should be kept out of other's rooms as much as possible. Thoughtful planning in assigning rooms can go a long way in creating an atmosphere of cooperativeness among the residents and in smoothing the relationships among residents.

Minor personality changes in which the resident tends to be forgetful or shows indifference regarding his or her personal hygiene may create additional nursing and administrative problems. However, they are not justification for transference to another facility. Consideration should be given to temporary restrictions if a resident becomes disturbing or abusive to others because of personal habits. However, if the resident develops severe mental illness, is severely depressed or manic to a degree that constitutes a threat to his or her own life or the lives of others, prompt consideration must be given to having him or her transferred to another facility with suitable staff and accommodations for protection. The administrator should seek advice and an evaluation from a duly qualified psychiatrist. As the ownership has the ultimate responsibility for the safety of residents, no one with the history of suicide attempts or attempts to harm others should remain in the facility. When a resident threatens suicide, severe emotional problems are confronting that resident, and the threats may become action. A considerable risk may be involved to keep such an individual in the facility for prolonged evaluation and treatment. It could lead to legal liability of the facility in the event the resident hurts himself or herself severely or harms others.

### To Family

Whatever the varied and complicated relationships of the resident to family members, they are an important factor in meeting his or her psychological needs and have a large impact on the ability of the resident to cope with his or her situation. These relationships can be particularly stressed during placement in the facility and the subsequent adjustment period.

When a relative is admitted to a nursing facility, a loss of a member from the family structure occurs, causing grief initially and at various times during the resident's stay. This grief can manifest itself in a variety of feelings: guilt and insecurity concerning the decision not to care for the relative at home, discomfort concerning the diagnosis and prognosis of the relative's illness and his or her awareness of these factors, relief that some of the burden of care has been shifted to the facility, and blame on the family member carrying through the final decision. These emotions, previous family relationships, the degree of the resident's mental and physical incapacity, circumstances surrounding admission, stress on the person dealing with the facility and balancing many other family demands, and relationships with the nursing facility staff are all variables affecting this complicated area of family and resident relationships.

Usually the admission is not a completely voluntary act but a compromise reached among the resident and the family. Old embittered feelings may resurface at this time. If the resident does not readily adjust to the institutional environment, he or she may be hostile and resentful toward the family, rejecting them as punishment for their desertion. The resident may strike out against the immediate environment (staff or administration) as well; both family and resident become anxious and fearful of the situation.

On the other hand, the resident frequently may seek reassurance of family love and concern by complaining about the care, facility or staff. Many need confidence that relatives will be available to help and offer support. As time and disease increase dependency on others for the simple activities of daily life, the resident may become frustrated at such loss of independence and fearful in this position of powerlessness. He or she will not directly challenge the authority on whom he or she depends, but will use relatives to voice complaints and fight the battles with the staff and administration. Regression, a childlike behavioral state associated with prolonged dependence on others, also may foster such manipulation.

As understanding and confidence in the roles of the nursing facility and family develop, residents will feel less need to play the family against the facility. The offer of support and empathy by staff can give both the family and resident an opportunity to ventilate their feelings toward more mutual understanding. Studies have indicated that relationships between the elderly and their adult children are improved, and family solidarity increases when a relative is put in a nursing facility. Admission indicates that a time limit exists in which to work out unfinished relationships.

## RESIDENT COUNSELING

Many people are living longer because of the advances in medical science; however, with the possibility of expanded life span, comes the problem of chronic diseases and their effects. A person who for many years has enjoyed a happy and healthy life may be stricken in older years with a crippling disease or injury. Generally, while suffering anxiety, depression, fear and other disturbing emotions, this person does not want to be pitied or made to feel no longer useful to society; he or she wants to remain active. Because of this phenomenon and lack of training and expensive equipment, families find it necessary to rely on professionals and facilities that have the necessary expertise and equipment to take rehabilitative measures with the elderly.

Resident and family counseling involves the administrator, nurses, social worker, activities director and others in the nursing facility. Initially, counseling is needed to assist with the resolution of feelings and concerns involved with placement in the facility. Both the resident and family must come to accept the role of the facility, the needs of the resident and the role of the family. As with all problems arising in the nursing

facility community, people must be allowed to vent their feelings and discuss their concerns with non-threatening patient staff members, who can explain the relative position of the facility and help residents and/or families to come to terms with these problems.

## Rehabilitation and Motivation

Rehabilitation cannot be effective unless the individual is so motivated. It has been estimated that rehabilitation is 95 percent resident motivation. A resident uninterested and/or unwilling to cooperate in rehabilitative measures will negate the most modern equipment and trained personnel. It is very important that the resident cooperate with efforts made on his or her behalf as he or she must contribute a lot to the rehabilitative goals to achieve success. Each resident needs to participate in and agree with these goals and feel that they are attainable. The older person does not like to be talked at and will accept rehabilitative efforts if assured that the staff is interested in him or her as an individual.

The therapists and all health care facility staff can help each resident become a functioning part of the health care facility community as far as he or she is able. Rehabilitation is prompted by the warmth and assurance of a genuine interest and concern. The amount of work it takes to properly motivate a person depends largely upon the individual's background, environment and type of handicap. The responsible staff member should be acquainted with the many aspects of each individual. Obtaining background information as to previous levels of functioning and physical activities from the resident, relatives and friends will help establish the interests and social needs of each person. Working with such realities to set individual goals has the added advantages of gaining resident confidence and support. Once an atmosphere of confidence is developed, residents undoubtedly will tell staff members about their fears, doubts or resentments, thereby releasing pent up emotions and allowing staff to know and help each person individually. Thus, good communication between residents and staff members is basic to learning about the residents in the facility and to their adjustments and rehabilitation.

Encouragement, another aspect of communication, plays an important role in rehabilitation of all residents. When one is incapacitated, independence cannot be achieved in one attempt but requires continuous effort.

An amputee, for example, is not encouraged to move to a chair, to the tub and to the room in one session; he or she learns to accomplish these feats one step at a time. The hemiplegic resident likewise is not taught to walk all at one time, first learning a sitting position and then interim goals to the final achievement. Encouraged by accomplishing intermediate goals, the resident will be less prone to discouragement and regression. The mentally defective resident may be a somewhat greater problem as he or she is usually unable to understand the reasons for rehabilitation. This means that special effort must be taken to motivate this kind of resident, and accomplishments must be praised no matter how small they seem.

## Remotivation Technique

Many modern health care facilities have recreational activities and therapy, TV, visitor programs, and church and club activities to involve the residents with outside agencies and people. However, even with all these programs some residents are confused, disoriented or do not react. How can they be motivated to get out of bed, to talk, to read or to participate in programs? Remotivation is the simplest level of reality orientation and seems to be an answer. The purpose of remotivation is to encourage residents to take their minds off of their own problems, to focus attention on simple features of everyday living and to develop an interest in their new environment. Before such a technique can be used effectively, an atmosphere of high morale must be created among residents.

The two phases of motivation toward better morale to be considered are self-respect and self-reliance or independence.

- **Self-respect**—This involves the desire of people to be respected, valued and recognized by others. If a resident does not have this acceptance, the first step in the rehabilitation process is to restore or establish his or her self-esteem. The personal appearance of the elderly resident becomes very important in this context. Staff personnel can express their interest by seeing to it that the female residents' hair is curled, the males' hair is groomed, and clothing is clean, attractive and well-fitted in accordance with the resident's wishes. Rooms and surroundings should be well-kept and the residents given opportunity to socialize.

- **Self-reliance**—A resident who has lost self-reliance because of a mental or physical handicap must learn to adapt to the new environment. This individual must be convinced that participation in former social activities can be maintained, though perhaps to a lesser degree in view of the disability, and new ones enjoyed. Development of self-confidence increases in direct proportion to the confidence the resident has in the staff and his or her own success in meeting goals. As one develops self-worth, he or she feels better and will reach out to participate in various programs and socialize more.

A remotivation technique seeks to remove attention from the present emotional situation by stimulating and exercising thought and discussion. After a series of meetings, hopefully, residents will take more interest in the immediate environment, developing ties with other participants and different outlooks on the value of their lives and worth. This technique can be learned by aides and need not entail a great expense to the facility. One attendant or nurse's aide conducts one or two 30-minute to 60-minute sessions a week involving a group of 2 to 10 people. A total of 12 sessions is held. Residents are encouraged (not forced) to participate. Five specific steps involved:

- **Climate of acceptance** (5 minutes)—The leader moves around the group, which is in a circle, speaking to each person individually and thanking him or her for attending. Each resident is encouraged to reply by commenting on weather, some pleasant incident or the resident's dress. This draws each person into the session with the hope of his or her participation.
- **Bridge to a world** (15 minutes)—Objective readings are presented to the group to link the participants to the outside world and into a realm of thought apart from the facility. The leader circles the group urging each person in turn to read a brief passage. Questions on different levels are asked to stimulate discussion of the idea expressed in the reading and include as many as possible.
- **Sharing the world we live in** (15 minutes)—Objective questions are asked requiring participants to look to experiences and expand the discussion to current situations and offer personal thoughts and opinions on the subject.

- **Work of the world** (15 minutes)—The leader encourages each resident to talk about personal experiences, work and similar situations in the outside world. What kind of work or activities does he or she do? How is a particular job done?
- **Residents are thanked for attending**—Appreciation is expressed for contributions to the discussion. Participants can be asked to suggest topics for future sessions and encouraged to continue to visit in smaller groups.

## Reminiscence Therapy

Reminiscence is another effective psychosocial intervention to alleviate depression and loneliness and to increase communication, spontaneity and sociability toward forming acquaintances and friendships, especially for the frail elderly where rehabilitation may not be possible to improve quality of life. It is used in one-to-one or group interaction. Groups can provide a network to encourage residents to leave the isolation of their rooms and to share past pleasures, experiences and accomplishments with others.

In the one-to-one situation, questions concerning childhood memories and earlier times and events can be asked while the nurse or nurse assistant is performing such tasks as bathing or feeding the individual or changing the bed. In small groups, residents sit in a circle and may wear a name tag to promote self-esteem and sociability, with the group leader. Meetings are once or twice a week and last about one hour. Sessions are structured by a review of the former session's topic, focus on the day's topic enhanced by supplemental materials (pictures of people, places and events from earlier years, old songs, old occupational and decorative items) to encourage memories, ground rules (take turns sharing), planned meeting times, and a sociable outgoing leader.

Leaders may be from several disciplines, including activity directors, volunteers, nurse assistants, nurses or university students. The leader will need to assess individual residents to assist those who would need help to adapt to a group setting. A good understanding of short- and long-term memory is needed. A leader stimulates reminiscing but does not probe or encourage strong feelings. If an individual feels more lonely or isolated, reminiscence needs to be discontinued. Reminiscence may help nurses to assess a resident's needs, cognitive functions, coping ability and emotional stability.

## Activity Programs

Activity programming takes in the concepts of recreational, occupational and social activities toward meeting the needs of the residents in the facility. These programs are developed to motivate the older person to continue to use learning capacity as much as able; they require detailed planning that reflects the desires, interests and abilities of the residents. Group activities can make the older person's life more meaningful and will be successful when support is given by the administrator, activity personnel and resident participation in the selection of programs. (See Chapter 6 on the activity department for more detail.)

### BIBLIOGRAPHY

Buren, J.E. 1967. *The psychology of aging.* New York: Prentice Hall.

Buckwalter, R.C. 1989. The depressed resident: what staff can do. *Provider*, August, 1989.

Burnside, Rodriguez, and Trevino. 1989. Reminiscence therapy offers many advantages. *Provider*, August, 1989.

Davis, W. 1994. *Introduction to health care administration.* Bossier City, LA: Professional Printing & Publishing.

Duffy, M., and G. Shuttlesworth. 1989. The resident's family: Adversary or advocate in long-term care? *Journal of Long-Term Care Administration*, Fall, 1989.

Gross, J. 1985. Update: Family involvement in long-term care. *Journal of Long-Term Care Administration*, Summer, 1995.

Kubler-Ross, E. 1969. *On death and dying.* New York: Macmillan Publishing.

Moss, J. 1987. Dealing with grief is not an easy task with nursing staff. *Contemporary LTC*, October, 1987.

*Volunteer guide.* 1993. Reno, NV: Publication Services.

# Appendix 8–A

## Glossary of Terms

**Alzheimer's Disease**—Presenile dementia characterized by confusion, memory failure, disorientation and inability to carry out purposeful movements.

**Delirium**—Acute mental disorder characterized by confusion, disorientation incoherence, fear, excitement and illusions.

**Delusional**—A belief maintained in the face of incontrovertible evidence to the contrary.

**Dementia**—Impairment of mental powers due to organic disease.

**Depression**—Mood disturbance characterized by feelings of sadness, despair and discouragement proportionate to personal loss. Also abnormal emotional state characterized by exaggerated feelings of sadness, melancholy, worthlessness and hopelessness out of proportion with reality. There are many kinds of depression.

**Endogenous Depression**—Depression due to internal factors (such as biochemical changes in the brain and genetic factors).

**Exogenous Depression**—Depression due to severe loss of psychosocial change.

**Hallucination**—A false sense of perception.

**Homocidal**—A threat to do grave harm to others.

**Melancholia**—Severe depression with dull effect and lack of interest in usually enjoyed activities.

**Neurosis**—Disorder (not due to disease or nervous system) of the psyche or psychic functions. May be caused by unresolved internal conflicts.

**Paranoia**—Psychosis characterized by delusions of persecution and frequent hallucinations.

**Phobia**—Abnormal fear of a specific object, experience or place.

**Psychosocial**—Mental health, social status and functional capacity within the community.

**Remotivation**—Use of specific techniques to stimulate interest, awareness and communication of withdrawn institutionalized persons.

**Senescent**—Growing old, aging.

**Senile Dementia**—Deteriorative mental state due to organic brain damage characterized by loss of memory.

**Senile Dementia—Alzheimer Type** (SDAT)—Alzheimer's disease.

**Senile Regression**—Gradual withdrawal; tendency to live in one's memories.

**Senility**—Disease related to changes affecting mental ability.

**Stress**—Any emotional, physical, social or other factor requiring a response or change.

**Suicidal**—Prone to taking one's own life.

**Trauma**—In psychiatry, an emotional shock leaving deep psychologic impression.

### Mental Health Specialists

**Psychiatrist**—A physician who diagnoses and treats mental disorders. Does psychotherapy and counseling.

**Psychoanalyst**—A psychiatrist who specializes in the use of psychoanalysis.

**Psychologist**—A specialist (not a physician) who studies the function of the mind and behavioral patterns and gives psychological tests. Treats mental and emotional disorders through counseling; cannot prescribe drugs.

**Social Worker**—Trained (bachelor's degree in social work at minimum) to counsel people on social and/or emotional problems.

# CHAPTER 9

# Environmental Management

## ENVIRONMENTAL MANAGEMENT

From the viewpoint of environmental management, the administrator needs a knowledge of the building, the agencies and regulations concerning construction, upkeep and preventive maintenance. The physical plant must be safe, clean and orderly. This involves safe basic housekeeping and maintenance techniques, adherence to state and federal standards, keeping essential resident care equipment in safe and proper operating condition, and development and implementation of fire and disaster plans.

A nursing facility must provide a safe, sanitary, functional and comfortable environment, being designed, constructed, equipped and maintained to protect the health and safety of residents, staff and the public. All housekeeping and maintenance personnel should be particularly aware of potential hazards that could cause falls, cuts or bruises. The engineering department is responsible for correcting any unsafe conditions observed or reported to them. The areas of regulation mandated by the federal government include the American Standards of the Physically Handicapped (ANSI), the Occupational Safety and Health Act (OSHA), the Life Safety Code (LSC) (these are covered extensively under regulatory management—Chapter 1) and Medicare and Medicaid requirements under the Code of Federal Regulations (CFR). Additionally, state and local standards may apply to the buildings and grounds. Sufficient housekeeping and maintenance personnel

and equipment are required to maintain a clean, orderly and safe environment.

## Housekeeping and Maintenance Departments

The executive housekeeper needs management skills and some formal education in institutional housekeeping. He or she is a full-time employee, reporting directly to the administrator. Duties and functions include: maintaining a policy and procedures manual; hiring, training, assigning tasks and supervising personnel; time scheduling and cleaning all areas of the facility; keeping the premises sanitary; coordinating and cooperating with other departments; and writing and retaining pertinent reports and records (such as attendance, inventories, supply and equipment requests, inspection, progress or budget). A full-time employee also must have specific orientation and in-service training on infection control and prevention, aseptic techniques and applicable provisions of state and local environmental protection laws. Housekeeping and cleaning tasks are not to be undertaken by nursing or other clinical personnel. Dietary personnel perform cleaning tasks within that department only to minimize cross-contamination between residential and dietary areas. Areas must be designated to store the equipment in the facility. Cleaning equipment should be stored in janitorial closets with areas of 4 feet by 6 feet on each floor or wing. A central storage area is designated for general housekeeping supplies used in common areas of the facility. Dietary cleaning supplies are to be stored in a separate area because the cleaning of foodservice areas is a separate function requiring special skills and should not be accomplished by general housekeeping personnel.

The maintenance or engineering department is responsible for maintenance of the power plant, buildings, tools and equipment, observation of safety and fire regulations, facility security and upkeep of the grounds. The plant engineer is a full-time department head reporting directly to the administrator and should be a qualified engineer or mechanic with training and experience in the operation of such basic equipment as boilers; heating, ventilation and air conditioning systems; water supply and sewage systems; electrical systems; and use of emergency generating equipment. Many states require that the engineer be licensed in the areas of boiler operation and refrigeration. General maintenance personnel must have training in areas of basic mechanics and the tools necessary to make minor repairs; minor carpentry, wall painting, repair and cleaning skills; and yard upkeep. For more extensive specialized work, independent contractors are hired. Electricians and plumbers are licensed and knowledgeable of their applicable national and local codes. It is important to keep "as built" plans, which are the blueprints by which the facility was constructed. These plans will assist the maintenance department in troubleshooting problems more quickly and, in a number of cases, help in deciding whether to bring in outside contractors to resolve problems.

### Environmental Design for the Elderly and Handicapped

The nursing facility must have the accommodations in accordance with ANSI A117.1 necessary to meet the needs of persons with semi-ambulatory, site, hearing, coordination and other disabilities.

Details of the ANSI Code, which are important in relation to the elderly and handicapped, were covered in detail in Chapter 1. Generally, particularly noteworthy guidelines are as follow:

1. Grounds should be graded to the same level as the primary entrance.

2. Widths and gradients of walks used by the residents and public should be designed for utilization by the handicapped.
3. A properly designated parking space should be available near the building allowing room for the physically handicapped to get out of an automobile and onto the surface suitable for wheeling and walking.
4. Ramps must be designed for negotiation by individuals in wheelchairs.
5. A primary entrance usable by persons in wheelchairs must be available.
6. Doors used by residents and the public must be of sufficient width and so equipped as to permit persons in wheelchairs to open them with a single effort.
7. Stairs should be of a height and design allowing handicapped individuals to negotiate without assistance.
8. Stairs must be equipped with handrails at least one of which extends past the top and bottom slope.
9. Nonslip floors on a common level are connected by a negotiable ramp on each story.
10. An appropriate number of toilet rooms, water fountains and public telephones should be accessible to and usable by the handicapped.
11. In multi-story buildings, elevators must be accessible to and usable by the handicapped at entrance level and all levels normally used by the public.
12. Appropriate means for the door should be found to identify rooms, facilities and hazardous areas.
13. The facility must provide simultaneous audible and visual warning signals.
14. Resident beds must be of heights that permit an individual in a wheelchair to get in and out of bed unassisted.
15. Other areas of particular importance are wheelchairs, crutches, accessible routes, protruding objects and services of grounds and floors.

### Physical Environment
### 42 CFR, Sec. 483.70, Ch. IV (10-1-98)

Those facilities receiving Medicare and Medicaid funds must comply with the following requirements relating to the physical environment.

## Life Safety From Fire

The facility must be designed, constructed, equipped and maintain to protect the health and safety of residents, personnel and the public. Except as noted below, the facility must meet the applicable provisions of the 1985 edition of the National Fire Protection Association.

1. A facility is considered to be in compliance with this requirement as long as it:
   a. On November 26, 1982, complied (with or without waivers) with the requirements of the 1967 or 1973 editions of the Life Safety Code and continues to remain in compliance with those additions of the code, or
   b. On May 9, 1988, complied (with or without waivers) with the 1981 edition of the Life Safety Code and continues to remain in compliance with that edition of the code.
2. After consideration of state survey agency findings, Health Care Financing Administration (HCFA) (or in the case of intermediate care facilities, the state survey agency) may waive the specific provisions of the Life Safety Code which if rigidly applied would result in unreasonable hardship upon the facility, but only if the waiver does not adversely affect the health and safety of the residents or personnel.
3. The provisions of the Life Safety Code do not apply in a state where HCFA finds that a fire and safety code imposed by state law adequately protects patients, residents and personnel in long-term care facilities.

## Emergency Power

An emergency electrical power system must supply power adequate at least for lighting all entrances and exits, equipment to maintain fire detection, alarm and extinguishing systems, and life support systems in the event the normal electrical supply is interrupted.

When life support systems are used, the facility must provide emergency electrical power with an emergency generator that is located on the premises.

## Space and Equipment

The facility must:

1. Provide sufficient space and equipment in dining, health services, recreation and program areas to enable staff to provide residents with needed services as required by these standards and as identified in each resident's plan of care.
2. Maintain all essential mechanical, electrical and resident care equipment in safe operating condition.

## Resident Rooms

Resident rooms must be designed and equipped for adequate nursing care, comfort and privacy of residents.

1. Bedrooms must:
   a. Accommodate no more than four residents.
   b. Provide at least 80 square feet per resident in multiple resident bedrooms and at least 100 square feet in single resident bedrooms.
   c. Have direct access to an exit corridor.
   d. Be designed or equipped to assure full visual privacy for each resident.
   e. In facilities initially certified after March 31, 1992, except in private rooms, each bed must have ceiling suspended curtains that extend around the bed to provide total visual privacy in combination with adjacent walls and curtains.
   f. Have at least one window to the outside.
   g. Have a floor at or above ground level.
2. The facility must provide each resident with:
   a. A separate bed of proper size and height for the convenience of the resident.
   b. A clean, comfortable mattress.
   c. Bedding appropriate to the weather and climate.
   d. Functional furniture appropriate to the resident's needs and individual closet space in the resident's bedroom with clothes racks and shelves accessible to the resident.
3. HCFA (or in the case of a nursing facility, the survey agency) may permit variations in requirements specified for the number of residents per room and space provisions in individual cases when the facility demonstrates in writing that the variations:
   a. Are in accordance with the special needs of the residents.

b. Will not adversely affect residents' health and safety.

### Toilet Facilities

Each resident room must be equipped with or located near toilet and bathing facilities.

### Resident Call System

The nurse's station must be equipped to receive resident calls through a communication system from:
1. Resident rooms.
2. Toilet and bathing facilities.

### Dining and Resident Activities

The facility must provide one or more rooms designated for resident dining and activities. These rooms must:

1. Be well lighted.
2. Be well ventilated with nonsmoking areas identified.
3. Be adequately furnished.
4. Have sufficient space to accommodate all activities.

### Lighting

The facility must provide resident rooms and other activity areas that are well lighted. The term well-lighted, according to the interpretative guidelines (42 CFR, Chap. 10, Part 430 to end, Sec. 488.115, 10-1-98) means "levels of illumination that are suitable to the tasks performed by the resident." This covers such activities as reading, dining, religious services, birthday and other parties, and other recreational games. The lighting should have no glare and no sharp contrasts of light and dark.

### Other Environmental Conditions

The facility must provide a safe, functional, sanitary and comfortable environment for residents, staff and the public. The facility must:

1. Establish procedures to ensure that water is available to essential areas when there is a loss of normal water supply.

2. Have adequate outside ventilation by means of windows, mechanical ventilation or a combination of the two.
3. Equip corridors with firmly secured handrails on each side.
4. Maintain an effective pest control program so that the facility is free of pests and rodents.

## ENVIRONMENTAL SECURITY, SAFETY AND ACCIDENT PREVENTION

**Security** is a broad term, referring to measures taken to ensure protection and safety of residents, staff and visitors. Security means more than physical protection and, therefore, includes a variety of other protective measures. Location of the nursing facility is an important factor to consider in security planning. Some of the measures to take for protection of the resident are:

1. Make sure the building and parking areas of the facility are well lighted.
2. Make sure that monitoring devices are being used to protect wandering residents. The courts have held that if a facility has a monitoring device and intentionally turns it off for staff convenience, liability may be attributed to the facility.
3. The use of security guards often are needed in high crime areas, especially during the evening hours. Regular rounds should be made by the security guard inside and outside the building. A close relationship with local law enforcement agencies is important.
4. Local law enforcement should be advised as to the security needs of the facility. A routine inspection by local police particularly during the night shift is encouraged.
5. Entrances to the facility should all be locked from the outside.
6. Potential hazards on the nursing facility grounds need to be identified and dealt with when possible.

Environmental safety also applies to all facility personnel, residents and visitors. Safety is especially significant in a nursing facility, considering the vulnerability of the residents who usually are unable to care for themselves during emergency (fire, disaster, evacuation) situations. Ordinarily diminished sensory abilities require more light, more audible speaking and alarms, and simple traffic patterns with visual and memory aids. Special consideration is needed for the physically handicapped. The entire staff needs to be aware of these aspects of aging and their ramifications. One of the greatest incidents of accidents in nursing facilities is the falling of ambulatory residents; most falling injuries occur near the bed. **Guidelines for special consideration for accident prevention** in the safety program include:

1. An in-service training program should be made available to all personnel using heavy equipment and/or special chemicals.
2. The use of wax on corridors and other floors should be discouraged. Throw rugs and stair treads must be secure.
3. Floors should be kept in smooth and unpitted condition.
4. All corridors and exits should be free from excess beds, bedside tables, wheelchairs, magazine racks and the like.
5. Corridors, stairways and resident areas must be well-lit.
6. Special attention should be paid to uncovered radiators or steam pipes in resident rooms or corridors.
7. Any frayed or defective wiring in resident rooms and other areas must be taken care of immediately.
8. Grab bars around baths and toilet fixtures must be checked periodically to see that they are secure.
9. Fire extinguishers must be serviced a minimum of once a year to ensure proper functioning and refilling. The date of inspection and the signature of the inspector must be recorded usually on a tag attached to each extinguisher.
10. The thermostatic control on main hot water heaters and tanks must be checked.
11. All food must be kept under cover and all refuse containers covered.
12. The evacuation and safety plan is available and distributed to all personnel. This plan is tested a minimum of four times a year per shift or according to state law.

It is recommended that the following policies concerning **accident prevention regarding residents** should be implemented:

1. Medications are to be kept under lock and key at all times; narcotics under double lock. Discontinue the use of medicine bottles with smudged labels. Discard all medicines with expired prescription dates.
2. When administering medications, the nurse must not place them at the bedside and leave the room. Medicine labels are to be checked three times (i.e., before pouring, while pouring and before returning to shelf) before the medication is given to the resident.
3. The names of residents with known allergies must be noted in a conspicuous place both at the nurses' station and on the outside of the resident's chart.
4. Chronic diseases (such as diabetes or arteriosclerosis) requiring a nurse's attention should be noted on the outside of the particular resident's chart.
5. Encourage the use of high-low beds in the facility. At night, all beds should be placed in a low position unless special instructions indicate otherwise; most accidents among residents are from falling.
6. A policy regarding the use of side rails should be in writing and distributed to all nursing personnel. Side rails should be used accordingly.
7. Small night lights should be in all residents' rooms.
8. Hot water bottles are to be covered, and the temperature checked before giving them to residents.
9. Residents are not left alone in a bath or shower without at least an aide nearby. Bathroom doors should not be locked.
10. Residents are not left outside the building with crutches or in a wheelchair unattended.

Policies concerning accident prevention **regarding equipment** should include:

1. Emergency equipment (such as oxygen, resuscitator or aspirator) should be readily available, and every nurse should know where it is stored and how to use it.
2. Routine inspections are made of vital equipment (oxygen tents, wheelchairs, stretchers or aspirators) to make sure they are in good working order.

3. Emergency drugs (anticoagulants or stimulants) must be available at all times.
4. When not in use, oxygen tanks are to be strapped to carriers or held against the wall of a storage area with chains away from steam pipes and radiators. Labels on all tanks indicate whether they are full, partially full or empty.
5. Housekeeping carts with cleaning solutions should have doors closed while in use in resident areas, or be covered with a sheet or other device.

Policies for accident prevention **relative to the staff** include:

1. A safety manual should be compiled and available to all personnel with a copy retained at each nursing station.
2. There must be sufficient staff to meet the needs of the residents.
3. All personnel are to be properly trained for any procedure they administer in the facility. Most accidents among the staff result from lifting.
4. Adequate supervision must be available at all times.

The **grounds** surrounding the facility include lawns, landscaping, parking lots and sidewalks. It is important that these areas are well kept, repaired and well-lit for security and safety purposes.

It is highly recommended that the facility establish a safety committee. Some of the duties would involve review of accident reports, investigation of accidents to determine high-risk areas and establishment of preventive measures to avoid future accidents. Employee safety education should include personnel in all departments and cover orientation to safety, body mechanics and avoiding back fatigue.

**Preventive Maintenance Programs**

Planned and organized maintenance programs play an important role in keeping essential mechanical, electrical and resident care equipment in proper working order. Such equipment includes refrigerators, freezers, dishwashers, stoves, ovens, air/heat systems, plumbing, water supply and the plant. A maintenance program should be initiated when new equipment is bought and installed. One of the most common organized methods of planned maintenance is the preventive main-tenance program. The type of equipment, instructions on how to use it and its location are very important. To support a good program in this area, the facility needs manufacturer's manuals on each piece of equipment to use as a guide as to how often the particular equipment should be checked and what should be done to keep it in top running order.

The first consideration in setting up a documented preventive maintenance program is a determination of what parts of the plant and what equipment should be included. Once this has been accomplished, there should be a schedule for examining each piece of equipment used in the facility. A checklist should be used at the time of inspection. The person inspecting the equipment will make notations as to each piece's condition, date and sign the report which is then filed in a place accessible to the maintenance engineer. If the equipment is working properly, a statement to that effect should be recorded. If the equipment is defective or needs repair, it should be taken out of service immediately, a work order written to request checking and repair, and the administrator notified so that this piece may be scheduled for immediate repair or replacement.

An effective preventive maintenance program has several advantages where the safety of residents is of primary importance to the facility. It assures that the residents will not be endangered or harmed by equipment that is not working properly. Such a program will enhance the quality of care because that care is not reduced by constant breakdown of related equipment. In the end, money spent for repairs will be decreased when problems are found and solved early. An operational preventive maintenance program may prevent lawsuits involving vicarious or corporate negligence.

The cooperation of the plant engineer and executive housekeeper is important in carrying out preventive maintenance. As opposed to the use of independent contractors, the facility will be well-advised to use its own personnel for several reasons:

1. The facility has direct control and supervision over the employee.
2. Employees are on the premises to render assistance in case of emergency.
3. The cost of operating the department is under control of the administration of the facility.

Some of the disadvantages to keep in mind when carrying out this program of utilization of the facility employees are:

1. The requirement of keeping parts, manuals, instructions, schematics and blueprints provided by the manufacturers on hand.
2. Employees will need to be knowledgeable about the operation and upkeep of the equipment and usually will not have specialized knowledge in some of the more technical areas.
3. The facility will be paying more in fringe benefits and salary.

If the facility uses its own personnel to maintain and repair its equipment, all relative information and handbooks should be kept in the office of the chief maintenance person where it is accessible to those who need to use them. Such employees must be familiar with the parts manuals, instructions, blueprints and schematics provided by the manufacturer when the equipment is originally purchased.

## INFECTION CONTROL

### Infection and Pest Control

The control of infection in a nursing facility is of primary importance. Because the housekeeping department has a major role regarding the prevention of infection, sanitation and safety within the facility, it must be staffed with personnel other than those in nursing. The facility must be kept clear of dirt, rubbish, offensive odors and safety hazards. Accepted detergent disinfectant cleaning agents should be used. Personnel must be free of communicable disease and practice hygienic methods in their particular tasks. The infection control program committee writes and controls communicable disease policy and procedures. The health status of both employees and the facility must be monitored by the quality assurance committee, which is responsible for supervising the maintenance of a clean and orderly environment.

### Water Supply

The water supply available to the facility must be tested and approved by the state and/or local department of health and must include adequate provision for fire protection. The water system must comply with any local water department requirements. The CFR mandates an adequate supply for the immediate needs of the residents in case of emergency; a reservoir need not be installed if community and/or civil defense resources are available.

From cold water service and hot water tanks, mains and branches should be run to supply all plumbing fixtures and equipment with protection against backflow. Toilets and urinals should be serviced with cold water only. Each main, branch main, riser and branch to a group of fixtures to the water system should be valved and pipes sized to supply water to all fixtures with a minimum pressure of 15 pounds to the top floor fixtures during maximum demand periods. Hot water and circulating pipes should be insulated, and cold water mains in occupied spaces, storerooms and food preparation areas also must be insulated to prevent condensation.

Plumbing fixtures in nursing facilities should be an approved nonabsorptive acid-resisting type. Flush valves must be designed for quiet operation with backflow preventers and silencers. All fixtures should be installed in an approved manner, preventing cross connection and backflow.

The temperature of hot water supplied to residents should comply with state requirements. The hot water storage tank(s) should have a capacity equal of 80 percent of the heater capacity. Tanks and heaters must be of an approved type, fitted with vacuum and relief valves and automatically regulated by control valves. All water heaters should be thermostatically controlled. Hot water tanks should be of corrosion-resistant materials or otherwise properly protected.

### Garbage and Waste Disposal

If community collection services are not available, a well-designed and well-operated system must be provided for prompt routine collection and disposal of all solid waste materials originating on the premises. Odor problems can be minimized and fire safety enhanced by frequent garbage collection. Provisions should be made to clean containers and store garbage in areas that are separate from those for food handling, preparation and storage. A rack one foot above the ground outside the building must be provided for storing garbage cans, garbage and trash while waiting to be picked up. Containers should have tight-fitting lids and be kept closed to discourage ingress of flies, rodents and other pests.

The handling, storage and disposal of waste that is hazardous to residents, employees and environment is regulated by OSHA and other agencies such as the Environmental Protection Agency or local health departments. Infectious waste must be collected in bags of regulation thickness, marked with the biohazard waste symbol and disposed of by an infectious waste disposal company.

### Incineration

Incinerators must be constructed to prevent the harboring of rodents, breeding of flies, smoke, odor and flying ash. If wet trash is to be burned, auxilliary fuel firing equipment to ensure complete combustion may be required. Compactors are helpful and replace the use of incinerators in some instances.

### Sewage

Every nursing facility must be provided with an adequate and satisfactory plumbing system for disposal of body wastes. This plumbing should discharge to an approved public sewer system whenever possible. If this is not available, an individual sewage disposal system built in accordance with the requirements of the state or local health authority must be constructed.

### Insect, Rodent and Pest Control

Nursing facilities must be constructed and maintained so that the premises are free from insects and rodents by maintenance personnel or by contract with a pest control company. The premises should be kept clean and free from debris which provides harborage for insects and rodents. Windows should be screened and ventilation openings equipped with covers that close automatically when the fan is not in operation. Doors and other openings also should be equipped or designed to minimize the ingress of flies and other insects.

Preventive measures concerning pests include checking items (such as TVs, chairs or radios) brought in by residents, educating residents and families that food in resident rooms needs to be in air-tight containers, and regular checking in lounge, vending and dining areas to see that spills and food particles are cleaned as soon as possible. Kitchen appliances need to be installed so as to facilitate cleaning around and under them.

Insecticides and rodenticides may be highly toxic and flammable and must be used and stored under carefully controlled conditions mostly away from resident and food service areas. Care must be exercised to prevent accidental or intentional ingestion.

### Linen and Laundry Handling

Linen and laundry should be handled, stored and processed so that the spread of infection will be controlled. Adequate supplies of linen—which is considered three times the number of beds—should be available at all times for the comfort and care of the residents. Soiled laundry should not be permitted to accumulate. It must be kept in well-ventilated areas away from clean storage areas, residents' rooms and other storage areas. Separate linen carts for transporting soiled and clean linen should be plainly marked. Contaminated linen should be stored in double bags, clearly marked and handled separately according to OSHA standards. Proper laundry formulas should be used in the washing of linen at a water temperature of 180° F, which is usually hot enough to destroy any bacteria. If linen is sent to an outside laundry, it must conform to a technique that will destroy bacteria.

### Wall, Floor and Ceiling Surfaces

These surfaces should be dry and nonporous so as not to harbor bacterial growth. Any carpet should consist of nonabsorbent pile and withstand frequent cleaning.

## Communicable Disease and Infection

Certain infections and communicable disease may be a problem at one time or another in the facility. Some of the more common communicable diseases are measles, scarlet fever, diphtheria, chicken pox, whooping cough, mumps, and meningitis. Residents who should be segregated include those with the following diseases: anthrax, typhoid fever, tuberculosis, malaria, influenza, pneumonia, syphilis and gonorrhea. An infections control committee responsible for investigating, controlling and preventing infections is required by the CFR.

If a resident is suspected of having a communicable disease, the proper laboratory tests should be performed to ascertain whether infection exists and, if so, the resident should be properly isolated and protected. Nursing procedural manuals should include written formal asceptic and isolation techniques that are reviewed annually by the quality assurance committee and followed by all personnel taking care of these residents. Some of the **general minimal principles** to be adhered to are:

1. All materials to be destroyed should be deposited in required bags or containers until they can be disposed of.
2. Linens and other items which have come into contact with the resident must be bundled separately, washed thoroughly and properly sterilized before being placed into general circulation again.
3. Use of disposable items (such as eating and drinking utensils and other items used to care for the resident) is encouraged.
4. Personnel and others who visit residents with communicable diseases should be properly gowned. Some health facilities use disposable gowns for this purpose.
5. A standing rule should be in place that if any contact is made with the resident, hands must be washed before and immediately after such contact. Running water must be available.

The following methods are recommended in caring for an **isolated bed resident**:

1. Place the resident in a separate room with outside ventilation and private toilet and handwashing facilities.
2. The equipment in the room (including bed, tray rack, bedside cabinet, bed lamp, mattress and mattress cover) must be of a type that can be easily cleaned.
3. Towels and washcloths should be changed on a daily basis; use of disposables is recommended.
4. Bed linens should be changed every day and sterile blankets used.
5. Disposable water pitchers, glasses, salt and pepper shakers, along with paper wipes, bags and sputum cups should be used.
6. If urinals or bed pans are not disposable, they should be cleaned after each use and sterilized.
7. The floors must be mopped and the furniture (including bed frames, tray stands, chairs and cabinets) and vehicles used to transport residents wiped with soap and water on a daily basis. Do not dry dust.

### Protection of Personnel and Visitors

Instruction lists explaining how to gown, how to act while with the resident and how to ungown and wash hands properly should be posted for nursing facility personnel and visitors. A supply of disposable gowns, caps, masks, and so on should be readily available. Visitors should have a place to hang their clothes and store personal belongings away from the isolated unit.

### Food Service

Food may be served from the general kitchen to the isolated resident, using disposable utensils if available. If disposable utensils are not used, the returned trays should be separated and properly sterilized. Persons handling the contaminated tray must be gowned and use rubber gloves. All excess food must be bagged and burned in the incinerator and none returned to the refrigerator. Dishes should be washed at 140° F and rinsed at 180° F.

### Discharge Units

When the resident leaves, all parts of the room and the equipment in the room must be thoroughly cleaned to prevent the harboring of germs and spread of infection:

1. Strip the bed and wash down the entire bed and springs.
2. Autoclave the mattress.
3. Sterilize the blankets.
4. Discard all papers, magazines, books, etc.
5. Clean and sterilize thermometers.
6. Sponge pillows and rubber pads with disinfectant; air dry.
7. Thoroughly wash walls and floors.

## Infection Control
### 42 CFR, Sec. 483.65, Ch. 4 (10-1-98)

Those facilities receiving Medicare and Medicaid funds must comply with the following requirements relating to infection control.

The facility must establish and maintain an infection control program designed to provide a safe, sanitary and comfortable environment and to help prevent the development and transmission of disease and infection.

### Infection Control Program

The facility must establish an infection control program under which it:

1. Investigates, controls and prevents infections in the facility.
2. Decides what procedures, such as isolation, should be applied to an individual resident.
3. Maintains a record of incidents and corrective actions related to infections.

### Preventing the Spread of Infection

When the infection control program determines that a resident needs isolation to prevent the spread of infection, the facility must isolate the resident.

The facility must prohibit employees with a communicable disease of infected skin lesions from direct contact with residents or their food, if direct contact will transmit the disease.

The facility must require staff to wash their hands after each direct contact for which handwashing is indicated by accepted professional practice.

### Linens

Personnel must handle, store, process and transport linens so as to prevent the spread of infection.

## Bloodborne Pathogens Standards

Concerning housekeeping procedures and infection control related to bloodborne pathogens and other potentially infectious materials, OSHA mandates the following procedures:

- **Equipment**—Work surfaces contaminated with blood spills or other potentially infectious materials must be decontaminated with disinfectant upon completion of procedures and at the end of the work shift. Protective coverings, waste cans and pails must be inspected and decontaminated on a regular basis. Broken glass is cleaned up with a brush or tongs.
- **Waste**—Contaminated sharps are disposed of in closable, puncture-resistant, leakproof, red or biohazard labeled containers. Other regulated waste (liquid or semiliquid blood, potentially infectious materials, items caked with blood) are placed in closable, leakproof, red or biohazard labeled bags or containers.
- **Laundry**—The facility is responsible for laundering contaminated materials, including employee lab coats and uniforms. The contaminated laundry is to be bagged immediately by personnel wearing gloves and removed to a designated area. Red bags with the biohazard symbol are to be used unless all employees use universal precautions and are trained to handle these bags. Such laundry is handled as little as possible with limited agitation by a washer and dryer in a designated area of the facility. It may be sent to a commercial laundry in red bags clearly marked with the biohazard symbol.

(For more detail, see OSHA-Enforced Standards, Chapter 1.)

## FIRE AND DISASTER PREPAREDNESS

The purpose of a fire and disaster plan is to have available emergency procedures and ensure that specific procedures are taken to protect the public, residents and employees in the event of disasters due to earthquake, flood or tornados. The facility also is required to have a fire prevention and control program by the Life Safety Code that contains standards established by the National Fire Protection Agency (NFPA). Individual state law that has adopted and enforces these standards and the CFR both require that the facility use the NFPA guidelines under the Life Safety Code. Nursing facilities should have good working relationships with the area hospitals, police agencies and community officials when designing their disaster plans. The fire and disaster plans should address both internal and external emergency situations; total emergency preparations for community emergencies is a must. Both programs must be operational and practiced at least quarterly by appropriate drills, testing and rehearsals.

## Staff Responsibility

In assigning areas of responsibility to the staff, the training and orientation of personnel will vary depending upon the locale of the facility. In some areas, tornados may be a concern; in others, flooding is a concern. The control of fires is of concern to all areas. Fire is said to be the most common disaster, and the primary cause of fire is smoking materials. The main cause of death in fire is smoke inhalation. According to authorities, employees should become familiar with the following areas:

- **Keeping the Occurrence of Fire at a Minimum**—The housekeeping department of a facility plays a major role in this area of concern. Some of the precautions housekeeping can take are to prevent trash accumulation and have adequate storage space, specially for flammable liquids. Employees using such fluids play an extremely important role in preventing fires.
- **Detecting Fire Early**—The proper operation of smoke detection and alarm systems is a very important part of fire safety and early detection. Alarm systems should be smoke and heat sensitive and both visible and audible. Alarm systems are both manually and automatically operated.
- **Controlling the Spread of Fire**—The NFPA guidelines specifically address the construction of the health care facility. The Medicare and Medicaid final requirements in the Code of Federal Regulations also address the Life Safety Code as it relates to fire.
- **Extinguishing the Fire**—There are various classes of fires and methods used to extinguish these fires. In-service programs should be held for facility personnel on the types of fires, applicable extinguishers, markings of these extinguishers and the proper way of extinguishing the fire. (For more detail, see the Life Safety Code section of this chapter.)
- **Making Certain All Residents Are Evacuated to a Safe Place**—The personnel of the facility play a key role in helping to move residents in case of fire or other disaster. Fire disaster plans are required by various state rules and regulations. In developing a fire disaster plan, it is wise to use the resources of the local fire department. The fire or disaster evacuation plan should be modified to meet the physical makeup of the facility. The emergency evacuation plan should include assigning responsibility to a specific person to take charge (usually the highest ranking person in the facility at the time), proper

use of alarm systems by all personnel employed, prompt and efficient transfer of casualties, efficient handling of records, appropriate means of stopping the spread of fire and notifying the attending physicians when residents are involved. Special emergency plans should be made for cardiac residents that contain appropriate operation procedures and policies, frequent rehearsals and drills by the staff.

### Community Resources

The facility must be located near a community for provision of appropriate access to fire protection, hospitals and medical services. A fire hydrant must be located within a minimum of 300 feet from the facility. The nursing facility is to be located near a health care facility capable of providing emergency care based on a mutual agreement.

### In-House Emergency Equipment

The CFR requires that a facility provide an emergency source of electrical power necessary to protect the health and safety of the residents in the event of interruption of the normal electrical supply. (For more detail, see the section on physical environment in this chapter.)

By incorporation of the Life Safety Code into the CFR, the facility is required to furnish fire extinguishers throughout the building at an interval of no more than 75 feet (Class A) or 50 feet (Classes B and C) from any point to reach the nearest extinguisher and should be located low enough for persons of short stature to use.

### Training Resources

The facility should have a disaster and emergency plan that is written, available and distributed to all employees. Training resources for this plan should comply with the Medicare and Medicaid final requirements in the Code of Federal Regulations relating to disaster preparedness.

### Evacuation Resources

The evacuation plan should take into consideration the various groups of persons involved in a nursing facility operation (i.e., residents, visitors or staff). The physical plant itself should have sufficient signs and directions as to evacuation of the building in case of emergency. The signs giving directions should be distinct, constructed of raised letters with high color contrast. Charts should be displayed prominently in all parts of the building as required by state and federal law.

## Disaster and Emergency Preparedness
### 42 CFR, Sec. 483.75(m), Ch. IV (10-1-98)

Those facilities receiving Medicare and Medicaid funds must comply with the following requirements relating to disaster preparedness.

### *Disaster and Emergency Preparedness*

The facility must have detailed written plans and procedures to meet all potential emergencies and disasters, such as fire, severe weather and missing residents.

The facility must train all employees in emergency procedures when they begin to work in the facility, periodically review the procedures with existing staff and carry out unannounced staff drills using those procedures.

## BIBLIOGRAPHY

Code of Federal Regulations, Bloodborne pathogens, Title 29, 1910.1031. December 1991.

Code of Federal Regulations, 42 CFR, Parts 430 to end, Sec. 488.115, 10-1-98, Public Health.

Feldman, E. 1987. *Housekeeping handbook for institutions, business and industry*. Frederick Fall, NY.

Kurth, J.M. 1984. *Essentials of housekeeping in health care facilities*. Rockville, MD: Aspen Systems Corp.

National Association of Boards of Examiners for Nursing Home Administrators. 1997. *NAB study guide*, 3rd ed. Washington, DC.

Spivac, M. 1984. *Institutional settings: An environmental design approach*. New York: Human Sciences Press.

# Appendix 9–A

# Glossary of Environmental Management Terms

**Accident**—An unintentional or unexpected injury or damage to a person, building or equipment.

**Accident Hazard**—Part of a physical plant that may cause safety problems (such as frayed wiring, defective floors or uncontrolled water temperatures).

**American National Standards Institute** (ANSI)—An agency that sets standards to ensure that buildings are accessible to and usable by the physically handicapped.

**Americans With Disabilities Act** (ADA; Public Law 101-366)—The most sweeping nondiscrimination legislation since the Civil Rights Act of 1964, it applies to most businesses and covers all individuals with a "physical or mental impairment that substantially limits one or more major life activities."

**As Built Plans**—Final blueprints by which a building is actually constructed.

**Automatic Control Device**—A mechanism used to prevent, for instance, the temperature of water from exceeding safe ranges or to monitor the water pressure in fire extinguishment systems.

**Blueprint**—A technical illustration of a building showing exact specifications and/or measurements.

**Class A Fire**—A fire involving ordinary combustible solid materials, such as wood, paper and fabrics.

**Class B Fire**—A fire involving flammable liquids, oil, grease, gasoline or paint.

**Class C Fire**—Electrical fires.

**Contingency Plans**—Plans providing procedures for various possible incidents, such as fire, hazardous weather, earthquakes, etc. The plans are a normal part of new employees' orientation.

**Disaster Plan**—A requirement of OBRA, calling for nursing facilities to have written plans and procedures for dealing with all potential disasters.

**18 Mesh Screen**—Screen providing protection from insects; 18 mesh means there are 18 squares within a square inch of material.

**Environmental Protection Agency** (EPA)—The federal EPA sets certain standards for waste disposal and hazardous emissions. There are also state EPAs with similar functions.

**Fluorescent Light**—Most commonly a tubular light providing bright, cool, non-glare lighting.

**Iatrogenic**—An illness or condition that is a result of treatment for another condition.

**Incandescent Light**—An ordinary light bulb.

**Life Safety Code**—A code for buildings and occupant safety published by the NFPA. Most nursing facilities are required by federal standard to follow this code.

**National Fire Protection Agency** (NFPA)—This organization provides codes for safety and specifications for fire safety and building construction.

**Nosocomial**—An infection acquired while in a health care facility. For example, staph infection.

**Planned Maintenance**—A specific scheduled servicing of equipment.

**Preventive Maintenance**—A type of planned maintenance designed to replace and repair to avoid breakdowns. It is based on the historical maintenance of similar equipment and theoretically will eliminate the need for repair or breakdown by anticipating when various components will wear out.

**Schematic**—A symbol drawing of a piece of equipment or appliance. It contains standard symbols and diagrams needed for the repair of equipment (especially electronic).

# APPENDIX A

# Minimum Data Set (MDS) for Nursing Facility Resident Assessment and Care Screening

Numeric Identifier_____

# MINIMUM DATA SET (MDS) — *VERSION 2.0*
### FOR NURSING HOME RESIDENT ASSESSMENT AND CARE SCREENING
### *BASIC ASSESSMENT TRACKING FORM*

**SECTION AA. IDENTIFICATION INFORMATION**

| **GENERAL INSTRUCTIONS** |
| --- |
| *Complete this information for submission with all full and quarterly assessments (Admission, Annual, Significant Change, State or Medicare required assessments, or Quarterly Reviews, etc.).* |

**1. RESIDENT NAME** ✱

a. (First)    b. (Middle Initial)    c. (Last)    d. (Jr./Sr.)

**2. GENDER** ✱

1. Male    2. Female

**3. BIRTHDATE** ✱

☐☐ — ☐☐ — ☐☐☐☐
Month   Day   Year

**4. RACE/ ✱ ETHNICITY**

1. American Indian/Alaskan Native
2. Asian/Pacific Islander
3. Black, not of Hispanic origin
4. Hispanic
5. White, not of Hispanic origin

**5. SOCIAL ✱ SECURITY AND ✱ MEDICARE NUMBERS** [C in 1st box if non Med. no.]

a. Social Security Number
☐☐☐ — ☐☐ — ☐☐☐☐

b. Medicare number (or comparable railroad insurance number)

**6. FACILITY PROVIDER NO.** ✱

a. State No.

b. Federal No.

**7. MEDICAID NO.** ["+" if pending, "N" if not a Medicaid ✱ recipient]

**8. REASONS FOR ASSESS- MENT**

[Note—Other codes do not apply to this form]
a. Primary reason for assessment
   1. Admission assessment (required by day 14)
   2. Annual assessment
   3. Significant change in status assessment
   4. Significant correction of prior full assessment
   5. Quarterly review assessment
   10. Significant correction of prior quarterly assessment
   0. *NONE OF ABOVE*
b. Codes for assessments required for Medicare PPS or the State
   *1. Medicare 5 day assessment*
   *2. Medicare 30 day assessment*
   *3. Medicare 60 day assessment*
   *4. Medicare 90 day assessment*
   *5. Medicare readmission/return assessment*
   *6. Other state required assessment*
   *7. Medicare 14 day assessment*
   *8. Other Medicare required assessment*

**9. SIGNATURES OF PERSONS COMPLETING THESE ITEMS:**

a. Signatures     Title     Date

b.     Date

✱ = Key items for computerized resident tracking

☐ = When box blank, must enter number or letter

[a.] = When letter in box, check if condition applies

Code "—" if information unavailable or unknown

## TRIGGER LEGEND

| | |
| --- | --- |
| **1** - Delirium | **10A** - Activities (Revise) |
| **2** - Cognitive Loss/Dementia | **10B** - Activities (Review) |
| **3** - Visual Function | **11** - Falls |
| **4** - Communication | **12** - Nutritional Status |
| **5A** - ADL-Rehabilitation | **13** - Feeding Tubes |
| **5B** - ADL-Maintenance | **14** - Dehydration/Fluid Maintenance |
| **6** - Urinary Incontinence and Indwelling Catheter | **15** - Dental Care |
| **7** - Psychosocial Well-Being | **16** - Pressure Ulcers |
| **8** - Mood State | **17** - Psychotropic Drug Use |
| **9** - Behavioral Symptoms | **17\*** - For this to trigger, O4a, b, or c must = 1-7 |
| | **18** - Physical Restraints |

**Form 39242R**

PRINTED IN U.S.A.

1 of 10

MDS 2.0   1/30/98

*Source:* © 1998 Briggs Corporation, Des Moines, IA 50306 (800) 247-2343. Copyright limited to addition of trigger system.

Resident _____     Numeric Identifier _____

## MINIMUM DATA SET (MDS) — *VERSION 2.0*
### FOR NURSING HOME RESIDENT ASSESSMENT AND CARE SCREENING
### *BACKGROUND (FACE SHEET) INFORMATION AT ADMISSION*

### SECTION AB. DEMOGRAPHIC INFORMATION

| 1. | DATE OF ENTRY | *Date the stay began. Note — Does not include readmission if record was closed at time of temporary discharge to hospital, etc. In such cases, use prior admission date.* |
|---|---|---|

☐☐ — ☐☐ — ☐☐☐☐
Month   Day   Year

| 2. | ADMITTED FROM (AT ENTRY) | 1. Private home/apt. with no home health services<br>2. Private home/apt. with home health services<br>3. Board and care/assisted living/group home<br>4. Nursing home<br>5. Acute care hospital<br>6. Psychiatric hospital, MR/DD facility<br>7. Rehabilitation hospital<br>8. Other |
|---|---|---|
| 3. | LIVED ALONE (PRIOR TO ENTRY) | 0. No    1. Yes    2. In other facility |
| 4. | ZIP CODE OF PRIOR PRIMARY RESIDENCE | ☐☐☐☐☐ |

| 5. | RESIDENTIAL HISTORY 5 YEARS PRIOR TO ENTRY | *(Check all settings resident lived in during 5 years prior to date of entry given in item AB1 above.)* | |
|---|---|---|---|
| | | Prior stay at this nursing home | a. |
| | | Stay in other nursing home | b. |
| | | Other residential facility — board and care home, assisted living, group home | c. |
| | | MH/psychiatric setting | d. |
| | | MR/DD setting | e. |
| | | *NONE OF ABOVE* | f. |

| 6. | LIFETIME OCCUPATION(S) (Put "/" between two occupations) | |
|---|---|---|

| 7. | EDUCATION (*Highest level completed*) | 1. No schooling      5. Technical or trade school<br>2. 8th grade/less   6. Some college<br>3. 9-11 grades       7. Bachelor's degree<br>4. High school       8. Graduate degree |
|---|---|---|
| 8. | LANGUAGE | *(Code for correct response)*<br>a. Primary Language<br>0. English    1. Spanish    2. French    3. Other |
| | | b. If other, specify ☐☐☐☐☐☐☐☐☐☐ |
| 9. | MENTAL HEALTH HISTORY | Does resident's RECORD indicate any history of mental retardation, mental illness, or developmental disability problem?<br>0. No          1. Yes |

| 10. | CONDITIONS RELATED TO MR/DD STATUS | *(Check all conditions that are related to MR/DD status that were manifested before age 22, and are likely to continue indefinitely)* | |
|---|---|---|---|
| | | Not applicable — no MR/DD (Skip to AB11) | a. |
| | | MR/DD with organic condition | b. |
| | | Down's syndrome | |
| | | Autism | c. |
| | | Epilepsy | d. |
| | | Other organic condition related to MR/DD | e. |
| | | MR/DD with no organic condition | f. |

| 11. | DATE BACKGROUND INFORMATION COMPLETED | |
|---|---|---|

☐☐ — ☐☐ — ☐☐☐☐
Month   Day   Year

### SECTION AC. CUSTOMARY ROUTINE

| 1. | CUSTOMARY ROUTINE<br><br>*(In year prior to DATE OF ENTRY to this nursing home, or year last in community if now being admitted from another nursing home)* | *(Check all that apply. If all information UNKNOWN, check last box only)* | |
|---|---|---|---|
| | | **CYCLE OF DAILY EVENTS** | |
| | | Stays up late at night (e.g., after 9 pm) | a. |
| | | Naps regularly during day (at least 1 hour) | b. |
| | | Goes out 1+ days a week | c. |
| | | Stays busy with hobbies, reading, or fixed daily routine | d. |
| | | Spends most of time alone or watching TV | e. |
| | | Moves independently indoors (with appliances, if used) | f. |
| | | Use of tobacco products at least daily | g. |
| | | *NONE OF ABOVE* | h. |
| | | **EATING PATTERNS** | |
| | | Distinct food preferences | i. |
| | | Eats between meals all or most days | j. |
| | | Use of alcoholic beverage(s) at least weekly | k. |
| | | *NONE OF ABOVE* | l. |
| | | **ADL PATTERNS** | |
| | | In bedclothes much of day | m. |
| | | Wakens to toilet all or most nights | n. |
| | | Has irregular bowel movement pattern | o. |
| | | Showers for bathing | p. |
| | | Bathing in PM | q. |
| | | *NONE OF ABOVE* | r. |
| | | **INVOLVEMENT PATTERNS** | |
| | | Daily contact with relatives/close friends | s. |
| | | Usually attends church, temple, synagogue (etc.) | t. |
| | | Finds strength in faith | u. |
| | | Daily animal companion/presence | v. |
| | | Involved in group activities | w. |
| | | *NONE OF ABOVE* | x. |
| | | **UNKNOWN — Resident/family unable to provide information** | y. |

**END**

### SECTION AD. FACE SHEET SIGNATURES
SIGNATURES OF PERSONS COMPLETING FACE SHEET:

| a. Signature of RN Assessment Coordinator | | | Date |
|---|---|---|---|
| b. Signatures | Title | Sections | Date |
| c. | | | Date |
| d. | | | Date |
| e. | | | Date |
| f. | | | Date |
| g. | | | Date |

☐ = When box blank, must enter number or letter

☐a. = When letter in box, check if condition applies

Code "—" if information unavailable or unknown

NOTE: Normally, the MDS Face Sheet is completed once, when an individual first enters the facility. However, the face sheet is also required if the person is reentering this facility after a discharge where return had not previously been expected. It is **not** completed following temporary discharges to hospitals or after therapeutic leaves/home visits.

Form 39242R

MDS 2.0   1/30/98

*Source:* © 1998 Briggs Corporation, Des Moines, IA 50306 (800) 247-2343. Copyright limited to addition of trigger system.

Resident _____  Numeric Identifier _____

# MINIMUM DATA SET (MDS) — *VERSION 2.0*
## FOR NURSING HOME RESIDENT ASSESSMENT AND CARE SCREENING
### *FULL ASSESSMENT FORM*
(Status in last 7 days, unless other time frame indicated)

## SECTION A. IDENTIFICATION AND BACKGROUND INFORMATION

| | | |
|---|---|---|
| 1. | RESIDENT NAME | a. (First)   b. (Middle Initial)   c. (Last)   d. (Jr./Sr.) |
| 2. | ROOM NUMBER | |
| 3. | ASSESS-MENT REFERENCE DATE | a. *Last day of MDS observation period*<br>Month — Day — Year<br>b. Original (0) or corrected copy of form (enter number of correction) |
| 4a. | DATE OF REENTRY | Date of reentry from most recent temporary discharge to a hospital in last 90 days (or since last assessment or admission if less than 90 days)<br>Month — Day — Year |
| 5. | MARITAL STATUS | 1. Never married   3. Widowed   5. Divorced<br>2. Married   4. Separated |
| 6. | MEDICAL RECORD NO. | |
| 7. | CURRENT PAYMENT SOURCES FOR N.H. STAY | *(Billing Office to indicate; check all that apply in last 30 days)*<br>Medicaid per diem — a.    VA per diem — f.<br>Medicare per diem — b.    Self or family pays for full per diem — g.<br>Medicare ancillary part A — c.    Medicaid resident liability or Medicare co-payment — h.<br>Medicare ancillary part B — d.    Private insurance per diem (including co-payment) — i.<br>CHAMPUS per diem — e.    Other per diem — j. |
| 8. | REASONS FOR ASSESS-MENT<br><br>*[Note—If this is a discharge or reentry assessment, only a limited subset of MDS items need be completed]* | a. Primary reason for assessment<br>1. Admission assessment (required by day 14)<br>2. Annual assessment<br>3. Significant change in status assessment<br>4. Significant correction of prior full assessment<br>5. Quarterly review assessment<br>6. Discharged—return not anticipated<br>7. Discharged—return anticipated<br>8. Discharged prior to completing initial assessment<br>9. Reentry<br>10. Significant correction of prior quarterly assessment<br>0. NONE OF ABOVE<br>b. Codes for assessments required for Medicare PPS or the State<br>1. Medicare 5 day assessment<br>2. Medicare 30 day assessment<br>3. Medicare 60 day assessment<br>4. Medicare 90 day assessment<br>5. Medicare readmission/return assessment<br>6. Other state required assessment<br>7. Medicare 14 day assessment<br>8. Other Medicare required assessment |
| 9. | RESPONSI-BILITY/ LEGAL GUARDIAN | *(Check all that apply)*<br>Legal guardian — a.    Durable power of attorney/financial — d.<br>Other legal oversight — b.    Family member responsible — e.<br>Durable power of attorney/health care — c.    Patient responsible for self — f.<br>NONE OF ABOVE — g. |
| 10. | ADVANCED DIRECTIVES | *(For those items with supporting documentation in the medical record, check all that apply)*<br>Living will — a.    Feeding restrictions — f.<br>Do not resuscitate — b.    Medication restrictions — g.<br>Do not hospitalize — c.    Other treatment restrictions — h.<br>Organ donation — d.    NONE OF ABOVE — i.<br>Autopsy request — e. |

## SECTION B. COGNITIVE PATTERNS

| | | |
|---|---|---|
| 1. | COMATOSE | *(Persistent vegetative state/no discernible consciousness)*<br>0. No   1. Yes *(If yes, skip to Section G)* |
| 2. | MEMORY | *(Recall of what was learned or known)*<br>a. Short-term memory OK—seems/appears to recall after 5 minutes<br>0. Memory OK   1. Memory problem 2<br>b. Long-term memory OK—seems/appears to recall long past<br>0. Memory OK   1. Memory problem 2 |

☐ = When box blank, must enter number or letter.

a. = When letter in box, check if condition applies

Code "—" if information unavailable or unknown

Form 39242R

| | | |
|---|---|---|
| 3. | MEMORY/ RECALL ABILITY | *(Check all that resident was normally able to recall during last 7 days)*<br>Current season — a.    That he/she is in a nursing home — d.<br>Location of own room — b.    NONE OF ABOVE are recalled — e.<br>Staff names/faces — c. |
| 4. | COGNITIVE SKILLS FOR DAILY DECISION-MAKING | *(Made decisions regarding tasks of daily life)*<br>0. INDEPENDENT—decisions consistent/reasonable<br>1. MODIFIED INDEPENDENCE—some difficulty in new situations only 2<br>2. MODERATELY IMPAIRED—decisions poor; cues/supervision required 2<br>3. SEVERELY IMPAIRED—never/rarely made decisions 2, 5B |
| 5. | INDICATORS OF DELIRIUM— PERIODIC DISOR-DERED THINKING/ AWARENESS | *(Code for behavior in the last 7 days.)* [Note: Accurate assessment requires conversations with staff and family who have direct knowledge of resident's behavior over this time.]<br>0. Behavior not present<br>1. Behavior present, not of recent onset<br>2. Behavior present, over last 7 days appears different from resident's usual functioning (e.g., new onset or worsening)<br>a. EASILY DISTRACTED—(e.g., difficulty paying attention; gets sidetracked) 2 = 1, 17*<br>b. PERIODS OF ALTERED PERCEPTION OR AWARENESS OF SURROUNDINGS—(e.g., moves lips or talks to someone not present; believes he/she is somewhere else; confuses night and day) 2 = 1, 17*<br>c. EPISODES OF DISORGANIZED SPEECH—(e.g., speech is incoherent, nonsensical, irrelevant, or rambling from subject to subject; loses train of thought) 2 = 1, 17*<br>d. PERIODS OF RESTLESSNESS—(e.g., fidgeting or picking at skin, clothing, napkins, etc.; frequent position changes; repetitive physical movements or calling out) 2 = 1, 17*<br>e. PERIODS OF LETHARGY—(e.g., sluggishness; staring into space; difficult to arouse; little body movement) 2 = 1, 17*<br>f. MENTAL FUNCTION VARIES OVER THE COURSE OF THE DAY—(e.g., sometimes better, sometimes worse; behaviors sometimes present, sometimes not) 2 = 1, 17* |
| 6. | CHANGE IN COGNITIVE STATUS | Resident's cognitive status, skills, or abilities have changed as compared to status of 90 days ago (or since last assessment if less than 90 days)<br>0. No change   1. Improved   2. Deteriorated 1, 17* |

## SECTION C. COMMUNICATION/HEARING PATTERNS

| | | |
|---|---|---|
| 1. | HEARING | *(With hearing appliance, if used)*<br>0. HEARS ADEQUATELY—normal talk, TV, phone<br>1. MINIMAL DIFFICULTY when not in quiet setting 4<br>2. HEARS IN SPECIAL SITUATIONS ONLY—speaker has to adjust tonal quality and speak distinctly 4<br>3. HIGHLY IMPAIRED/absence of useful hearing 4 |
| 2. | COMMUNI-CATION DEVICES/ TECH-NIQUES | *(Check all that apply during last 7 days)*<br>Hearing aid, present and used — a.<br>Hearing aid, present and not used regularly — b.<br>Other receptive comm. techniques used (e.g., lip reading) — c.<br>NONE OF ABOVE — d. |
| 3. | MODES OF EXPRESSION | *(Check all used by resident to make needs known)*<br>Speech — a.    Signs/gestures/sounds — d.<br>Writing messages to express or clarify needs — b.    Communication board — e.<br>American sign language or Braille — c.    Other — f.<br>NONE OF ABOVE — g. |
| 4. | MAKING SELF UNDER-STOOD | *(Expressing information content—however able)*<br>0. UNDERSTOOD<br>1. USUALLY UNDERSTOOD—difficulty finding words or finishing thoughts 4<br>2. SOMETIMES UNDERSTOOD—ability is limited to making concrete requests 4<br>3. RARELY/NEVER UNDERSTOOD 4 |
| 5. | SPEECH CLARITY | *(Code for speech in the last 7 days)*<br>0. CLEAR SPEECH—distinct, intelligible words<br>1. UNCLEAR SPEECH—slurred, mumbled words<br>2. NO SPEECH—absence of spoken words |
| 6. | ABILITY TO UNDER-STAND OTHERS | *(Understanding verbal information content—however able)*<br>0. UNDERSTANDS<br>1. USUALLY UNDERSTANDS—may miss some part/intent of message 2, 4<br>2. SOMETIMES UNDERSTANDS—responds adequately to simple, direct communication 2, 4<br>3. RARELY/NEVER UNDERSTANDS 2, 4 |
| 7. | CHANGE IN COMMUNI-CATION/ HEARING | Resident's ability to express, understand, or hear information has changed as compared to status of 90 days ago (or since last assessment if less than 90 days)<br>0. No change   1. Improved   2. Deteriorated 17* |

TRIGGER LEGEND
1 - Delirium
2 - Cognitive Loss/Dementia
4 - Communication
5B - ADL Maintenance
17* - Psychotropic Drugs
(For this to trigger, O4a, b, or c must = 1-7)

PRINTED IN U.S.A.

MDS 2.0   1/30/98

*Source:* © 1998 Briggs Corporation, Des Moines, IA 50306 (800) 247-2343. Copyright limited to addition of trigger system.

Resident _____

## SECTION D. VISION PATTERNS

| 1. | VISION | *(Ability to see in adequate light and with glasses if used)* | |
|---|---|---|---|
| | | 0. *ADEQUATE*—sees fine detail, including regular print in newspapers/books | |
| | | 1. *IMPAIRED*—sees large print, but not regular print in newspapers/books **3** | |
| | | 2. *MODERATELY IMPAIRED*—limited vision; not able to see newspaper headlines, but can identify objects **3** | |
| | | 3. *HIGHLY IMPAIRED*—object identification in question, but eyes appear to follow objects **3** | |
| | | 4. *SEVERELY IMPAIRED*—no vision or sees only light, colors, or shapes; eyes do not appear to follow objects | |
| 2. | VISUAL LIMITATIONS/ DIFFICULTIES | Side vision problems—decreased peripheral vision (e.g., leaves food on one side of tray, difficulty traveling, bumps into people and objects, misjudges placement of chair when seating self) **3** | a. |
| | | Experiences any of following: sees halos or rings around lights; sees flashes of light; sees "curtains" over eyes | b. |
| | | *NONE OF ABOVE* | c. |
| 3. | VISUAL APPLIANCES | Glasses; contact lenses; magnifying glass | |
| | | 0. No      1. Yes | |

## SECTION E. MOOD AND BEHAVIOR PATTERNS

| 1. | INDICATORS OF DEPRESSION, ANXIETY, SAD MOOD | *(Code for indicators observed in last 30 days, irrespective of the assumed cause)* <br> 0. Indicator not exhibited in last 30 days <br> 1. Indicator of this type exhibited up to five days a week <br> 2. Indicator of this type exhibited daily or almost daily (6, 7 days a week) | |
|---|---|---|---|

**VERBAL EXPRESSIONS OF DISTRESS**

a. Resident made negative statements—e.g., "Nothing matters; Would rather be dead; What's the use; Regrets having lived so long; Let me die" 1 or 2 = **8**

b. Repetitive questions—e.g., "Where do I go; What do I do?" 1 or 2 = **8**

c. Repetitive verbalizations—e.g., calling out for help ("God help me") 1 or 2 = **8**

d. Persistent anger with self or others—e.g., easily annoyed, anger at placement in nursing home; anger at care received 1 or 2 = **8**

e. Self deprecation—e.g., "I am nothing; I am of no use to anyone" 1 or 2 = **8**

f. Expressions of what appear to be unrealistic fears—e.g., fear of being abandoned, left alone, being with others 1 or 2 = **8**

g. Recurrent statements that something terrible is about to happen—e.g., believes he or she is about to die, have a heart attack 1 or 2 = **8**

h. Repetitive health complaints—e.g., persistently seeks medical attention, obsessive concern with body functions 1 or 2 = **8**

i. Repetitive anxious complaints/concerns (non-health related)—e.g., persistently seeks attention/reassurance regarding schedules, meals, laundry/clothing, relationship issues 1 or 2 = **8**

**SLEEP-CYCLE ISSUES**

j. Unpleasant mood in morning 1 or 2 = **8**

k. Insomnia/change in usual sleep pattern 1 or 2 = **8**

**SAD, APATHETIC, ANXIOUS APPEARANCE**

l. Sad, pained, worried facial expressions—e.g., furrowed brows 1 or 2 = **8**

m. Crying, tearfulness 1 or 2 = **8**

n. Repetitive physical movements—e.g., pacing, hand wringing, restlessness, fidgeting, picking 1 or 2 = **8, 17\***

**LOSS OF INTEREST**

o. Withdrawal from activities of interest—e.g., no interest in longstanding activities or being with family/friends 1 or 2 = **7, 8**

p. Reduced social interaction 1 or 2 = **8**

| 2. | MOOD PERSISTENCE | One or more indicators of depressed, sad or anxious mood were not easily altered by attempts to "cheer up", console, or reassure the resident over last 7 days <br> 0. No mood     1. Indicators present,     2. Indicators present, <br> indicators     easily altered **8**     not easily altered **8** | |
|---|---|---|---|
| 3. | CHANGE IN MOOD | Resident's mood status has changed as compared to status of 90 days ago (or since last assessment if less than 90 days) <br> 0. No change     1. Improved     2. Deteriorated **1, 17\*** | |
| 4. | BEHAVIORAL SYMPTOMS | *(A) Behavioral symptom frequency in last 7 days* <br> 0. Behavior not exhibited in last 7 days <br> 1. Behavior of this type occurred 1 to 3 days in last 7 days <br> 2. Behavior of this type occurred 4 to 6 days, but less than daily <br> 3. Behavior of this type occurred daily <br> *(B) Behavioral symptom alterability in last 7 days* <br> 0. Behavior not present OR behavior was easily altered <br> 1. Behavior was not easily altered | (A)  (B) |

a. WANDERING (moved with no rational purpose, seemingly oblivious to needs or safety) A = 1, 2, or 3 = **9, 11**

b. VERBALLY ABUSIVE BEHAVIORAL SYMPTOMS (others were threatened, screamed at, cursed at) A = 1, 2, or 3 = **9**

c. PHYSICALLY ABUSIVE BEHAVIORAL SYMPTOMS (others were hit, shoved, scratched, sexually abused) A = 1, 2, or 3 = **9**

d. SOCIALLY INAPPROPRIATE/DISRUPTIVE BEHAVIORAL SYMPTOMS (made disruptive sounds, noisiness, screaming, self-abusive acts, sexual behavior or disrobing in public, smeared/threw food/feces, hoarding, rummaged through others' belongings) A = 1, 2, or 3 = **9**

e. RESISTS CARE (resisted taking medications/injections, ADL assistance, or eating) A = 1, 2, or 3 = **9**

---

Numeric Identifier _____

| 5. | CHANGE IN BEHAVIORAL SYMPTOMS | Resident's behavior status has changed as compared to **status** of 90 days ago (or since last assessment if less than 90 days) <br> 0. No change     1. Improved **9**     2. Deteriorated **1, 17\*** | |
|---|---|---|---|

## SECTION F. PSYCHOSOCIAL WELL-BEING

| 1. | SENSE OF INITIATIVE/ INVOLVEMENT | At ease interacting with others | a. |
|---|---|---|---|
| | | At ease doing planned or structured activities | b. |
| | | At ease doing self-initiated activities | c. |
| | | Establishes own goals **7** | d. |
| | | Pursues involvement in life of facility (e.g., makes/keeps friends; involved in group activities; responds positively to new activities; assists at religious services) | e. |
| | | Accepts invitations into most group activities | f. |
| | | *NONE OF ABOVE* | g. |
| 2. | UNSETTLED RELATIONSHIPS | Covert/open conflict with or repeated criticism of staff **7** | a. |
| | | Unhappy with roommate **7** | b. |
| | | Unhappy with residents other than roommate **7** | c. |
| | | Openly expresses conflict/anger with family/friends **7** | d. |
| | | Absence of personal contact with family/friends | e. |
| | | Recent loss of close family member/friend | f. |
| | | Does not adjust easily to change in routines | g. |
| | | *NONE OF ABOVE* | h. |
| 3. | PAST ROLES | Strong identification with past roles and life status **7** | a. |
| | | Expresses sadness/anger/empty feeling over lost roles/status **7** | b. |
| | | Resident perceives that daily routine (customary routine, activities) is very different from prior pattern in the community **7** | c. |
| | | *NONE OF ABOVE* | d. |

## SECTION G. PHYSICAL FUNCTIONING AND STRUCTURAL PROBLEMS

| 1. | (A) ADL SELF-PERFORMANCE—*(Code for resident's PERFORMANCE OVER ALL SHIFTS during last 7 days—Not including setup)* |
|---|---|

0. *INDEPENDENT*—No help or oversight—OR—Help/oversight provided only 1 or 2 times during last 7 days

1. *SUPERVISION*—Oversight, encouragement or cueing provided 3 or more times during last 7 days—OR—Supervision (3 or more times) plus physical assistance provided only 1 or 2 times during last 7 days

2. *LIMITED ASSISTANCE*—Resident highly involved in activity; received physical help in guided maneuvering of limbs or other nonweight bearing assistance 3 or more times—OR—More help provided only 1 or 2 times during last 7 days

3. *EXTENSIVE ASSISTANCE*—While resident performed part of activity, over last 7-day period, help of following type(s) provided 3 or more times: <br> —Weight-bearing support <br> —Full staff performance during part (but not all) of last 7 days

4. *TOTAL DEPENDENCE*—Full staff performance of activity during entire 7 days

8. *ACTIVITY DID NOT OCCUR* during entire 7 days

(B) ADL SUPPORT PROVIDED—*(Code for MOST SUPPORT PROVIDED OVER ALL SHIFTS during last 7 days; code regardless of resident's self-performance classification)*

0. No setup or physical help from staff    3. Two+ persons physical assist
1. Setup help only    8. ADL activity itself did not
2. One person physical assist      occur during entire 7 days

| | | | (A) SELF-PERF | (B) SUPPORT |
|---|---|---|---|---|
| a. | BED MOBILITY | How resident moves to and from lying position, turns side to side, and positions body while in bed <br> A = 1 = **5A**; A = 2, 3, or 4 = **5A, 16**; A = 8 = **16** | | |
| b. | TRANSFER | How resident moves between surfaces—to/from: bed, chair, wheelchair, standing position (EXCLUDE to/from bath/toilet) <br> A = 1, 2, 3, or 4 = **5A** | | |
| c. | WALK IN ROOM | How resident walks between locations in his/her room <br> A = 1, 2, 3, or 4 = **5A** | | |
| d. | WALK IN CORRIDOR | How resident walks in corridor on unit <br> A = 1, 2, 3, or 4 = **5A** | | |
| e. | LOCOMOTION ON UNIT | How resident moves between locations in his/her room and adjacent corridor on same floor. If in wheelchair, self-sufficiency once in chair  A = 1, 2, 3, or 4 = **5A** | | |
| f. | LOCOMOTION OFF UNIT | How resident moves to and returns from off unit locations (e.g., areas set aside for dining, activities, or treatments). If facility has only one floor, how resident moves to and from distant areas on the floor. If in wheelchair, self-sufficiency once in chair <br> A = 1, 2, 3, or 4 = **5A** | | |
| g. | DRESSING | How resident puts on, fastens, and takes off all items of street clothing, including donning/removing prosthesis <br> A = 1, 2, 3, or 4 = **5A** | | |
| h. | EATING | How resident eats and drinks (regardless of skill). Includes intake of nourishment by other means (e.g., tube feeding, total parenteral nutrition) A = 1, 2, 3, or 4 = **5A** | | |
| i. | TOILET USE | How resident uses the toilet room (or commode, bedpan, urinal); transfers on/off toilet, cleanses, changes pad, manages ostomy or catheter, adjusts clothes <br> A = 1, 2, 3, or 4 = **5A** | | |
| j. | PERSONAL HYGIENE | How resident maintains personal hygiene, including combing hair, brushing teeth, shaving, applying makeup, washing/drying face, hands, and perineum (EXCLUDE baths and showers) A = 1, 2, 3, or 4 = **5A** | | |

**TRIGGER LEGEND**

| | |
|---|---|
| 1 - Delirium | 8 - Mood State |
| 3 - Visual Function | 9 - Behavior Symptoms |
| 5A - ADL Rehabilitation | 11 - Falls |
| 7 - Psychosocial Well-Being | 17\* - Psychotropic Drugs |
| | (\*For this to trigger, O4a, b, or c must = 1-7) |

*Source:* © 1998 Briggs Corporation, Des Moines, IA 50306 (800) 247-2343. Copyright limited to addition of trigger system.

Resident _____     Numeric Identifier _____

| 2. | BATHING | How resident takes full-body bath/shower, sponge bath, and transfers in/out of tub/shower (EXCLUDE washing of back and hair). *Code for most dependent in self-performance and support.* — 5A<br>(A) BATHING SELF-PERFORMANCE codes appear below.<br>0. Independent—No help provided<br>1. Supervision—Oversight help only<br>2. Physical help limited to transfer only<br>3. Physical help in part of bathing activity<br>4. Total dependence<br>8. Activity itself did not occur during entire 7 days<br>*(Bathing support codes are as defined in Item 1, code B above)* |
|---|---|---|

(A) (B)

| 3. | TEST FOR BALANCE<br>(See training manual) | *(Code for ability during test in the last 7 days)*<br>0. Maintained position as required in test<br>1. Unsteady, but able to rebalance self without physical support<br>2. Partial physical support during test; or stands (sits) but does not follow directions for test<br>3. Not able to attempt test without physical help |
|---|---|---|

| | |
|---|---|
| a. Balance while standing | |
| b. Balance while sitting—position, trunk control 1, 2, or 3 = 17* | |

| 4. | FUNCTIONAL LIMITATION IN RANGE OF MOTION<br>(see training manual) | *(Code for limitations during last 7 days that interfered with daily functions or placed resident at risk of injury)*<br>*(A) RANGE OF MOTION*  *(B) VOLUNTARY MOVEMENT*<br>0. No limitation    0. No loss<br>1. Limitation on one side  1. Partial loss<br>2. Limitation on both sides  2. Full loss |
|---|---|---|

(A) (B)

| | |
|---|---|
| a. Neck | |
| b. Arm—Including shoulder or elbow | |
| c. Hand—Including wrist or fingers | |
| d. Leg—Including hip or knee | |
| e. Foot—Including ankle or toes | |
| f. Other limitation or loss | |

| 5. | MODES OF LOCOMOTION | *(Check all that apply during last 7 days)* |
|---|---|---|

| | | | |
|---|---|---|---|
| Cane/walker/crutch | a. | Wheelchair primary mode of locomotion | d. |
| Wheeled self | b. | | |
| Other person wheeled | c. | NONE OF ABOVE | e. |

| 6. | MODES OF TRANSFER | *(Check all that apply during last 7 days)* |
|---|---|---|

| | | | |
|---|---|---|---|
| Bedfast all or most of time 16 | a. | Lifted mechanically | d. |
| Bed rails used for bed mobility or transfer | b. | Transfer aid (e.g., slide board, trapeze, cane, walker, brace) | e. |
| Lifted manually | c. | NONE OF ABOVE | f. |

| 7. | TASK SEGMENTATION | Some or all of ADL activities were broken into subtasks during last 7 days so that resident could perform them<br>0. No    1. Yes |
|---|---|---|

| 8. | ADL FUNCTIONAL REHABILITATION POTENTIAL | Resident believes he/she is capable of increased independence in at least some ADLs 5A | a. |
|---|---|---|---|
| | | Direct care staff believe resident is capable of increased independence in at least some ADLs 5A | b. |
| | | Resident able to perform tasks/activity but is very slow | c. |
| | | Difference in ADL Self-Performance or ADL Support, comparing mornings to evenings | d. |
| | | NONE OF ABOVE | e. |

| 9. | CHANGE IN ADL FUNCTION | Resident's ADL self-performance status has changed as compared to status of 90 days ago (or since last assessment if less than 90 days)<br>0. No change   1. Improved   2. Deteriorated |
|---|---|---|

## SECTION H. CONTINENCE IN LAST 14 DAYS

| 1. | CONTINENCE SELF-CONTROL CATEGORIES<br>*(Code for resident's PERFORMANCE OVER ALL SHIFTS)*<br>0. CONTINENT—Complete control *(includes use of indwelling urinary catheter or ostomy device that does not leak urine or stool)*<br>1. USUALLY CONTINENT—BLADDER, incontinent episodes once a week or less; BOWEL, less than weekly<br>2. OCCASIONALLY INCONTINENT—BLADDER, 2 or more times a week but not daily; BOWEL, once a week<br>3. FREQUENTLY INCONTINENT—BLADDER, tended to be incontinent daily, but some control present (e.g., on day shift); BOWEL, 2-3 times a week<br>4. INCONTINENT—Had inadequate control. BLADDER, multiple daily episodes; BOWEL, all (or almost all) of the time |
|---|---|

| a. | BOWEL CONTINENCE | Control of bowel movement, with appliance or bowel continence programs, if employed 1, 2, 3 or 4 = 16 | |
|---|---|---|---|
| b. | BLADDER CONTINENCE | Control of urinary bladder function (if dribbles, volume insufficient to soak through underpants), with appliances (e.g., foley) or continence programs, if employed 2, 3 or 4 = 6 | |

| 2. | BOWEL ELIMINATION PATTERN | Bowel elimination pattern regular—at least one movement every three days | a. | Diarrhea | c. |
|---|---|---|---|---|---|
| | | | | Fecal impaction 17* | d. |
| | | Constipation 17* | b. | NONE OF ABOVE | e. |

| 3. | APPLIANCES AND PROGRAMS | Any scheduled toileting plan | a. | Did not use toilet room/commode/urinal | f. |
|---|---|---|---|---|---|
| | | Bladder retraining program | b. | Pads/briefs used 6 | g. |
| | | External (condom) catheter 6 | c. | Enemas/irrigation | h. |
| | | Indwelling catheter 6 | d. | Ostomy present | i. |
| | | Intermittent catheter 6 | e. | NONE OF ABOVE | j. |

| 4. | CHANGE IN URINARY CONTINENCE | Resident's urinary continence has changed as compared to status of 90 days ago (or since last assessment if less than 90 days)<br>0. No change    1. Improved    2. Deteriorated |
|---|---|---|

## SECTION I. DISEASE DIAGNOSES

Check only those diseases that have a relationship to current ADL status, cognitive status, mood and behavior status, medical treatments, nursing monitoring, or risk of death. (Do not list inactive diagnoses.)

| 1. | DISEASES | *(If none apply, CHECK the NONE OF ABOVE box)* | | | |
|---|---|---|---|---|---|
| | | ENDOCRINE/METABOLIC/NUTRITIONAL | | Hemiplegia/Hemiparesis | v. |
| | | Diabetes mellitus | a. | Multiple sclerosis | w. |
| | | Hyperthyroidism | b. | Paraplegia | x. |
| | | Hypothyroidism | c. | Parkinson's disease | y. |
| | | HEART/CIRCULATION | | Quadriplegia | z. |
| | | Arteriosclerotic heart disease (ASHD) | d. | Seizure disorder | aa. |
| | | Cardiac dysrhythmias | e. | Transient ischemic attack (TIA) | bb. |
| | | Congestive heart failure | f. | Traumatic brain injury | cc. |
| | | Deep vein thrombosis | g. | PSYCHIATRIC/MOOD | |
| | | Hypertension | h. | Anxiety disorder | dd. |
| | | Hypotension 17* | i. | Depression 17* | ee. |
| | | Peripheral vascular disease 16 | j. | Manic depression (bipolar disease) | ff. |
| | | Other cardiovascular disease | k. | Schizophrenia | gg. |
| | | MUSCULOSKELETAL | | PULMONARY | |
| | | Arthritis | l. | Asthma | hh. |
| | | Hip fracture | m. | Emphysema/COPD | ii. |
| | | Missing limb (e.g., amputation) | n. | SENSORY | |
| | | Osteoporosis | o. | Cataracts 3 | jj. |
| | | Pathological bone fracture | p. | Diabetic retinopathy | kk. |
| | | NEUROLOGICAL | | Glaucoma 3 | ll. |
| | | Alzheimer's disease | q. | Macular degeneration | mm. |
| | | Aphasia | r. | OTHER | |
| | | Cerebral palsy | s. | Allergies | nn. |
| | | Cerebrovascular accident (stroke) | t. | Anemia | oo. |
| | | Dementia other than Alzheimer's disease | u. | Cancer | pp. |
| | | | | Renal failure | qq. |
| | | | | NONE OF ABOVE | rr. |

| 2. | INFECTIONS | *(If none apply, CHECK the NONE OF ABOVE box)* | | | |
|---|---|---|---|---|---|
| | | Antibiotic resistant infection (e.g., Methicillin resistant staph) | a. | Septicemia | g. |
| | | | | Sexually transmitted diseases | h. |
| | | Clostridium difficile (c. diff.) | b. | Tuberculosis | i. |
| | | Conjunctivitis | c. | Urinary tract infection in last 30 days 14 | j. |
| | | HIV infection | d. | Viral hepatitis | k. |
| | | Pneumonia | e. | Wound infection | l. |
| | | Respiratory infection | f. | NONE OF ABOVE | m. |

| 3. | OTHER CURRENT OR MORE DETAILED DIAGNOSES AND ICD-9 CODES | Dehydration 276.5 = 14 | |
|---|---|---|---|
| | | a. _____ | • |
| | | b. _____ | • |
| | | c. _____ | • |
| | | d. _____ | • |
| | | e. _____ | • |

## SECTION J. HEALTH CONDITIONS

| 1. | PROBLEM CONDITIONS | *(Check all problems present in last 7 days unless other time frame is indicated)* | | | |
|---|---|---|---|---|---|
| | | INDICATORS OF FLUID STATUS | | Dizziness/Vertigo 11, 17* | f. |
| | | Weight gain or loss of 3 or more pounds within a 7 day period 14 | a. | Edema | g. |
| | | | | Fever 14 | h. |
| | | Inability to lie flat due to shortness of breath | b. | Hallucinations 17* | i. |
| | | | | Internal bleeding 14 | j. |
| | | Dehydrated; output exceeds input 14 | c. | Recurrent lung aspirations in last 90 days 17* | k. |
| | | Insufficient fluid; did NOT consume all/almost all liquids provided during last 3 days 14 | d. | Shortness of breath | l. |
| | | | | Syncope (fainting) 17* | m. |
| | | | | Unsteady gait 17* | n. |
| | | OTHER | | Vomiting | o. |
| | | Delusions | e. | NONE OF ABOVE | p. |

TRIGGER LEGEND
3 - Visual Function
5A - ADL Rehabilitation
6 - Urinary Incontinence/Indwelling Catheter
11 - Falls
14 - Dehydration/Fluid Maintenance
16 - Pressure Ulcers
17* - Psychotropic Drugs
    (*For this to trigger, O4a, b, or c must = 1-7)

Form 39242R

MDS 2.0  1/30/98

*Source:* © 1998 Briggs Corporation, Des Moines, IA 50306 (800) 247-2343. Copyright limited to addition of trigger system.

Resident _____                                    Numeric Identifier _____

| 2. | PAIN SYMPTOMS | (Code the **highest level** of pain present **in the last 7 days**) |
|---|---|---|
| | | **a. FREQUENCY** with which resident complains or shows evidence of pain<br>0. No pain *(skip to J4)*<br>1. Pain less than daily<br>2. Pain daily | **b. INTENSITY** of pain<br>1. Mild pain<br>2. Moderate pain<br>3. Times when pain is horrible or excruciating |

| 3. | PAIN SITE | (If pain present, **check all sites that apply in last 7 days**) | | | |
|---|---|---|---|---|---|
| | | Back pain | a. | Incisional pain | f. |
| | | Bone pain | b. | Joint pain (other than hip) | g. |
| | | Chest pain while doing usual activities | c. | Soft tissue pain (e.g., lesion, muscle) | h. |
| | | Headache | d. | Stomach pain | i. |
| | | Hip pain | e. | Other | j. |

| 4. | ACCIDENTS | (Check all that apply) | | | |
|---|---|---|---|---|---|
| | | Fell in past 30 days **11, 17\*** | a. | Hip fracture in last 180 days **17\*** | c. |
| | | Fell in past 31-180 days **11, 17\*** | b. | Other fracture in last 180 days | d. |
| | | | | *NONE OF ABOVE* | e. |

| 5. | STABILITY OF CONDITIONS | Conditions/diseases make resident's cognitive, ADL, mood or behavior patterns unstable—(fluctuating, precarious, or deteriorating) | a. |
|---|---|---|---|
| | | Resident experiencing an acute episode or a flare-up of a recurrent or chronic problem | b. |
| | | End-stage disease, 6 or fewer months to live | c. |
| | | *NONE OF ABOVE* | d. |

## SECTION K. ORAL/NUTRITIONAL STATUS

| 1. | ORAL PROBLEMS | Chewing problem | a. |
|---|---|---|---|
| | | Swallowing problem **17\*** | b. |
| | | Mouth pain **15** | c. |
| | | *NONE OF ABOVE* | d. |

| 2. | HEIGHT AND WEIGHT | Record **(a.)** height in inches and **(b.)** weight in pounds. Base weight on most recent measure in last 30 days; measure weight consistently in accord with standard facility practice—e.g., in a.m. after voiding, before meal, with shoes off, and in nightclothes. |
|---|---|---|
| | | **a. HT (in.)**            **b. WT (lb.)** |

| 3. | WEIGHT CHANGE | a. Weight loss—5% or more in **last 30 days**; or 10% or more in **last 180 days**<br>0. No            1. Yes **12** |
|---|---|---|
| | | b. Weight gain—5% or more in **last 30 days**; or 10% or more in **last 180 days**<br>0. No            1. Yes |

| 4. | NUTRITIONAL PROBLEMS | Complains about the taste of many foods **12** | a. | Leaves 25% or more of food uneaten at most meals **12** | c. |
|---|---|---|---|---|---|
| | | Regular or repetitive complaints of hunger | b. | *NONE OF ABOVE* | d. |

| 5. | NUTRITIONAL APPROACHES | (Check all that apply in last 7 days) | | | |
|---|---|---|---|---|---|
| | | Parenteral/IV **12, 14** | a. | Dietary supplement between meals | f. |
| | | Feeding tube **13, 14** | b. | Plate guard, stabilized built-up utensil, etc. | g. |
| | | Mechanically altered diet **12** | c. | On a planned weight change program | h. |
| | | Syringe (oral feeding) **12** | d. | *NONE OF ABOVE* | i. |
| | | Therapeutic diet **12** | e. | | |

| 6. | PARENTERAL OR ENTERAL INTAKE | **(Skip to Section L if neither 5a nor 5b is checked)**<br>a. Code the proportion of **total calories** the resident received through parenteral or tube feedings in the **last 7 days**<br>0. None            3. 51% to 75%<br>1. 1% to 25%            4. 76% to 100%<br>2. 26% to 50% |
|---|---|---|
| | | b. Code the average fluid intake per day by IV or tube in **last 7 days**<br>0. None            3. 1001 to 1500 cc/day<br>1. 1 to 500 cc/day            4. 1501 to 2000 cc/day<br>2. 501 to 1000 cc/day            5. 2001 or more cc/day |

## SECTION L. ORAL/DENTAL STATUS

| 1. | ORAL STATUS AND DISEASE PREVENTION | Debris (soft, easily movable substances) present in mouth prior to going to bed at night **15** | a. |
|---|---|---|---|
| | | Has dentures or removable bridge | b. |
| | | Some/all natural teeth lost—does not have or does not use dentures (or partial plates) **15** | c. |
| | | Broken, loose, or carious teeth **15** | d. |
| | | Inflamed gums (gingiva); swollen or bleeding gums; oral abscesses; ulcers or rashes **15** | e. |
| | | Daily cleaning of teeth/dentures or daily mouth care—by resident or staff Not ✓ – **15** | f. |
| | | *NONE OF ABOVE* | g. |

## SECTION M. SKIN CONDITION

| 1. | ULCERS (Due to any cause) | (Record the number of ulcers at each ulcer stage—regardless of cause. If none present at a stage, record "0" (zero). Code all that apply during last 7 days. Code 9 = 9 or more.) [Requires full body exam.] | Number at Stage |
|---|---|---|---|
| | | a. **Stage 1.** A persistent area of skin redness (without a break in the skin) that does not disappear when pressure is relieved. | |
| | | b. **Stage 2.** A partial thickness loss of skin layers that presents clinically as an abrasion, blister, or shallow crater. | |
| | | c. **Stage 3.** A full thickness of skin is lost, exposing the subcutaneous tissues—presents as a deep crater with or without undermining adjacent tissue. | |
| | | d. **Stage 4.** A full thickness of skin and subcutaneous tissue is lost, exposing muscle or bone. | |

| 2. | TYPE OF ULCER | (For each type of ulcer, code for the **highest stage in the last 7 days** using scale in item M1—i.e., 0=none; stages 1, 2, 3, 4) |
|---|---|---|
| | | a. Pressure ulcer—any lesion caused by pressure resulting in damage of underlying tissue 1 - **16**; 2, 3, or 4 - **12, 16** |
| | | b. Stasis ulcer—open lesion caused by poor circulation in the lower extremities |

| 3. | HISTORY OF RESOLVED ULCERS | Resident had an ulcer that was resolved or cured in **LAST 90 DAYS**<br>0. No            1. Yes **16** |
|---|---|---|

| 4. | OTHER SKIN PROBLEMS OR LESIONS PRESENT | (Check all that apply during last 7 days) | |
|---|---|---|---|
| | | Abrasions, bruises | a. |
| | | Burns (second or third degree) | b. |
| | | Open lesions other than ulcers, rashes, cuts (e.g., cancer lesions) | c. |
| | | Rashes—e.g., intertrigo, eczema, drug rash, heat rash, herpes zoster | d. |
| | | Skin desensitized to pain or pressure **16** | e. |
| | | Skin tears or cuts (other than surgery) | f. |
| | | Surgical wounds | g. |
| | | *NONE OF ABOVE* | h. |

| 5. | SKIN TREATMENTS | (Check all that apply during last 7 days) | |
|---|---|---|---|
| | | Pressure relieving device(s) for chair | a. |
| | | Pressure relieving device(s) for bed | b. |
| | | Turning/repositioning program | c. |
| | | Nutrition or hydration intervention to manage skin problems | d. |
| | | Ulcer care | e. |
| | | Surgical wound care | f. |
| | | Application of dressings (with or without topical medications) other than to feet | g. |
| | | Application of ointments/medications (other than to feet) | h. |
| | | Other preventative or protective skin care (other than to feet) | i. |
| | | *NONE OF ABOVE* | j. |

| 6. | FOOT PROBLEMS AND CARE | (Check all that apply during last 7 days) | |
|---|---|---|---|
| | | Resident has one or more foot problems—e.g., corns, calluses, bunions, hammer toes, overlapping toes, pain, structural problems | a. |
| | | Infection of the foot—e.g., cellulitis, purulent drainage | b. |
| | | Open lesions on the foot | c. |
| | | Nails/calluses trimmed during last 90 days | d. |
| | | Received preventative or protective foot care (e.g., used special shoes, inserts, pads, toe separators) | e. |
| | | Application of dressings (with or without topical medications) | f. |
| | | *NONE OF ABOVE* | g. |

## SECTION N. ACTIVITY PURSUIT PATTERNS

| 1. | TIME AWAKE | (Check appropriate time periods over last 7 days) Resident awake all or most of time (i.e., naps no more than one hour per time period) in the: | | | |
|---|---|---|---|---|---|
| | **10B** only if BOTH N1a = ✓ and N2 = 0 | Morning **10B** | a. | Evening | c. |
| | | Afternoon | b. | *NONE OF ABOVE* | d. |

**(IF RESIDENT IS COMATOSE, SKIP TO SECTION O)**

| 2. | AVERAGE TIME INVOLVED IN ACTIVITIES | (When awake and not receiving treatments or ADL care) |
|---|---|---|
| | | 0. Most—more than 2/3 of time **10B**            2. Little—less than 1/3 of time **10A**<br>1. Some—from 1/3 to 2/3 of time            3. None **10A** |

| 3. | PREFERRED ACTIVITY SETTINGS | (Check all settings in which activities are **preferred**) | | | |
|---|---|---|---|---|---|
| | | Own room | a. | | |
| | | Day/activity room | b. | Outside facility | d. |
| | | Inside NH/off unit | c. | *NONE OF ABOVE* | e. |

| 4. | GENERAL ACTIVITY PREFERENCES (Adapted to resident's current abilities) | (Check all PREFERENCES whether or not activity is currently available to resident) | | | |
|---|---|---|---|---|---|
| | | Cards/other games | a. | Trips/shopping | g. |
| | | Crafts/arts | b. | Walking/wheeling outdoors | h. |
| | | Exercise/sports | c. | Watching TV | i. |
| | | Music | d. | Gardening or plants | j. |
| | | Reading/writing | e. | Talking or conversing | k. |
| | | Spiritual/religious activities | f. | Helping others | l. |
| | | | | *NONE OF ABOVE* | m. |

**TRIGGER LEGEND**
| | | |
|---|---|---|
| 10A - Activities (Revise) | 13 - Feeding Tubes | 17\* - Psychotropic Drugs |
| 10B - Activities (Review) | 14 - Dehydration/Fluid Maintenance | (\*For this to trigger, O4a, b, or c must = 1-7) |
| 11 - Falls | 15 - Dental Care | |
| 12 - Nutritional Status | 16 - Pressure Ulcers | |

**Form 39242R**

PRINTED IN U.S.A.

MDS 2.0   1/30/98

Resident _____    Numeric Identifier _____

| 5. | PREFERS CHANGE IN DAILY ROUTINE | Code for resident preferences in daily routines |
|---|---|---|
| | | 0. No change  1. Slight change  2. Major change |
| | | a. Type of activities in which resident is currently involved 1 or 2 = **10A** |
| | | b. Extent of resident involvement in activities 1 or 2 = **10A** |

## SECTION O. MEDICATIONS

| 1. | NUMBER OF MEDICATIONS | *(Record the number of different medications used in the last 7 days; enter "0" if none used)* | |
|---|---|---|---|
| 2. | NEW MEDICA-TIONS | *(Resident currently receiving medications that were initiated during the last 90 days)* 0. No  1. Yes | |
| 3. | INJECTIONS | *(Record the number of DAYS injections of any type received during the last 7 days; enter "0" if none used)* | |
| 4. | DAYS RECEIVED THE FOLLOWING MEDICATION | *(Record the number of DAYS during last 7 days; enter "0" if not used. Note—enter "1" for long-acting meds used less than weekly)* | |

(NOTE: For **17** to actually be triggered, O4a, b, or c MUST = 1-7 AND at least one additional item marked **17\*** must be indicated. See sections B, C, E, G, H, I, J, and K.)

| a. Antipsychotic 1-7 = **17** | d. Hypnotic | |
|---|---|---|
| b. Antianxiety 1-7 = **11, 17** | e. Diuretic 1-7 = **14** | |
| c. Antidepressant 1-7 = **11, 17** | | |

## SECTION P. SPECIAL TREATMENTS AND PROCEDURES

| 1. | SPECIAL TREAT-MENTS, PROCE-DURES, AND PROGRAMS | a. SPECIAL CARE—*Check treatments or programs received during the last 14 days* | |
|---|---|---|---|

**TREATMENTS**

| Chemotherapy | a. | Ventilator or respirator **PROGRAMS** | l. |
|---|---|---|---|
| Dialysis | b. | Alcohol/drug treatment program | m. |
| IV medication | c. | Alzheimer's/dementia special care unit | n. |
| Intake/output | d. | Hospice care | o. |
| Monitoring acute medical condition | e. | Pediatric unit | p. |
| Ostomy care | f. | Respite care | q. |
| Oxygen therapy | g. | Training in skills required to return to the community (e.g., taking medications, house work, shopping, transportation, ADLs) | r. |
| Radiation | h. | | |
| Suctioning | i. | | |
| Tracheostomy care | j. | | |
| Transfusions | k. | NONE OF ABOVE | s. |

b. THERAPIES—*Record the number of days and total minutes each of the following therapies was administered (for at least 15 minutes a day) in the last 7 calendar days (Enter 0 if none or less than 15 min. daily) [Note—count only post admission therapies]*

(A) = # of days administered for 15 minutes or more
(B) = total # of minutes provided in last 7 days

| | DAYS (A) | MIN (B) |
|---|---|---|
| a. Speech-language pathology and audiology services | | |
| b. Occupational therapy | | |
| c. Physical therapy | | |
| d. Respiratory therapy | | |
| e. Psychological therapy (by any licensed mental health professional) | | |

| 2. | INTERVEN-TION PROGRAMS FOR MOOD, BEHAVIOR, COGNITIVE LOSS | *(Check all interventions or strategies used in last 7 days—no matter where received)* | |
|---|---|---|---|
| | | Special behavior symptom evaluation program | a. |
| | | Evaluation by a licensed mental health specialist in last 90 days | b. |
| | | Group therapy | c. |
| | | Resident-specific deliberate changes in the environment to address mood/behavior patterns—e.g., providing bureau in which to rummage | d. |
| | | Reorientation—e.g., cueing | e. |
| | | NONE OF ABOVE | f. |

| 3. | NURSING REHABILI-TATION/ RESTOR-ATIVE CARE | *Record the NUMBER OF DAYS each of the following rehabilitation or restorative techniques or practices was provided to the resident for more than or equal to 15 minutes per day in the last 7 days (Enter 0 if none or less than 15 min. daily.)* | |
|---|---|---|---|

| a. Range of motion (passive) | | f. Walking | |
|---|---|---|---|
| b. Range of motion (active) | | g. Dressing or grooming | |
| c. Splint or brace assistance | | h. Eating or swallowing | |
| **TRAINING AND SKILL PRACTICE IN:** | | i. Amputation/ prosthesis care | |
| d. Bed mobility | | j. Communication | |
| e. Transfer | | k. Other | |

| 4. | DEVICES AND RESTRAINTS | *(Use the following codes for last 7 days:)* |
|---|---|---|
| | | 0. Not used |
| | | 1. Used less than daily |
| | | 2. Used daily |
| | | Bed rails |
| | | a. —Full bed rails on all open sides of bed |
| | | b. —Other types of side rails used (e.g., half rail, one side) |
| | | c. Trunk restraint 1 = **11, 18**; 2 = **11, 16, 18** |
| | | d. Limb restraint 1 or 2 = **18** |
| | | e. Chair prevents rising 1 or 2 = **18** |

| 5. | HOSPITAL STAY(S) | Record number of times resident was admitted to hospital with an overnight stay in last 90 days (or since last assessment if less than 90 days). (Enter 0 if no hospital admissions) | |
|---|---|---|---|
| 6. | EMERGENCY ROOM (ER) VISIT(S) | Record number of times resident visited ER without an overnight stay in last 90 days (or since last assessment if less than 90 days). (Enter 0 if no ER visits) | |
| 7. | PHYSICIAN VISITS | In the LAST 14 DAYS (or since admission if less than 14 days in facility) how many days has the physician (or authorized assistant or practitioner) examined the resident? (Enter 0 if none) | |
| 8. | PHYSICIAN ORDERS | In the LAST 14 DAYS (or since admission if less than 14 days in facility) how many days has the physician (or authorized assistant or practitioner) changed the resident's orders? Do not include order renewals without change. (Enter 0 if none) | |
| 9. | ABNORMAL LAB VALUES | Has the resident had any abnormal lab values during the last 90 days (or since admission)? 0. No  1. Yes | |

## SECTION Q. DISCHARGE POTENTIAL AND OVERALL STATUS

| 1. | DISCHARGE POTENTIAL | a. Resident expresses/indicates preference to return to the community 0. No  1. Yes | |
|---|---|---|---|
| | | b. Resident has a support person who is positive toward discharge 0. No  1. Yes | |
| | | c. Stay projected to be of a short duration—discharge projected within 90 days (do not include expected discharge due to death) | |
| | | 0. No  2. Within 31-90 days | |
| | | 1. Within 30 days  3. Discharge status uncertain | |
| 2. | OVERALL CHANGE IN CARE NEEDS | Resident's overall self sufficiency has changed significantly as compared to status of 90 days ago (or since last assessment if less than 90 days) | |
| | | 0. No change | |
| | | 1. Improved—receives fewer supports, needs less restrictive level of care | |
| | | 2. Deteriorated—receives more support | |

## SECTION R. ASSESSMENT INFORMATION

| 1. | PARTICI-PATION IN ASSESSMENT | a. Resident: 0. No  1. Yes | |
|---|---|---|---|
| | | b. Family: 0. No  1. Yes  2. No family | |
| | | c. Significant other: 0. No  1. Yes  2. None | |

2. SIGNATURES OF PERSONS COMPLETING THE ASSESSMENT:

a. Signature of RN Assessment Coordinator (sign on above line)

b. Date RN Assessment Coordinator signed as complete [ ][ ] — [ ][ ] — [ ][ ][ ][ ]
Month   Day   Year

| c. Other Signatures | Title | Sections | Date |
|---|---|---|---|
| d. | | | Date |
| e. | | | Date |
| f. | | | Date |
| g. | | | Date |
| h. | | | Date |

**TRIGGER LEGEND**
10A - Activities (Revise)
11 - Falls
14 - Dehydration/Fluid Maintenance
16 - Pressure Ulcers
17 - Psychotropic Drugs
17\* - For this to trigger, O4a, b, or c must = 1-7
18 - Physical Restraints

*Source:* © 1998 Briggs Corporation, Des Moines, IA 50306 (800) 247-2343. Copyright limited to addition of trigger system.

Resident _____    Numeric Identifier _____

| SECTION S. SOUTH DAKOTA SPECIFIC INFORMATION | |
|---|---|
| **1. PASARR**<br><br>*(complete ONLY for initial admission, readmission, or significant change MDS)* | A PASARR evaluation was conducted due to the evidence of known or suspected:<br><br>a. Mental illness    a.<br><br>b. Mental retardation or developmental disability   b.<br><br>c. Usage of psychotropic medications   c.<br><br>d. PASARR is exempt due to a confirmed diagnosis of Alzheimer's or Dementia and there is NO evidence of MR/DD   d.<br><br>e. *NONE OF ABOVE*   e. |
| **2. PNEUMOVAX VACCINATION** | Has the resident received a pneumovax vaccination in the last 90 days?<br><br>0. No    1. Yes (If Yes, give date)<br>☐☐ — ☐☐ — ☐☐☐☐ |
| **3. INFLUENZA VACCINATION** | Has the resident received an influenza vaccination in the last 90 days?<br><br>0. No    1. Yes (If Yes, give date)<br>☐☐ — ☐☐ — ☐☐☐☐ |
| **4. DISCHARGE PLANNING NEEDS** | Complete this item if Section Q.1. a or b are coded as 1, if Q.1.c is coded as a 1 or 2, or if Section Q.2. is coded as 1. Check all interventions or strategies that would need to occur or be necessary to prepare the resident for discharge.<br><br>a. assisting resident or support person to plan for discharge   a.<br>b. self-medication education or assistance   b.<br>c. establish or arrange a pain management program   c.<br>d. assistance obtaining medications   d.<br>e. education regarding self-care techniques   e.<br>f. education of caregiver(s)   f.<br>g. assistance with meals/nutrition   g.<br>h. adaptive or durable medical equipment in the discharge setting   h.<br>i. home and community services case management   i.<br>j. adult protective services   j.<br>k. homemaker services   k.<br>l. adult day care   l. |
| **5a. DOCUMENT NUMBER** | ☐☐☐ |
| **5b. CORRECTION DOCUMENT NUMBER** | ☐☐☐ |

| SECTION T. THERAPY SUPPLEMENT FOR MEDICARE PPS | | |
|---|---|---|
| **1. SPECIAL TREAT-MENTS AND PROCE-DURES** | a. RECREATION THERAPY—*Enter number of days and total minutes of recreation therapy administered (for at least 15 minutes a day) in the last 7 days (Enter 0 if none)*<br><br>(A) = # of days administered for 15 minutes or more<br>(B) = total # of minutes provided in last 7 days | DAYS    MINS.<br>(A)    (B)<br>☐☐   ☐☐☐☐ |
| | *Skip unless this is a Medicare 5 day or Medicare readmission/return assessment*<br><br>b. ORDERED THERAPIES—*Has physician ordered any of following therapies to begin in FIRST 14 days of stay—physical therapy, occupational therapy, or speech pathology service?*<br>0. No      1. Yes<br><br>*If not ordered, skip to item 2*<br><br>c. Through day 15, provide an estimate of the number of days when at least 1 therapy service can be expected to have been delivered.<br><br>d. Through day 15, provide an estimate of the number of therapy minutes (across the therapies) that can be expected to be delivered. | |
| **2. WALKING WHEN MOST SELF-SUFFICIENT** | *Complete item 2 if ADL self-performance score for TRANSFER (G.1.b.A) is 0, 1, 2, or 3 AND at least one of the following are present:*<br><br>• Resident received physical therapy involving gait training (P.1.b.c)<br>• Physical therapy was ordered for the resident involving gait training (T.1.b)<br>• Resident received nursing rehabilitation for walking (P.3.f)<br>• Physical therapy involving walking has been discontinued within the past 180 days<br><br>*Skip to item 3 if resident did not walk in last 7 days*<br><br>*(FOR FOLLOWING FIVE ITEMS, BASE CODING ON THE EPISODE WHEN THE RESIDENT WALKED THE FARTHEST WITHOUT SITTING DOWN. INCLUDE WALKING DURING REHABILITATION SESSIONS.)*<br><br>a. **Farthest distance walked** without sitting during this episode.<br>  0. 150+ feet     3. 10-25 feet<br>  1. 51-149 feet   4. Less than 10 feet<br>  2. 26-50 feet<br><br>b. **Time walked** without sitting down during this episode.<br>  0. 1-2 minutes    3. 11-15 minutes<br>  1. 3-4 minutes    4. 16-30 minutes<br>  2. 5-10 minutes   5. 31+ minutes<br><br>c. **Self-Performance in walking** during this episode.<br>  0. *INDEPENDENT*—No help or oversight<br>  1. *SUPERVISION*—Oversight, encouragement or cueing provided<br>  2. *LIMITED ASSISTANCE*—Resident highly involved in walking; received physical help in guided maneuvering of limbs or other nonweight-bearing assistance<br>  3. *EXTENSIVE ASSISTANCE*—Resident received weight-bearing assistance while walking<br><br>d. **Walking support provided** associated with this episode (code regardless of resident's self-performance classification).<br>  0. No setup or physical help from staff<br>  1. Setup help only<br>  2. One person physical assist<br>  3. Two+ persons physical assist<br><br>e. **Parallel bars** used by resident in association with this episode.<br>  0. No      1. Yes | |
| **3. CASE MIX GROUP** | Medicare ☐☐☐☐☐    State ☐☐☐☐☐ | |

Resident _____ Numeric Identifier _____

## SECTION U. MEDICATIONS

List all medications that the resident **received** during the last 7 days. Include scheduled medications that are used regularly, but less than weekly.

1. **Medication Name and Dose Ordered.** Record the name of the medication and dose ordered.
2. **Route of Administration (RA).** Code the Route of Administration using the following list:

| | | |
|---|---|---|
| 1 = by mouth (PO) | 5 = subcutaneous (SQ) | 8 = inhalation |
| 2 = sublingual (SL) | 6 = rectal (R) | 9 = enteral tube |
| 3 = intramuscular (IM) | 7 = topical | 10 = other |
| 4 = intravenous (IV) | | |

3. **Frequency (Freq.).** Code the number of times per day, week, or month the medication is administered using the following list:

| | | |
|---|---|---|
| PR = (PRN) as necessary | 2D = (BID) two times daily | QO = every other day |
| 1H = (QH) every hour | (includes every 12 hours) | 4W = four times each week |
| 2H = (Q2H) every two hours | 3D = (TID) three times daily | 5W = five times each week |
| 3H = (Q3H) every three hours | 4D = (QID) four times daily | 6W = six times each week |
| 4H = (Q4H) every four hours | 5D = five times daily | 1M = (Q month) once every month |
| 6H = (Q6H) every six hours | 1W = (Q week) once each week | 2M = twice every month |
| 8H = (Q8H) every eight hours | 2W = two times every week | C = continuous |
| 1D = (QD or HS) once daily | 3W = three times every week | O = other |

4. **Amount Administered (AA).** Record the number of tablets, capsules, suppositories, or liquid (any route) **per dose** administered to the resident. Code 999 for topicals, eye drops, inhalants and oral medications that need to be dissolved in water.
5. **PRN-number of days (PRN-n).** If the frequency code for the medication is "PR," record the number of times during the last 7 days each PRN medication was given. Code STAT medications as PRNs given once.
6. **NDC Codes.** Enter the National Drug Code for each medication given. Be sure to enter the correct NDC code for the drug name, strength, and form. The NDC code must match the drug dispensed by the pharmacy.

| 1. Medication Name and Dose Ordered | 2. RA | 3. Freq | 4. AA | 5. PRN-n | 6. NDC Codes |
|---|---|---|---|---|---|
| | | | | | |
| | | | | | |
| | | | | | |
| | | | | | |
| | | | | | |
| | | | | | |
| | | | | | |
| | | | | | |
| | | | | | |
| | | | | | |
| | | | | | |
| | | | | | |
| | | | | | |
| | | | | | |
| | | | | | |
| | | | | | |
| | | | | | |
| | | | | | |

*Source:* © 1998 Briggs Corporation, Des Moines, IA 50306 (800) 247-2343. Copyright limited to addition of trigger system.

## SECTION V. RESIDENT ASSESSMENT PROTOCOL SUMMARY  Numeric Identifier_____

| Resident's Name: | Medical Record No.: |
|---|---|

1. Check if RAP is triggered.
2. For each triggered RAP, use the RAP guidelines to identify areas needing further assessment. Document relevant assessment information regarding the resident's status.

   • Describe:
   —Nature of the condition (may include presence or lack of objective data and subjective complaints).
   —Complications and risk factors that affect your decision to proceed to care planning.
   —Factors that must be considered in developing individualized care plan interventions.
   —Need for referrals/further evaluation by appropriate health professionals.

   • Documentation should support your decision-making regarding whether to proceed with a care plan for a triggered RAP and the type(s) of care plan interventions that are appropriate for a particular resident.

   • Documentation may appear anywhere in the clinical record (e.g., progress notes, consults, flowsheets, etc.).

3. Indicate under the Location of RAP Assessment Documentation column where information related to the RAP assessment can be found.
4. For each triggered RAP, indicate whether a new care plan, care plan revision, or continuation of current care plan is necessary to address the problem(s) identified in your assessment. The Care Planning Decision column must be completed within 7 days of completing the RAI (MDS and RAPs).

| A. RAP Problem Area | (a) Check if Triggered | Location and Date of RAP Assessment Documentation | (b) Care Planning Decision—check if addressed in care plan |
|---|---|---|---|
| 1. DELIRIUM | | | |
| 2. COGNITIVE LOSS | | | |
| 3. VISUAL FUNCTION | | | |
| 4. COMMUNICATION | | | |
| 5. ADL FUNCTIONAL/ REHABILITATION POTENTIAL | | | |
| 6. URINARY INCONTINENCE AND INDWELLING CATHETER | | | |
| 7. PSYCHOSOCIAL WELL-BEING | | | |
| 8. MOOD STATE | | | |
| 9. BEHAVIORAL SYMPTOMS | | | |
| 10. ACTIVITIES | | | |
| 11. FALLS | | | |
| 12. NUTRITIONAL STATUS | | | |
| 13. FEEDING TUBES | | | |
| 14. DEHYDRATION/FLUID MAINTENANCE | | | |
| 15. ORAL/DENTAL CARE | | | |
| 16. PRESSURE ULCERS | | | |
| 17. PSYCHOTROPIC DRUG USE | | | |
| 18. PHYSICAL RESTRAINTS | | | |

B. _____   2. ☐☐ – ☐☐ – ☐☐☐☐
   1. Signature of RN Coordinator for RAP Assessment Process          Month    Day       Year

   _____   4. ☐☐ – ☐☐ – ☐☐☐☐
   3. Signature of Person Completing Care Planning Decision           Month    Day       Year

# Areas From Which NAB Examination Questions Will Be Taken

**RESIDENT CARE MANAGEMENT (34%, 51 QUESTIONS)**

**Nursing Services (6%, 9 Questions)— Chapters 6, 7, 8 and 9**

- Aging process (psychological), pp. 265–268
- Aging process (physiological), pp. 225–230
- Definition, concept and basic principles of nursing, pp. 197–201
- Basic principles of restorative nursing, pp. 235–236
- Basic principles of rehabilitation, pp. 203–204
- Basic principles of infection control, pp. 287–288
- Basic principles of drug administration, pp. 214–216
- Basic pharmacological terminology, p. 260
- Resident care needs, pp. 235–246
- Resident Assessment Instrument (RAI) and interdisciplinary care plan requirements and process, pp. 240–242, 248
- Professional ethics of licensed personnel, p. 236
- Admissions, transfers and discharges, pp. 236, 239
- Techniques of auditing care outcomes, pp. 246–248

**Social Service Program (4%, 6 Questions)— Chapters 6, 7 and 8**

- Resident and family council formation and function, p. 273

- Resident admissions, transfers and discharges, pp. 236, 240
- Social, emotional, psychological, spiritual and financial needs of residents and their families, pp. 270–272
- Basic principles of family consultation, pp. 270–272
- Dynamics of interpersonal relationships, pp. 269–270
- Role of social worker, pp. 179–183
- Grieving process, pp. 266–267
- Death and dying, pp. 273–274
- Resident Assessment Instrument (RAI) and interdisciplinary care plan requirements, pp. 236–237, 240–242, 243
- Resident rights, pp. 184–196
- Advance medical directives (living wills, DNR and DNI) , pp. 176–178
- Resident legal service needs, pp. 175–183
- Personalization of equipment, pp. 274–275

**Food Service Program (4%, 6 Questions)— Chapters 6 and 7**

- Basic nutritional requirements, p. 244
- Basic principles of food preparation and presentation, pp. 212–213
- Effects of dining experience on residents, p. 210
- Frequency of meals, p. 213
- Types of therapeutic diets, pp. 212–213

- Principles of dietary sanitation, including dishwashing technique and water temperature, p. 213
- Role of registered dietitian, pp. 210–212
- Role of director of food service, pp. 210–212
- Food service delivery, pp. 212–213
- Food serving and storage (holding, serving and storage temperatures, p. 212
- Types of nutrition supplements, p. 212
- Types of adaptive feeding equipment, p. 212
- Resident Assessment Instrument (RAI) and interdisciplinary care plan requirements, pp. 236–237, 240–242, 248

## Medical Services (5%, 7–8 Questions)—Chapters 6 and 7

- Basic medical terminology, pp. 250–263
- Provision of basic consultant specialty medical services (podiatry, psychiatry, psychology), pp. 237–238
- Role of physician in the facility, pp. 237, 244–245
- Frequency of physician visits, p. 245
- Provision of dental services, pp. 245–246
- Provision of emergency medical services, pp. 238, 245
- Physician/resident relationships, p. 245
- Quality assurance, pp. 236–237, 242–248
- Resident Assessment Instrument (RAI) and interdisciplinary care plan requirements, pp. 236–237, 240–242, 248
- Information needed from the facility by the physician, p. 237

## Therapeutic Recreation/Activity Programs (4%, 6 Questions)—Chapters 2, 6, 7 and 8

- Basic therapeutic recreational/activity needs of residents, p. 278
- Role of recreational/activity therapist, p. 217
- Volunteer resources, pp. 221–223
- Available resources (community, volunteer), p. 40
- Resident Assessment Instrument (RAI) and interdisciplinary care plan requirements, pp. 240–242

## Medical Records Program (4%, 6 Questions)—Chapters 6 and 7

- Basic medical record-keeping systems, including automation and retention, pp. 205–210

- Role of medical records managers, pp. 205–206
- Clinical medical record content and format, pp. 236–237, 239
- Federal documentation requirements, including Resident Assessment Instrument (RAI), pp. 240–242, 248
- Safeguarding clinical record information (procedures, safety considerations), p. 205

## Pharmaceutical Programs (4%, 6 Questions)—Chapters 6 and 7

- Basic drug administration terminology, pp. 259, 260
- Regulations for handling, administration, labeling of drugs and biologicals, record-keeping and drug destruction, pp. 214–217, 238
- Systems of inventory controls, pp. 214–215
- Role of pharmacist and/or consultant pharmacist, p. 213

## Rehabilitation Program (4%, 6 Questions)—Chapters 6, 7 and 8

- Basic resident rehabilitation needs, pp. 235–236, 276–278
- Roles of all rehabilitation service disciplines, pp. 203–205, 235–236
- Resident Assessment Instrument (RAI) and interdisciplinary care plan requirements related to rehabilitation, pp. 236–237

## PERSONNEL MANAGEMENT (23%, 35 QUESTIONS)

## Communication between Management and All Staff (8%, 12 Questions)—Chapters 1, 3 and 4

- Effective and clear written and verbal communications to personnel, pp. 82–85
- Conducting group meetings (departmental staff meetings), p. 83
- Using basic negotiating techniques, pp. 131–132

## Recruitment, Evaluation and Retention of Individuals (6%, 9 Questions)—Chapter 4

- Grievance procedures, pp. 111, 188
- Employee interview procedures, pp. 118, 120

- Facility staffing needs, p. 118
- Job descriptions, p. 136
- Recruiting procedures, pp. 118–119
- Employment history and verification procedures, p. 120
- Basic staff development procedures, pp. 123–124
- Audit procedures to evaluate the effectiveness of training, p. 124
- Procedures to analyze absenteeism and turnover, p. 121
- Staff disciplinary procedures, pp. 115–116
- Staff recognition and appreciation techniques, pp. 116–117
- Performance-based employee evaluation procedures, pp. 121–122
- How to develop wage scales, pp. 122–123

### Personnel Policies (5%, 6–8 Questions)—Chapters 1, 4 and 9

- Labor laws, pp. 124–127
- Civil rights laws, p. 2
- Federal rules and regulations, including family medical leave act, military leave, etc., pp. 108–109
- NLRB rules and regulations, pp. 126–127
- Federal and case law requirements for personnel files, p. 108
- Work rules (smoking, breaks, no tipping), pp. 114–116
- Employee benefits policies, pp. 111–113
- Performance-based evaluation procedures, pp. 121–122
- Staff grievance procedures, pp. 111, 118
- Staff disciplinary procedures, pp. 115–116
- Unemployment compensation rules and procedures, p. 109
- Safety procedures, pp. 284–287, 290–292
- Basic management-union contracts, pp. 127–131

### Employee Health and Safety Programs (5%, 6–8 Questions)—Chapters 2, 4 and 9

- Basic safety training programs, pp. 289–290
- Federal rules and regulations, governing employee health and safety, p. 283
- Employee benefits insurance programs, pp. 111–113

- Workers compensation rules and procedures, p. 109
- Injury prevention procedures, pp. 284–287, 290–292
- Relationship between employee health status and job performance, pp. 285–288

## FINANCIAL MANAGEMENT (16%, 24 QUESTIONS)

### Budget (7%, 10–11 Questions)—Chapter 5

- Programs and services offered by the facility, p. 139
- Budgeting methods and financial planning, pp. 153–155
- Basic accounting and bookkeeping methods, pp. 139–145
- Financial statements, pp. 145, 146–147
- Reimbursement mechanisms (Medicare, Medicaid, managed care) and revenue sources, pp. 142–143
- Facility's capital needs, pp. 153–154
- Regulatory requirements for budgeting, pp. 153–155
- Need for reserve profit, pp. 154–155

### Monitor Fiscal Performance (5%, 7–8 Questions)—Chapter 5

- Internal controls, p. 165
- Inventory controls, p. 152
- Purchasing procedures and controls, p. 149
- Financial resources, p. 139
- Financial ratios, pp. 152–153
- Financial analysis methods, pp. 153–154
- Fixed versus variable costs, pp. 166, 170

### Audit and Reporting Systems (4%, 6 Questions)—Chapters 5 and 6

- Cash flow procedures, needs and trends, pp. 154–155
- Financial reports, p. 145
- Payroll procedures and documentation, p. 151
- Regulatory accounting requirements, pp. 145–153
- Collections procedures, p. 150

- Billing procedures, pp. 149–150
- Resident banking procedures and account management, p. 150
- Account aging, pp. 149–150
- Accounts payable control system, p. 149

## ENVIRONMENTAL MANAGEMENT (13%, 19–20 QUESTIONS)

### Maintaining and Improving Buildings, Grounds and Equipment (3%, 3–5 Questions)— Chapters 3 and 9

- Preventive maintenance systems, pp. 286–287
- Equipment and operating manuals, pp. 285–286
- Retention of blueprints, approved "built drawings," and original building documents, pp. 282, 286–287
- Environmental design needs of nursing home residents, p. 282
- Physical plant needs, pp. 279–280
- Implementing equipment and replacement program, p. 281
- Existence of all local, state and federal codes, rules and regulations for buildings, grounds, equipment and maintenance, pp. 282–284
- Establishing maintenance procedures, pp. 284–285

### Environment for Residents, Staff and Visitors (4%, 6 Questions)—Chapters 6 and 9

- Waste management (biomedical waste), pp. 285–286
- Basic housekeeping concepts and procedures, p. 288
- Basic sanitation concepts and procedures, pp. 287–288
- Basic infection control concepts and procedures, pp. 287–290
- Pest control, pp. 286–289
- All local, state and federal rules and regulations, pp. 281, 284

### Safety Program (3–4%, 5–6 Questions)— Chapters 3 and 9

- Safe housekeeping and maintenance practices, pp. 281–282
- Basic concepts regarding safety devices, pp. 282–284
- Potential hazards, pp. 279–290
- Required lighting, pp. 283, 284
- Security measures, pp. 284–285
- Hazardous communication standard, p. 282
- Existence of local, state and federal codes, rules and regulations affecting environment health, welfare and safety rules and regulations, pp. 280–290

### Emergency Program (3%, 4–5 Questions)— Chapter 9

- Existence of local, state and federal rules and regulations affecting fire, disaster and emergencies, p. 290
- Elements of fire and disaster programs, pp. 288–290
- National Fire Protection Association (NFPA) guidelines (life safety codes), p. 288
- Community emergency resources, p. 289
- In-house emergency equipment, p. 289
- Training resources, p. 290
- Evacuation resources, p. 290
- Emergency procedures, p. 290
- Natural disaster preparedness, p. 291

## GOVERNANCE AND MANAGEMENT (14%, 21 QUESTIONS)

### Policies and Procedures (2%, 3 Questions)— Chapters 1, 3, 4, 5 and 6

- Government agencies, p. 1
  — Medicare, pp. 157–158
  — Medicaid, pp. 89–83
  — Labor Laws, pp. 124–127
  — OSHA, pp. 21–31

— Residents Bill of Rights, pp. 175–176, 184–196
— Civil Rights Law, p. 2
- Professional licensing and certification boards and applicable rules and regulations, pp. 6–9
- Types of governing entities (ownership, boards), pp. 52–57
- Mission statement and philosophy, p. 89
- Bylaws, p. 61
- Responsibilities of and to the governing entity, pp. 91–92
- Legal liability of the facility, pp. 155–157
- Legal liability of administration, pp. 58–59
- Ethical policies of the governing entity, p. 92
- Professional ethics of the nursing home administrator, pp. 94–95

**Facility Program, Policy and Procedure Evaluation (2%, 3 Questions)–Chapters 2, 3 and 7**

- Community, social, educational and consumer organizations, pp. 37–41
- Role of ethics committee, p. 236
- Management principles and philosophies, pp. 64–68
- Information collection procedures, pp. 85–86
- Basic computer operations related to facility management, pp. 85–86

**Monitor and Evaluate Quality of Care and Quality of Life (3%, 4–5 Questions)—Chapters 2, 3 and 6**

- Basic techniques of conflict resolution, pp. 69, 85
- Grievance procedures for residents and family, pp. 111, 118
- Residents' rights, pp. 175–176, 184–196
- Roles of the resident ombudsman, p. 248
- Residents and responsible parties' participation in care planning process, pp. 235–246

- Oral and written communications practices, pp. 82–83
- Community, social, educational and consumer organizations, pp. 37–45

**Integration of Residents' Rights into Facility's Operations (3%, 5 Questions)—Chapter 7**

- Internal and external reporting procedures, pp. 236–237
- Monitoring systems, procedures and information, pp. 246–248

**Risk Management Program (2%, 3 Questions)—Chapter 5**

- Risk management principles, including legal liability issues, pp. 155–157

**Program to Inform Residents and the Community of Services Offered (1%, 1–2 Questions)—Chapter 3**

- Basic public relations and marketing techniques, pp. 86–87

**Integration Between Facility and Other Community Resources (1%, 1–2 Questions)—Chapters 2 and 6**

- Basic contracts and agreeements, pp. 45–46, 179, 180–182

*Note:* Percentages shown relate directly to number of questions in each area.

# INDEX

# About the Author

Peter J. Buttaro is an attorney at law and a health care administration educator. He received his AB in psychology from Syracuse University in Syracuse, NY, his masters degree in health care administration from Northwestern University in Chicago, IL and his doctor of law from Suffolk Law School in Boston, MA.

Mr. Buttaro has taught long-term care administration and legal aspects of health care administration at Northeastern University in Boston, MA and at Presentation College in Aberdeen, SD. He has been a guest lecturer and has presented workshops nationally at leading universities and state health care associations. He has authored three books: *Principles of Long-Term Health Care Administration, Step-by-Step Guide to a Higher Score on the NAB Exam* and *Legal Guide for Long-Term Care Administrators*. Over the past 25 years, these books have been used as basic texts in university and college programs and individually for national licensure of nursing home administrators.

Mr. Buttaro is a fellow of the American College of Health Care Executives and a subscribing member of the National Board of Examiners for Long Term Care Administrators. He is past president of the board of directors of the Benedictine Living Centers, who own and operate nursing homes and related facilities in several midwestern states.